AF595111

Current Challenges and Advances in Atherosclerosis

Current Challenges and Advances in Atherosclerosis

Editor

Tomoaki Ishigami

MDPI • Basel • Beijing • Wuhan • Barcelona • Belgrade • Manchester • Tokyo • Cluj • Tianjin

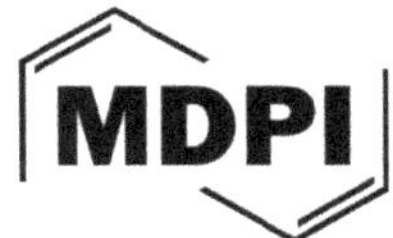

Editor
Tomoaki Ishigami
Department of Cardiology,
Yokohama City University Hospital
Japan

Editorial Office
MDPI
St. Alban-Anlage 66
4052 Basel, Switzerland

This is a reprint of articles from the Topical Collection published online in the open access journal *Journal of Clinical Medicine* (ISSN 2077-0383) (available at: https://www.mdpi.com/journal/jcm/topical collections/athersoclerosis research?authAll=true).

For citation purposes, cite each article independently as indicated on the article page online and as indicated below:

LastName, A.A.; LastName, B.B.; LastName, C.C. Article Title. *Journal Name* **Year**, *Volume Number*, Page Range.

ISBN 978-3-0365-7730-2 (Hbk)
ISBN 978-3-0365-7731-9 (PDF)

Contents

About the Editor

Tomoaki Ishigami

Tomoaki Ishigami was born in Tokyo, Japan. He obtained his medical degree and Ph.D. from Yokohama City University, Yokohama, Japan. Following this, he moved to the Eccles Institute of Human Genetics, Howard Hughes Medical Institute, University of Utah in the USA, where he worked as a post-doctoral fellow. His primary research interest is elucidating the molecular pathophysiology of salt-sensitive hypertension and atherosclerosis. Prof. Ishigami and colleagues developed a "high-sensitivity, high-throughput immunoglobulin auto-antibody screening system" using cell-free technology that can detect IgG-type antibodies against self-components with high sensitivity in atherosclerotic patients.(Ishigami T, et al. FASEB J, 2013) Prof. Ishigami and colleagues also conducted experiments using ApoE knockout mice, with the aim of clarifying the molecular biological mechanisms by which lifestyle habits induce atherosclerosis. As a result of the activation and conditioning of splenic B2 cells, they infiltrate PVAT, and an experiment was conducted to clarify the effect of B2 cell depletion on atherosclerosis. Using anti-CD23 antibody treatment, it was found to significantly suppress aortic plaque area and aortic annulus plaque area, as well as significantly suppress serum IgG/IgG3. (Chen L, Ishigami T, et al. eBioMedicine, 2016) Lubiprostone, a chloride channel activator, has the effect of improving the intestinal barrier function, and administration to ApoE knockout mice can also suppress atherosclerosis. (Arakawa K, Ishigami T, et al. Plos One, 2019).

Preface to "Current Challenges and Advances in Atherosclerosis"

Atherosclerosis is a systemic disorder which is of major interest in both basic science and clinical medicine in order to achieve healthy longevity worldwide. Atherosclerosis generally develops without any signs and symptoms, eventually resulting in various kinds of catastrophic cardiovascular events, such as ischemic heart disease, ischemic stroke, and rupture of major vessel aneurysms. Scientists working on the biological facets of atherosclerosis have recently focused on the persistent inflammation in vessel walls from intimal to adventitial tissues. Although inflammation is indeed a dominant pathological phenomenon in atherosclerosis, it has been recognized that there is no simple answer to the question of whether inflammation promotes or delays atherosclerosis. Atherosclerosis is a complex disease that involves several different cell types, such as lymphocytes, macrophages, monocytes, dendric cells, and their molecular products. Chronic inflammation in atherosclerosis can be accompanied by immunological changes, including auto-immune disorders. For example, our recent studies have shown that multiple auto-antibodies are found in the sera of subjects with atherosclerosis via inventory high-throughput auto-antibody screening techniques using cell-free technologies. Nevertheless, the immune system is even more complicated, with many cell types, hundreds of cytokines, and literally millions of different antigens, making research into atherosclerosis more complicated. Macrophages, which are differentiated from monocytes, one of the components of blood cells, phagocytize denatured LDL cholesterol on the vascular wall, become foamy cells, accumulate under the vascular endothelium, and cause atherosclerotic plaque formation. This forms the primary lesion, the fatty streak. Some of the aggregated foam cells undergo cell death over time, release denatured lipids in the cytoplasm, and increase in volume while forming a lipid core (necrotic core). The lipid core is surrounded by immune response cells, such as T cells, monocytes, macrophages, dendritic cells, and fibroblasts, to form atherosclerotic plaques. Enlarged lipid cores are at risk of rupture due to stresses on the vascular endothelium, such as blood pressure and shear stress from blood flow. The vulnerability of atherosclerotic plaques is thought to be determined by the formation of a fibrous cap around the plaque and the antagonism of degradation of fibrous components by protease, peptidase, etc., secreted by cells.

Fatal and non-fatal myocardial infarctions and cerebral infarctions, collectively referred to as cardiovascular events, result from accidental plaque rupture. As a result of plaque rupture, plaque components leak into the vascular lumen, causing local thrombus formation and subsequent activation of the fibrinolytic system. When the force of thrombus formation brought about by the qualitative and quantitative abnormalities of denatured lipids leaking from the lipid core exceeds the force of the endogenous fibrinolytic system, the thrombus occupies the finite space of the vascular lumen. As a result, blood flow with the thrombus is interrupted, and infarction of important organs occurs. Plaque rupture is accidental and unpredictable, and medical treatment starting from plaque rupture is a post-event response. Regarding the occurrence of cardiovascular events, there is only a therapeutic strategy that controls the risk and lowers the probability of atherosclerotic accidents, and a fundamental, radical therapeutic approach is required.

Among the immune cells and inflammatory cells involved in atherosclerosis, B cells have not necessarily been recognized to play a central role so far. Looking back at the history of atherosclerosis research, we can see that research on B cells is progressing. Arteries have a three-layered structure consisting of the intima, media, and adventitia. In 1915, at the very early stage of atherosclerosis research, Sir Clifford Allbutt investigated the relationship between atherosclerosis and B cells infiltrating the tunica adventitia, which can be traced back to the description of "round cell growth in the adventitia in atherosclerosis is correlated with absorption of depraved matter from the diseased intima." ([Diseases of the Artery]). The "round cells" infiltrating the adventitia described in this article were also reported in 1956 and 1962, and were found to be mainly B cells. Recent studies have shown that the activation of B cells in the adventitia is important in controlling atherosclerosis. Hamze et al. used microdissection techniques to analyze individual lymphocytes in coronary arteries. (J Immunol. 2013;191:3006-16.) They found that the majority of B cells reside in the adventitia of coronary arteries. In human and rodent models of atherosclerosis, B cells are present in the adventitia and form the tertiary lymph node tissue (ATLO, Artery Tertiary Lymphoid Organ). PVAT (perivascular adipose tissue), which is adjacent to the adventitia of arteries, contains complex and diverse cellular components, such as macrophages, T cells, and B cells, named FALCs (Fat-Associated Lymphoid Clusters). FALCs are in close proximity to the adventitial ATLO and may play a role in the establishment of atherosclerosis. Inflammation in atherosclerosis is not a transient inflammation. We reported that as a result of the activation and conditioning of B2 cells in the spleen, they infiltrate PVAT, and become the starting point of the pathology related to the onset of atherosclerosis. (Chen L, Ishigami T, et al. eBioMedicine, 2016) A high-fat, high-calorie diet causes changes in intestinal bacteria, dysbiosis, a decrease in intestinal barrier function, and activation of splenic B2 cells. Activated B2 cells can serve as a hypothetical biological model of atherosclerosis, in which they infiltrate the aortic adipose tissue and secrete IgG/IgG3 antibodies to promote atherosclerosis.

B cells infiltrate the PVAT from the very early stage of atherosclerosis, form FALCs, and form ATLO, a tertiary lymphoid tissue, in the adventitia. This may be the origin of immune response in atherosclerotic plaques in the endothelium/intima. The humoral immune response mediated by atherosclerotic B cells derives from antibody production and specific activation of B cell subtypes in the spleen. If this reaction, which can be said to be the biological starting point of atherosclerosis, can be controlled, it may become an option for the treatment of atherosclerosis.

This Special Issue, entitled "Current Challenges and Advances in Atherosclerosis", will focus on recent challenges and advances in the field of atherosclerosis by global expert scientists and clinicians to elucidate the complicated features of atherosclerosis and translational attempts for both medical and scientifical frontiers.

Tomoaki Ishigami
Editor

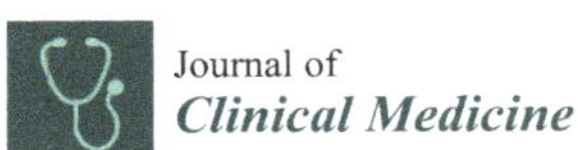
Journal of
Clinical Medicine

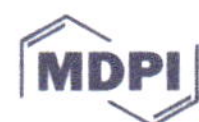

Article

Severity by National Institute of Health Stroke Scale Score and Clinical Features of Stroke Patients with Patent Foramen Ovale Stroke and Atrial Fibrillation

Kaito Abe [1,2], Fumiya Hasegawa [1,2], Ryota Nakajima [1], Hidetoshi Fukui [1], Moto Shimada [1,2], Takahiro Miyazaki [1,2], Hiroshi Doi [1,2], Goro Endo [1], Kaori Kanbara [1,2], Yasuyuki Mochida [1,2], Jun Okuda [1,2], Nobuya Maeda [3], Akira Isoshima [4], Koichi Tamura [2] and Tomoaki Ishigami [2,*]

1 Department of Cardiology, Omori Red Cross Hospital, 4-30-1 Chuo, Ota-Ward, Tokyo 143-8527, Japan; kaitoabemed@gmail.com (K.A.); e103061a@gmail.com (F.H.); cisvjikoryota@gmail.com (R.N.); fukubobu777@yahoo.co.jp (H.F.); petapetapeta@live.jp (M.S.); taka.miyazaki.55@gmail.com (T.M.); doihiroshi6120@yahoo.co.jp (H.D.); goro.08.29.09054261798@docomo.ne.jp (G.E.); kkanbara.circ@gmail.com (K.K.); yasmochi90@gmail.com (Y.M.); jokudajun@yahoo.co.jp (J.O.)

2 Department of Medical Science and Cardiorenal Medicine, Yokohama City University, 3-9 Fukuura Kanazawa-Ward, Yokohama City 236-0004, Japan; tamukou@yokohama-cu.ac.jp

3 Department of Neurology, Omori Red Cross Hospital, 4-30-1 Chuo, Ota-Ward, Tokyo 143-8527, Japan; nobmaeda@khf.biglobe.ne.jp

4 Department of Neurosurgery, Omori Red Cross Hospital, 4-30-1 Chuo, Ota-Ward, Tokyo 143-8527, Japan; a-isoshima@omori.jrc.or.jp

* Correspondence: tommmish@hotmail.com or tommmis@yokohama-cu.ac.jp; Tel.: +81-45-787-2635 (ext. 6312); Fax: +81-45-701-3738

Citation: Abe, K.; Hasegawa, F.; Nakajima, R.; Fukui, H.; Shimada, M.; Miyazaki, T.; Doi, H.; Endo, G.; Kanbara, K.; Mochida, Y.; et al. Severity by National Institute of Health Stroke Scale Score and Clinical Features of Stroke Patients with Patent Foramen Ovale Stroke and Atrial Fibrillation. *J. Clin. Med.* **2021**, *10*, 332. https://doi.org/10.3390/jcm10020332

Received: 30 December 2020
Accepted: 14 January 2021
Published: 18 January 2021

Publisher's Note: MDPI stays neutral with regard to jurisdictional claims in published maps and institutional affiliations.

Abstract: The comparative severity of patent foramen ovale (PFO)-related stroke in patients without atrial fibrillation (AF) and AF-related stroke in patients without PFO is unknown. Therefore, we compared the severity of PFO-related stroke and AF-related stroke. Twenty-six patients who underwent transesophageal echocardiography (TEE) were diagnosed with cardioembolic stroke from July 2018 to March 2020. Cases with AF detected by electrocardiograms or thrombus in the left atrium or left atrial appendage on TEE were included in the AF-related stroke group. Cases with a positive microbubble test on the Valsalva maneuver during TEE, and with no other factors that could cause stroke, were included in the PFO-related stroke group. This study was designed as a single-center, small population pilot study. The stroke severity of the two groups by the National Institute of Health Stroke Scale (NIHSS) score was compared by statistical analysis. Of the 26 cases, five PFO-related stroke patients and 21 AF-related stroke patients were analyzed. The NIHSS score was 2.2 ± 2.8 and 11.5 ± 9.2 (p-value < 0.01), the rate of hypertension was 20.0% and 85.7% (p-value = 0.01), and the HbA1c value was 5.5 ± 0.2% and 6.3 ± 1.3% (p-value = 0.02) in the PFO-related and AF-related stroke groups, respectively. Compared with AF-related stroke patients, stroke severity was low in PFO-related stroke patients.

Keywords: patent foramen ovale and stroke; atrial fibrillation and stroke; cryptogenic stroke; severity of stroke; National Institute of Health Stroke Scale score

1. Introduction

Stroke results in substantial disability and sometimes causes death [1]. The TOAST classification denotes five subtypes of ischemic stroke: (1) large-artery atherosclerosis, (2) cardioembolism, (3) small-vessel occlusion, (4) stroke of other determined etiology, and (5) stroke of undetermined etiology [2]. Cardioembolic stroke accounts for 15–30% of ischemic strokes [3].

In up to 40% of patients with acute ischemic stroke, there is a stroke of undetermined etiology in TOAST classification (5); this stroke has been labeled as cryptogenic stroke [1,2,4,5]. Major cardioembolic risk sources include atrial fibrillation (AF), recent myocardial infarction, previous myocardial infarction (left ventricular aneurysm), intracardiac thrombus, tumors, rheumatic valve disease, aortic arch atheromatous plaques, endocarditis, and mechanical valve prosthesis, whereas minor or unclear risk sources include patent foramen ovale (PFO), atrial septal aneurysm (ASA), and giant Lambl's excrescences [3]. Evaluation of stroke sources is important for preventing second stroke events.

In the general population, 0.4–1% have AF, and the prevalence increases to 9% in the population aged 80 years or older [6]. The CHADS2 and CHA2DS2-VASc risk scores show the frequent occurrence of stroke and embolism, ranging from 0 (low risk) to 18% event/year (high-risk) among patients with AF [7,8].

For the management of AF, anticoagulant therapy, catheter ablation, and antiarrhythmic drugs are well-established [9]. Recently, transcatheter left atrial appendage closure has been used as a primary therapy for AF patients with contraindications for using chronic oral anticoagulation to prevent stroke [10].

PFO is caused by incomplete fusion of the septum primum and secundum after birth in the cranial portion of the fossa ovalis, and is a common anatomical variant found in about 25% of the general population [11,12]. Stroke with PFO occurs when a systemic venous thrombus travels directly into the systemic arterial circulation [1]. The proportion of stroke patients with PFO is 21–63% [11]. According to a report, cryptogenic stroke patients with PFO were younger and less likely to have conventional vascular risk factors than cryptogenic stroke patients without PFO [11].

Recently, the DEFENSE, REDUCE, and CLOSE trials demonstrated the superiority of PFO closure over medical management [13–15]. In cryptogenic stroke, detection of PFO is important to select an adequate secondary stroke prevention therapy. Transesophageal echocardiography (TEE) is the gold standard for PFO detection. The microbubble test with Valsalva maneuver is recommended for detecting PFO on TEE to avoid the increasing false negative rate of up to 20% when the Valsalva maneuver is not performed [3,16].

It is known that the severity of ischemic stroke patients with PFO, including patients with AF, is lower than that of patients without PFO, including patients with AF [17]; however, whether the severity of PFO-related stroke in patients without AF is lower than that of AF-related stroke in patients without PFO is unknown. Thus, the purpose of this analysis was to evaluate the severity of PFO-related stroke and AF-related stroke, and to identify the characteristics of both stroke types.

2. Materials and Methods

2.1. Study Design and Patient Population

We performed a single-center (Omori Red Cross Hospital) retrospective study on consecutive patients with cardioembolic stroke, including suspected cases on magnetic resonance imaging, who underwent TEE between July 2018 and March 2020.

Patients with AF diagnosed from history, electrocardiogram (ECG) at admission, 24 h-holter ECG monitoring, ECG monitoring in the ward, or patients with thrombi including smoke-like echo with a swirling motion of blood in the left atrium (LA) or left atrial appendage (LAA), which is known to be a marker of a prothrombotic state, were classified as AF-related stroke patients [18]. Patients with PFO without AF were classified as PFO-related stroke patients.

Patients with mobile aortic plaque were defined as Class V in the Katz Index [19], patients after valve replacement and those with cardiac tumor, infectious endocarditis, Lambl's excrescence on the aortic valve, or those diagnosed with atherosclerotic stroke by neurologists after TEE were excluded from this study. Patients with PFO between the right atrium (RA) and LA diagnosed only by the color Doppler method without passage of microbubbles were excluded from this study.

2.2. Evaluations

The diagnosis of ischemic stroke was made by neurologists with known experience in cerebrovascular diseases. TEE was performed and evaluated by cardiologists who were well-experienced in echocardiology. TEE was performed with either Vivid E95 (GE Healthcare, Tokyo, Japan) or ALOKA Prosoundα10 (ALOKA, Tokyo, Japan).

2.3. Baseline Study Assessment

We collected data on patient characteristics (age, sex, height, body weight, and smoking habit); vascular risk factors; the administration ratio of antiplatelet therapy or oral anticoagulant therapy before stroke onset; blood tests (aspartate transaminase (AST), alanine aminotransferase (ALT), lactate dehydrogenase (LDH), alkaline phosphatase (ALP), total bilirubin (T-bil), brain natriuretic peptide (BNP), hemoglobin, HbA1c, D-dimer, low-density lipoprotein (LDL), high-density lipoprotein (HDL), triglycerides (TGs), creatinine (Cre), estimated glomerular filtration rate (eGFR), and creatinine clearance (CCR) (Cockcroft–Gault equation)); HAS-BLED score to assess bleeding risk in AF patients from hypertension, abnormal renal/liver function, stroke, bleeding history or predisposition, labile INR, elderly (>65 years old), and concomitant drugs/alcohol use [20]; National Institute of Health Stroke Scale (NIHSS) [21]; the risk of paradoxical embolism (RoPE) score to assess the likelihood of the cryptogenic stroke being related to PFO based on the scoring items of age, hypertension, diabetes, history of stroke or transient ischemic attack, smoking habit, and cortical infarct on imaging [11]; ECG; 24 h-holter ECG monitoring; ECG monitoring in the hospital ward; thrombus, including smoke-like echo in LA or LAA by TEE; and left ventricular ejection fraction (LVEF) by transthoracic echocardiography.

The TEE was performed under light sedation with propofol. The LA or LAA thrombi were evaluated in all patients by TEE. For all patients who underwent TEE, an intravenous microbubble test during the Valsalva maneuver was performed. In the GORE-REDUCE trial [14], the classification of PFO size was based on the maximum number of microbubbles during the first three cardiac cycles; 0 microbubbles were classified as no shunt, one to five microbubbles as small, six to 25 microbubbles as moderate, and more than 25 microbubbles as large. PFO was diagnosed by the microbubble test using the Valsalva maneuver technique between the RA and LA. Complex PFO was classified as PFO with ASA, or with a long tunnel length of over 8 mm, or with the eustachian valve [22]. Some AF-related stroke patients with LA or LAA thrombi skipped the microbubble test.

2.4. Statistical Analysis

JMP Pro version 15 software (SAS Institute Japan Inc., Tokyo, Japan) was used for statistical analysis. Data are expressed as mean ± standard deviation for continuous variables and as frequencies and percentages for categorical variables. Baseline characteristics were compared using the Student's *t* test or Welch's *t* test for continuous variables and Fisher's exact test for categorical variables. A p-value < 0.05 was considered statistically significant.

3. Results

3.1. Stroke Classification

A total of 82 patients were enrolled from July 2018 to March 2020. AF-related stroke was noted in 21 (25.6%) patients, atherosclerotic stroke in 21 (25.6%), PFO-related stroke in five (6.1%), cardioembolic stroke without AF in 13 (15.9%), others (systemic lupus erythematosus, hyperemia, vasculitis, lacunar infarction) in four (4.9%), and cryptogenic stroke in 18 (22.0%) (Figure 1). Cardioembolic stroke without AF included patients with post-valve replacement (four patients), cardiac tumor (two patients), infectious endocarditis (one patient), Lambl's excrescence on the aortic valve (two patients), old myocardial infarction (one patient), and patients with PFO between the RA and LA diagnosed only by the color Doppler method without passage of microbubbles (three patients).

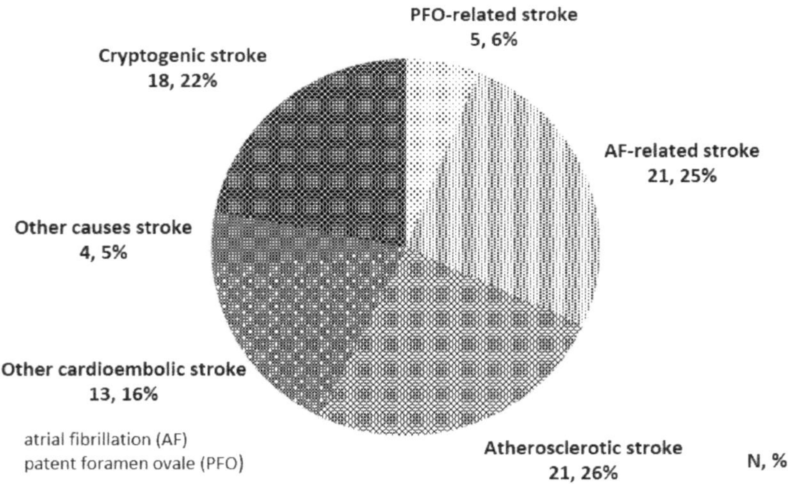

Figure 1. Stroke classification of this study.

3.2. Study Population and Patient Features

Among the 21 AF-related stroke patients, 20 (95.2%) patients had AF and 10 (47.6%) had LA or LAA thrombus, whereas the PFO-related stroke patients had no AF or thrombus in the LA or LAA. The ratio of comorbidity with hypertension in AF-related stroke patients was higher than that in PFO-related stroke patients (85.7%, 20.0%, *p*-value = 0.01). The NIHSS score in AF-related stroke patients was more severe than that in PFO-related stroke patients (11.5 ± 9.2, 2.2 ± 2.8, *p*-value < 0.01). Age, height, body weight, LVEF, and HAS-BLED score were not significantly different between the groups. The comorbidity ratio of dyslipidemia, diabetes, old myocardial infarction, or past stroke history had no significant differences between the two groups. The administration ratio of antiplatelet therapy or oral anticoagulant therapy before stroke onset had no significant differences between the two groups (Table 1).

Table 1. Baseline patient characteristics of PFO-related stoke and AF-related stroke.

Characteristics		PFO-Related Stroke	AF-Related Stroke	*p*-Value
		(*n* = 5)	(*n* = 21)	
Age	y.o	58.2 ± 23.4	77.9 ± 7.6	n.s *
Sex (Male)	*n* (%)	4 (80%)	14 (66.7%)	n.s †
Height	cm	166.4 ± 7.3	162.0 ± 8.0	n.s
Body Weight	kg	59.9 ± 10.7	58.9 ± 11.0	n.s
Smoking Habit	*n* (%)	5 (100%)	11 (52.4%)	n.s †
Hypertension	*n* (%)	1 (20%)	18 (85.7%)	0.01 †
Dyslipidemia	*n* (%)	3 (60%)	11 (52.4%)	n.s †
Diabetes	*n* (%)	0 (0%)	7 (33.3%)	n.s †
OMI	*n* (%)	0 (0%)	2 (9.5%)	n.s †
History of Stroke	*n* (%)	0 (0%)	2 (9.5%)	n.s †
PFO	*n* (%)	5 (100%)	0 (0%)	<0.01 †
AF	*n* (%)	0 (0%)	20 (95.2%)	<0.01 †
LA/LAA thrombus	*n* (%)	0 (0%)	10 (47.6%)	n.s †
LVEF	%	69.0 ± 5.2	66.0 ± 8.4	n.s

Table 1. *Cont.*

Characteristics		PFO-Related Stroke	AF-Related Stroke	p-Value
		(n = 5)	(n = 21)	
Antiplatet Therapy	n (%)	2 (40%)	7 (33.3%)	n.s †
Anticoagulant Therapy	n (%)	0 (0%)	4 (19%)	
DOAC	n (%)		3 (14.3%)	
Warfarin	n (%)		1 (4.8%)	
HAS-BLED Score		2.2 ± 1.6	3.3 ± 0.9	n.s
NIHSS Score		2.2 ± 2.8	11.5 ± 9.2	<0.01 *

Atrial fibrillation (AF), direct oral anticoagulants (DOAC), left atrium (LA), left atrial appendage (LAA), left ventricular ejection fraction (LVEF), National Institute of Health Stroke Scale (NIHSS), old myocardial infarction (OMI), patent foramen ovale (PFO), years old (y.o); * Welch's *t* test, † Fisher's exact test.

HbA1c values in AF-related stroke patients were higher than that in PFO-related stroke patients (6.3% ± 1.3%, 5.5% ± 0.2%, *p*-value = 0.02). BNP, D-dimer, hemoglobin, LDL, HDL, TG, Cre, eGFR, CCR, AST, ALT, T-bil, and ALP were not significantly different between the groups (Table 2).

Table 2. Baseline patient blood test parameters of PFO-related stoke and AF-related stroke.

Blood Test Parameters		PFO-Related Stroke	AF-Related Stroke	p-Value
		(n = 5)	(n = 21)	
BNP	pg/mL	39.5 ± 28.1	155.4 ± 189.0	n.s *
D-dimer	ug/mL	3.7 ± 5.6	2.0 ± 2.4	n.s *
Hb	g/dL	14.4 ± 1.3	13.8 ± 2.0	n.s
HbA1c	%	5.5 ± 0.2	6.3 ± 1.3	0.02 *
LDL	mg/dL	116.0 ± 32.0	110.3 ± 42.4	n.s
HDL	mg/dL	67.2 ± 25.6	57.5 ± 17.4	n.s
TG	mg/dL	112.6 ± 55.6	125.1 ± 98.7	n.s
Cre	mg/dL	0.84 ± 0.2	1.01 ± 0.5	n.s
eGFR	ml/min/1.73 m2	73.8 ± 17.4	58.9 ± 20.6	n.s
CCR	ml/min	83.2 ± 35.5	56.5 ± 23.7	n.s
AST	IU/l	19.0 ± 4.7	23.4 ± 5.8	n.s
ALT	IU/l	15.6 ± 2.7	15.5 ± 6.4	n.s
LDH	IU/l	178.0 ± 18.4	231.0 ± 45.2	0.02
T-bil	mg/dL	0.62 ± 0.23	0.77 ± 0.32	n.s
ALP	IU/l	182.4 ± 70.8	237.4 ± 95.3	n.s

Atrial fibrillation (AF), alkaline phosphatase (ALP), alanine aminotransferase (ALT), aspartate transaminase (AST), brain natriuretic peptide (BNP), creatinine clearance (CCR) (Cockcroft–Gault equation), creatinine (Cre), estimated glomerular filtration rate (eGFR), hemoglobin (Hb), high-density lipoprotein (HDL), lactate dehydrogenase (LDH), low-density lipoprotein (LDL), patent foramen ovale (PFO), total bilirubin (T-bil), triglycerides (TG); * Welch's *t* test.

3.3. PFO Characteristics of This Study

Among the five PFO-related stroke patients, one patient had a small shunt PFO, two patients had moderate shunt PFO, and two patients had a large shunt PFO. Of the five PFO-related stroke patients, four patients had complex PFO; all complex PFOs had a long PFO tunnel, and had no eustachian valve or ASA. The RoPE score was 4.8 ± 2.4, the average PFO attributable fraction was 36.0 ± 37.3%, and the estimated two years stroke recurrence rate was 12.2 ± 7.2% in this PFO population by RoPE score to assess the likelihood of the cryptogenic stroke being related to PFO (Table 3) [11].

Table 3. PFO characteristics, PFO attributable fraction, and estimated two years stroke recurrence rate by RoPE score.

PFO Characteristics		PFO-Related Stroke (n = 5)
PFO Size		
Small	n	1
Moderate	n	2
Large	n	2
Rope Score		4.8 ± 2.4
PFO-Attributable Fraction	%	36.0 ± 37.3
Estimated Two Years Stroke Recurrence Rate	%	12.2 ± 7.2

The classification of PFO size: 0 microbubbles were classified as no shunt, one to five microbubbles as small, six to 25 microbubbles as moderate, and more than 25 microbubbles as large.; patent foramen ovale (PFO), risk of paradoxical embolism (RoPE).

4. Discussion

The novelty of this study is that it is a PFO group diagnosed by TEE with the highly diagnostic Valsalva maneuver technique, and that it includes the severity of stroke between PFO-related stroke in patients without AF and AF-related stroke in patients without PFO.

Severity comparison by the NIHSS showed that AF-related stroke was more severe than PFO-related stroke. Previous studies [17] also reported that PFO-related stroke was less severe than strokes in the other groups; it was expected that AF-related stroke would be more severe, which was also revealed in our study. Regarding administration of oral medication before stroke onset, antiplatelet therapy was administered to two (40%) patients in the PFO-related stroke group. In the AF-related stroke group, anticoagulation therapy was administered to four (19.0%) patients and antiplatelet therapy to seven (33.3%). It may be necessary to consider the effect of these pre-medications on the severity of stroke.

Generally, it is said that PFO-related stroke patients are younger and have less cardiovascular risk; this study also showed that the ratio of comorbidity of hypertension and high HbA1c in blood tests was significantly lower in the PFO-related stroke patients compared to AF-related stroke patients. Although there was no significant difference in other factors, the age, ratio of comorbidity of dyslipidemia, diabetes, and ratio of smoking habits tended to be low in the PFO-related stroke group, which was similar to the existing report [11]. In particular, the average age of the PFO-related stroke patients was 58.2 years, which is younger than that of the AF-related stroke patients (77.9 years), and it is necessary to consider that the fact that there are few cardiovascular risk factors may also contribute to the low severity of stroke in the PFO-related stroke patients. For younger patients, functional improvement after stroke can be expected, and observation of long prognosis is also important.

It has been reported that the probability of stroke due to PFO is 88%, and the recurrence rate after two years is 2% in the group with the highest RoPE Score [11]. The PFO attributable stroke rate in this study is not high at 36.0%, but the average recurrence probability after two years by the RoPE score is estimated to be high at 12.2%. Therefore, secondary prevention therapies, such as antiplatelet therapy, anticoagulant therapy, or a PFO occluder device, seemed to be important in decreasing the recurrence rate of strokes.

This study has some limitations. This study is a pilot study not registered in clinical trials with an international clinical trials register. As this was a retrospective analysis at a single institution, it is necessary to consider the influence of the small population, five PFO-related stroke patients and 21 AF-related stroke patients. Statistical results may not be sufficient, as power analysis has not been performed in this study. It is also necessary to consider the influence of population bias, such as pre-test probability, because it is a group of cases in which neurologists suspected cardioembolic stroke and who needed TEE. In addition, there is a possibility that latent AF and PFO may be involved in cases of stroke other than cardioembolic stroke diagnosed by neurologists. Since patient prognosis was not observed in this study, it is necessary to observe their prognosis after medical interventions. We need to be careful in interpreting the results of this study.

There were 18 (22.0%) cases in the stroke group with unknown causes in the analysis target, and four of them were suspected of being cardioembolic stroke by the neurologist, but definitive clinical findings were unclear. It seems necessary to evaluate the comorbidity of AF with an implantable electrocardiograph.

In this analysis, TEE with the Valsalva maneuver technique was performed for PFO detection; therefore, PFO detection in this study was highly credible. However, it is said that there are detection limits of this method; hence, it seems that there is a possibility of wrongly classifying other strokes into the cryptogenic stroke group.

In addition, even in the group diagnosed with cryptogenic stroke, the detection rate of thrombus in LA/LAA may have decreased, because at the time of TEE, antiplatelet therapy or anticoagulant therapy had already been performed. In this study, after stroke, anticoagulant therapy was administered to three patients, and antiplatelet therapy was administered to one patient in the PFO-related stroke group. In the AF-related stroke group, anticoagulant therapy was administered to all patients. Of these, anticoagulation therapy alone was administered to 19 (90.5%) patients, and a combination of antiplatelet therapy and anticoagulant therapy was administered to two (9.5%) patients. Therefore, it is necessary to observe the secondary preventive effect on the recurrence rate in the future.

5. Conclusions

Compared with AF-related stroke patients, stroke severity, the comorbidity of hypertension rate, and the value of HbA1c were low in PFO-related stroke patients.

Author Contributions: Conceptualization, K.A.; methodology, K.A.; software, K.A. and T.I.; validation, K.A., F.H., R.N., H.F., M.S., T.M., H.D., G.E., K.K., Y.M., J.O., N.M., A.I., K.T. and T.I.; formal analysis, K.A. and T.I.; investigation, K.A. and T.I.; resources, K.A., F.H., R.N., H.F., M.S., T.M., H.D., G.E., K.K., Y.M., J.O., N.M. and A.I.; data curation, K.A. and T.I.; writing—original draft preparation, K.A.; writing—review and editing, K.T. and T.I.; visualization, K.A. and T.I.; supervision, N.M., A.I., K.T. and T.I.; project administration, K.A. and T.I.; All authors have read and agreed to the published version of the manuscript.

Funding: This research received no external funding.

Institutional Review Board Statement: The study was conducted according to the guidelines of the Declaration of Helsinki, and approved by the ethical committee of Omori Red Cross Hospital (protocol code: No.20-5, 26 May 2020).

Informed Consent Statement: Informed consent was obtained from all subjects involved in the study.

Data Availability Statement: The data presented in this study are available on request from the corresponding author.

Acknowledgments: We are grateful to departments of neurology, neurosurgery, and cardiology staffs for stroke patients' care.

Conflicts of Interest: The authors declare no conflict of interest.

References

1. Mir, H.; Siemieniuk, R.A.C.; Ge, L.C.; Foroutan, F.; Fralick, M.; Syed, T.; Lopes, L.C.; Kuijpers, T.; Mas, J.-L.; Vandvik, P.O.; et al. Patent foramen ovale closure, antiplatelet therapy or anticoagulation in patients with patent foramen ovale and cryptogenic stroke: A systematic review and network meta-analysis incorporating complementary external evidence. *BMJ Open* **2018**, *8*, e023761. [CrossRef] [PubMed]
2. Adams, H.P.; Bendixen, B.H.; Kappelle, L.J.; Biller, J.; Love, B.B.; Gordon, D.L.; Marsh, E.E. Classification of subtype of acute ischemic stroke. Definitions for use in a multicenter clinical trial. TOAST. Trial of Org 10172 in Acute Stroke Treatment. *Stroke* **1993**, *24*, 35–41. [CrossRef] [PubMed]
3. Pepi, M.; Evangelista, A.; Nihoyannopoulos, P.; Flachskampf, F.A.; Athanassopoulos, G.; Colonna, P.; Habib, G.; Ringelstein, E.B.; Sicari, R.; Zamorano, J.L.; et al. Recommendations for echocardiography use in the diagnosis and management of cardiac sources of embolism: European Association of Echocardiography (EAE) (a registered branch of the ESC). *Eur. J. Echocardiogr.* **2010**, *11*, 461–476. [CrossRef]

4. Osteraas, N.D.; Vargas, A.; Cherian, L.; Song, S. Role of PFO Closure in Ischemic Stroke Prevention. *Curr. Treat. Options Cardiovasc. Med.* **2019**, *21*, 63. [CrossRef]
5. Benjamin, E.J.; Blaha, M.J.; Chiuve, S.E.; Cushman, M.; Das, S.R.; Deo, R.; de Ferranti, S.D.; Floyd, J.; Fornage, M.; Gillespie, C.; et al. Heart Disease and Stroke Statistics-2017 Update: A Report From the American Heart Association. *Circulation* **2017**, *135*, e146–e603. [CrossRef] [PubMed]
6. Go, A.S.; Hylek, E.M.; Phillips, K.A.; Chang, Y.; Henault, L.E.; Selby, J.V.; Singer, D.E. Prevalence of diagnosed atrial fibrillation in adults: National implications for rhythm management and stroke prevention: The AnTicoagulation and Risk Factors in Atrial Fibrillation (ATRIA) Study. *JAMA* **2001**, *285*, 2370–2375. [CrossRef]
7. Gage, B.F.; Waterman, A.D.; Shannon, W.; Boechler, M.; Rich, M.W.; Radford, M.J. Validation of clinical classification schemes for predicting stroke: Results from the National Registry of Atrial Fibrillation. *JAMA* **2001**, *285*, 2864–2870. [CrossRef]
8. Lip, G.Y.H.; Nieuwlaat, R.; Pisters, R.; Lane, D.A.; Crijns, H.J.G.M. Refining clinical risk stratification for predicting stroke and thromboembolism in atrial fibrillation using a novel risk factor-based approach: The euro heart survey on atrial fibrillation. *Chest* **2010**, *137*, 263–272. [CrossRef]
9. Ono, K.; Iwasaki, Y.; Shimizu, W.; Akao, M.; Ikeda, T.; Ishii, K.; Inden, Y.; Kusano, K.; Kobayashi, Y.; Koretsune, Y.; et al. JCS/JHRS 2020 Guideline on Pharmacotherapy of Cardiac Arrhythmias. Available online: https://www.j-circ.or.jp/cms/wp-content/uploads/2020/01/JCS2020_Ono.pdf (accessed on 28 August 2020).
10. Majule, D.N.; Jing, C.; Rutahoile, W.M.; Shonyela, F.S. The Efficacy and Safety of the WATCHMAN Device in LAA Occlusion in Patients with Non-Valvular Atrial Fibrillation Contraindicated to Oral Anticoagulation: A Focused Review. *Ann. Thorac. Cardiovasc. Surg.* **2018**, *24*, 271–278. [CrossRef]
11. Kent, D.M.; Ruthazer, R.; Weimar, C.; Mas, J.-L.; Serena, J.; Homma, S.; Di Angelantonio, E.; Di Tullio, M.R.; Lutz, J.S.; Elkind, M.S.V.; et al. An index to identify stroke-related vs incidental patent foramen ovale in cryptogenic stroke. *Neurology* **2013**, *81*, 619–625. [CrossRef]
12. Homma, S.; Sacco, R.L. Patent foramen ovale and stroke. *Circulation* **2005**, *112*, 1063–1072. [CrossRef] [PubMed]
13. Lee, P.H.; Song, J.-K.; Kim, J.S.; Heo, R.; Lee, S.; Kim, D.-H.; Song, J.-M.; Kang, D.-H.; Kwon, S.U.; Kang, D.-W.; et al. Cryptogenic Stroke and High-Risk Patent Foramen Ovale: The DEFENSE-PFO Trial. *J. Am. Coll. Cardiol.* **2018**, *71*, 2335–2342. [CrossRef] [PubMed]
14. Søndergaard, L.; Kasner, S.E.; Rhodes, J.F.; Andersen, G.; Iversen, H.K.; Nielsen-Kudsk, J.E.; Settergren, M.; Sjöstrand, C.; Roine, R.O.; Hildick-Smith, D.; et al. Patent Foramen Ovale Closure or Antiplatelet Therapy for Cryptogenic Stroke. *N. Engl. J. Med.* **2017**, *377*, 1033–1042. [CrossRef] [PubMed]
15. Mas, J.-L.; Derumeaux, G.; Guillon, B.; Massardier, E.; Hosseini, H.; Mechtouff, L.; Arquizan, C.; Béjot, Y.; Vuillier, F.; Detante, O.; et al. Patent Foramen Ovale Closure or Anticoagulation vs. Antiplatelets after Stroke. *N. Engl. J. Med.* **2017**, *377*, 1011–1021. [CrossRef] [PubMed]
16. Rodrigues, A.C.; Picard, M.H.; Carbone, A.; Arruda, A.L.; Flores, T.; Klohn, J.; Furtado, M.; Lira-Filho, E.B.; Cerri, G.G.; Andrade, J.L. Importance of adequately performed Valsalva maneuver to detect patent foramen ovale during transesophageal echocardiography. *J. Am. Soc. Echocardiogr.* **2013**, *26*, 1337–1343. [CrossRef]
17. Consoli, D.; Paciaroni, M.; Galati, F.; Aguggia, M.; Melis, M.; Malferrari, G.; Consoli, A.; Vidale, S.; Bosco, D.; Cerrato, P.; et al. Prevalence of Patent Foramen Ovale in Ischaemic Stroke in Italy: Results of SISIFO Study. *Cerebrovasc. Dis.* **2015**, *39*, 162–169. [CrossRef]
18. Sahin, O.; Savas, G. Relationship between presence of spontaneous echo contrast and platelet-to-lymphocyte ratio in patients with mitral stenosis. *Echocardiography* **2019**, *36*, 924–929. [CrossRef]
19. Katz, E.S.; Tunick, P.A.; Rusinek, H.; Ribakove, G.; Spencer, F.C.; Kronzon, I. Protruding aortic atheromas predict stroke in elderly patients undergoing cardiopulmonary bypass: Experience with intraoperative transesophageal echocardiography. *J. Am. Coll. Cardiol.* **1992**, *20*, 70–77. [CrossRef]
20. Pisters, R.; Lane, D.A.; Nieuwlaat, R.; De Vos, C.B.; Crijns, H.J.G.M.; Lip, G.Y.H. A Novel User-Friendly Score (HAS-BLED) To Assess 1-Year Risk of Major Bleeding in Patients with Atrial Fibrillation. *Chest* **2010**, *138*, 1093–1100. [CrossRef]
21. Brott, T.; Adams, H.P.; Olinger, C.P.; Marler, J.R.; Barsan, W.G.; Biller, J.; Spilker, J.; Holleran, R.; Eberle, R.; Hertzberg, V. Measurements of acute cerebral infarction: A clinical examination scale. *Stroke* **1989**, *20*, 864–870. [CrossRef]
22. Vitarelli, A.; Mangieri, E.; Capotosto, L.; Tanzilli, G.; D'Angeli, I.; Toni, D.; Azzano, A.; Ricci, S.; Placanica, A.; Rinaldi, E.; et al. Echocardiographic findings in simple and complex patent foramen ovale before and after transcatheter closure. *Eur. Heart J. Cardiovasc. Imaging* **2014**, *15*, 1377–1385. [CrossRef] [PubMed]

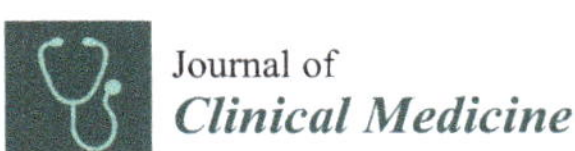
Journal of
Clinical Medicine

MDPI

Review

The Types and Proportions of Commensal Microbiota Have a Predictive Value in Coronary Heart Disease

Lin Chen [1,2], Tomoaki Ishigami [1,*], Hiroshi Doi [1], Kentaro Arakawa [1] and Kouichi Tamura [1]

[1] Department of Medical Science and Cardio-Renal Medicine, Graduate School of Medicine, Yokohama City University, Kanagawa 236-0027, Japan; linchen@njmu.edu.cn (L.C.); doihiroshi6120@yahoo.co.jp (H.D.); hiroking@gamma.ocn.ne.jp (K.A.); tamukou@yokohama-cu.ac.jp (K.T.)

[2] Department of Cardiology, Sir Run Run Hospital, Nanjing Medical University, Nanjing 210029, China

* Correspondence: tommmish@yokohama-cu.ac.jp; Tel.: +81-45-787-2635

Abstract: Previous clinical studies have suggested that commensal microbiota play an important role in atherosclerotic cardiovascular disease; however, a synthetic analysis of coronary heart disease (CHD) has yet to be performed. Therefore, we aimed to investigate the specific types of commensal microbiota associated with CHD by performing a systematic review of prospective observational studies that have assessed associations between commensal microbiota and CHD. Of the 544 published articles identified in the initial search, 16 publications with data from 16 cohort studies (2210 patients) were included in the analysis. The combined data showed that Bacteroides and Prevotella were commonly identified among nine articles (n = 13) in the fecal samples of patients with CHD, while seven articles commonly identified Firmicutes. Moreover, several types of commensal microbiota were common to atherosclerotic plaque and blood or gut samples in 16 cohort studies. For example, Veillonella, Proteobacteria, and Streptococcus were identified among the plaque and fecal samples, whereas Clostridium was commonly identified among blood and fecal samples of patients with CHD. Collectively, our findings suggest that several types of commensal microbiota are associated with CHD, and their presence may correlate with disease markers of CHD.

Keywords: commensal microbiota; coronary heart disease; systematic review

Citation: Chen, L.; Ishigami, T.; Doi, H.; Arakawa, K.; Tamura, K. The Types and Proportions of Commensal Microbiota Have a Predictive Value in Coronary Heart Disease. *J. Clin. Med.* **2021**, *10*, 3120. https://doi.org/10.3390/jcm10143120

Academic Editors: Maciej Banach, Francesco Giallauria and Massimo Mancone

Received: 10 March 2021
Accepted: 24 June 2021
Published: 15 July 2021

1. Introduction

In recent years, coronary heart disease (CHD) has remained the leading cause of death worldwide, while statins and other pharmacological agents for coronary secondary prevention have failed to completely protect people against CHD, despite their widespread use [1–3]. Given the unmet need for effective therapies, there has been increasing interest in targeting novel pathways that underlie the pathogenesis of CHD and in establishing a precise system to track its development. Additionally, to observe the progression of the disease, there is an increasingly important clinical value in discovering a predictive biomarker for CHD. Although the molecular mechanisms responsible for the development of CHD are not completely understood, recent studies have highlighted the critical role of commensal microbiota in CHD [4–6], with alterations in the gut microbiota being linked to CHD progression [4]. However, a synthetic analysis of the predictive value of specific types of commensal microbes in CHD patients has not yet been performed. In particular, a cross-site comparison of the types of microbes in the blood, gut, and atherosclerotic plaques of these patient is essential, given the high level of variability observed in the microbiota between different subjects and studies [7–11]. Therefore, in this analysis, we aimed to combine the results from published clinical trials to compare the types, proportions, and sources of commensal microbes in CHD. Our findings revealed several types of commensal microbes common to the atherosclerotic plaques, blood, or gut samples in patients with CHD, and the expression of some specific types of commensal microbes could be used as predictive or disease biomarkers of CHD in the future.

2. Materials and Methods

2.1. Search Strategy

We searched several electronic databases (PubMed, Embase, Web of Science, Cochrane Library, and ClinicalTrials.gov) up until 8 March 2020 for prospective, observational clinical studies that have investigated commensal microbes in patients with CHD. We used broad search terms (Additional File 1) describing aspects of 'Gastrointestinal Microbiome' and 'Coronary Disease'. These terms were used in combination with "AND" or "OR". This literature review was performed independently by two investigators, with a third resolving any disputes as needed. The detailed search strategy of PubMed: used: ("Coronary Disease") or (Coronary Diseases) or (Disease, Coronary) or (Diseases, Coronary) or (Coronary Heart Disease) or (Coronary Heart Diseases) or (Disease, Coronary Heart) or (Diseases, Coronary Heart) or (Heart Disease, Coronary) or (Heart Diseases, Coronary) and ("Gastrointestinal Microbiome") or (Gastrointestinal Microbiomes) or (Microbiome, Gastrointestinal) or (Gut Microbiome) or (Gut Microbiomes) or (Microbiome, Gut) or (Gut Microflora) or (Microflora, Gut) or (Gut Microbiota) or (Gut Microbiotas) or (Microbiota, Gut) or (Gastrointestinal Flora) or (Flora, Gastrointestinal) or (Gut Flora) or (Flora, Gut) or (Gastrointestinal Microbiota) or (Gastrointestinal Microbiotas) or (Microbiota, Gastrointestinal) or (Gastrointestinal Microbial Community) or (Gastrointestinal Microbial Communities) or (Microbial Community, Gastrointestinal) or (Gastrointestinal Microflora) or (Microflora, Gastrointestinal) or (Gastric Microbiome) or (Gastric Microbiomes) or (Microbiome, Gastric) or (Intestinal Microbiome) or (Intestinal Microbiomes) or (Microbiome, Intestinal) or (Intestinal Microbiota) or (Intestinal Microbiotas) or (Microbiota, Intestinal) or (Intestinal Microflora) or (Microflora, Intestinal) or (Intestinal Flora) or (Flora, Intestinal) or (Enteric Bacteria) or (Bacteria, Enteric) and (risk*[Title/Abstract] or risk*[MeSH:noexp] or risk *[MeSH:noexp] or cohort studies[MeSH Terms] or group*[Text Word]). We then used a similar approach with Embase, Web of Science, Cochrane Library, and ClinicalTrials.gov. Following the PICOS (Participants, Interventions, Comparisons, Outcomes and Study design) principle, the key search terms included (P) patients with CHD; (I) detection of the gene of microbiota; (C/O) compare the types of commensal microbiota between the CHD group and the control group; (S) case-control studies or cohort study.

2.2. Study Selection

Prospective, observational, controlled studies that assessed changes in populations of commensal microbes were included if they conducted baseline measurements in a population with CHD, including those with atherosclerosis or acute coronary syndrome (ACS) or chronic CHD (defined as a history of myocardial infarction (MI), percutaneous coronary intervention (PCI), coronary artery bypass grafting (CABG), or a diagnosis confirmed through coronary angiography). Publications without detailed data were excluded from this study. When multiple publications were based on the same source study, we included the publication that had the larger sample size or more relative data.

2.3. Data Extraction

The following data from each study were extracted: the first author's name, publication year, country of the conducted study, sample size, population, source of commensal microbes (atherosclerotic plaque or blood or fecal samples), region from which the genetic expression was quantified, and the specific types of commensal microbes demonstrating statistically significant changes in expression, whether increased or decreased, in CHD.

2.4. Data Synthesis and Analysis

The commensal microbes demonstrating statistically significant changes in expression in fecal, blood, or atherosclerotic plaque samples from the 16 included studies were sorted and classified according to the degree to which the populations were increased or decreased. Subsequently, an overall comparison of the gut, blood, and atherosclerotic plaque microbiota was performed, and any microbiota demonstrating a change among at least two publications for each of the three sample types was recorded. Furthermore, interstudy comparisons of atherosclerotic plaque, blood, and gut microbiota were also performed, and the microbiota that were common to at least two body sites were recorded.

3. Results

3.1. Study Selection

The search process and study selection (presented in Figure 1) identified 544 records of interest. Among these, 163 were excluded for being repetitive, and 353 additional articles were excluded from the analysis because they were review articles, published protocols, lab studies, animal studies, or articles deemed not to be of relevance based on their titles and abstracts. The full texts of the 28 remaining articles were obtained. Several studies were subsequently excluded because they did not meet the predefined inclusion criteria, including those with no relevant outcome data (three articles) and those reporting on unrelated topics (two articles). Four studies were excluded due to insufficient information pertaining to the inclusion criteria, and a second article by the same authors was found to be a repetitive report based on a partial dataset. In total, 16 publications, reporting on 16 cohort studies, were selected for inclusion in the analysis [11–26].

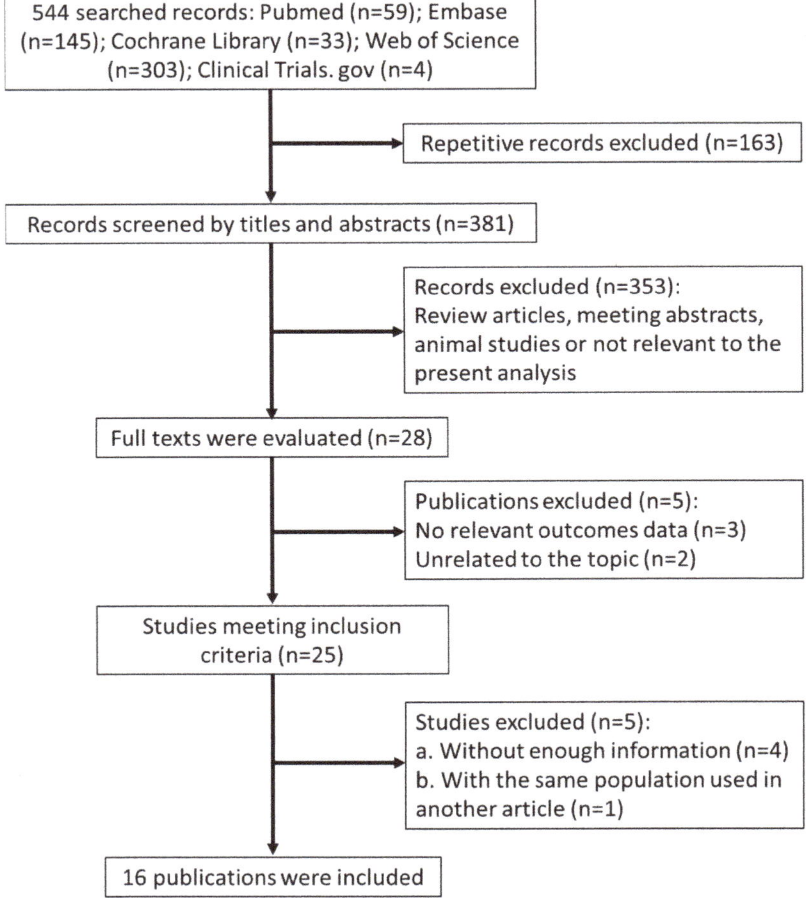

Figure 1. Flow diagram of the study selection.

3.2. Characteristics of Included Studies

Ultimately, 16 cohort studies, published from 2011 to 2020, were included in the analysis. These studies reported on the characterization of commensal microbe profiles in CHD patients and analyzed changes in commensal microbe populations in fecal, blood, or atherosclerotic plaque samples. These studies are summarized in Table 1.

Table 1. Characteristics of included studies.

Study	Country of Origin	Population	Sample Size	Type of Sample			Region of Gene Quantification
				Fecal Samples	Plaque Samples	Blood Samples	
Tuomisto S, 2019 [13]	Finland	CHD	67	√	√		DNA
Liu HH, 2019 [14]	China	CAD	201	√			V3-V4 of 16S rRNA
Emoto T, 2016 [15]	Japan	CAD	119	√			16S rDNA
Cui L, 2017 [16]	China	CHD	64	√			V3-V5 of 16S rRNA
Yoshida N, 2018 [17]	Japan	CAD	60	√			V3-V4 of 16S rRNA
Amar J, 2019 [18]	France	MI	201			√	V3-V4 of 16S rDNA
Emoto T, 2017 [19]	Japan	CAD	69	√			16S rDNA
Toya T, 2020 [20]	USA	Advanced CAD	106	√			V3-V5 of 16S rDNA
Zhu Q, 2018 [21]	China	CAD	168	√			V4 of 16S rRNA
Gao J, 2020 [22]	China	ACS	90	√			V4 of 16S rDNA
Zheng YY, 2020 [23]	China	CAD	309	√			V3-V4 of 16S rRNA
Koren O, 2011 [11]	USA	Atherosclerosis	30		√		V1-V2 of 16S rRNA
Alhmoud T, 2019 [24]	USA	ACS	38	√			V3-V4 of 16S rRNA
Jie Z, 2017 [25]	China	ACVD	405	√			DNA
Li CW, 2016 [26]	China	CAD	206			√	16S rRNA
Pisano E, 2019 [27]	Italy	CAD	77	√	√		16S rRNA

ACS, acute coronary syndrome; ACVD, atherosclerotic cardiovascular disease; CAD, coronary artery disease; CHD, coronary heart disease; MI, myocardial infarction.

In total, this systematic review included data collected from 2210 participants. Three of the studies were conducted in the United States of America, three in Japan, one in Finland, one in France, one in Italy, and seven in China. Three studies reported on patients with ACS, 12 included patients with chronic CHD, and one included patients with atherosclerosis. Thirteen studies analyzed changes in commensal microbes in fecal samples, two of which also analyzed changes in plaque samples, one study reported on changes in the microbiota of plaque alone, while two reported on changes in blood alone (Table 1).

3.3. Overall Comparison of the Gut, Blood, and Atherosclerotic Plaque Microbiota

We surveyed changes in the atherosclerotic plaque, blood, and gut (feces) bacterial communities to look for commonalities among the studies. The microbiota commonly identified by three publications in patients' plaque samples were classified as Streptococcus, whereas the microbiota commonly identified among nine papers in patient fecal samples were classified as Bacteroides and Prevotela, regardless of the direction of change (increased or decreased) (Tables 2 and 3). After taking the trend of change into consideration, we found that Streptococcus was increased in five studies, whereas Lachnospiraceae was decreased in four studies in the fecal samples of patients (Table 4). Unfortunately, we did not observe any similarities in microbiota between two papers in patient blood samples, which may have been due to only two contributing to the comparisons of bacterial populations in the blood (Table 5). Collectively, these results support the notion that several common types of commensal microbiota that exist in the atherosclerotic plaque, blood, and gut (feces) are associated with CHD.

Table 2. Microbiota commonly identified by at least two publications in the atherosclerotic plaque samples of those with coronary heart disease.

Microbiota in Plaque Samples	No. of Publications (n = 3)
Veillonella; Staphylococcus; Burkholderia; Propionibacterium; Corynebacterium; Proteobacteria	2
Streptococcus	3

The column on the right indicates the number of publications for which the microbiota were identified in plaque samples.

Table 3. Microbiota commonly identified by at least two publications in the fecal samples of those with coronary heart disease.

Microbiota in Fecal Samples	No. of Publications (n = 13)
Enterococcus; Catenisphaera; Coriobacteriaceae; Akkermansla; Veillonella; Erysipelotrichaceae bacterium	2
Proteobacteria; Fusobacteria; Escherichia	3
Lachnospiraceae; Ruminococcaceae; Roseburia; Faecalibacterium	4
Streptococcus	5
Enterobacteriaceae; Lactobacillales	6
Firmicutes	7
Bacteroides; Prevotela	9

The column on the right indicates the number of publications for which the microbiota were identified in fecal samples.

Table 4. Changes in microbiota populations in fecal samples of CHD patients.

Microbiota in Fecal Samples	Increase	Decrease	No. of Publications (n = 13)
Catenisphaera; Coriobacteriaceae	√		2
Fusobacteria; Escherichia	√		3
Lachnospiraceae		√	4
Streptococcus	√		5

The columns in the middle and on the right indicate the direction of change in the expression of microbiota populations in the feces of patients with coronary heart disease (CHD), and the number of publications reporting the change.

Table 5. Microbiota commonly identified in blood samples.

The Change of Microbiota	
Increase	Sphingobacteria, hymenobacter, virgisporangium, micromonosporaceae, bauldia, rhizobiales, Pseudomonadaceae, Rahnella, Serratia, Pseudomonas
Decrease	Caulobacteraceae, Clostridiales, Microbacteriaceae, Neisseriaceae, Brevundimonas, Chryseobacterium, Gordonia, Microbacterium

The columns at the right indicate the microbiota that were found in blood samples from two papers.

3.4. Comparisons of Atherosclerotic Plaque, Blood, and Gut Microbiotas between Studies

One of the main purposes of this study was to search for microbial communities that were commonly observed between gut and atherosclerotic plaque samples, or between gut and blood samples of those with CHD. Although all three sites typically express distinct microbial communities, the comparison of the overall bacterial community compositions revealed commonalities in the microbiota between the atherosclerotic plaque and fecal samples, and between the blood and fecal samples. However, no specific microbial communities were present in all three sample types. Table 6 summarizes the microbial communities that were identified in fecal samples and at least one other sample type in at least two studies. Clostridiales populations were observed in both the blood and fecal samples of patients, whereas Veillonella, Proteobacteria, and Streptococcus communities were identified in atherosclerotic plaque and gut samples in at least two studies. Interestingly, only Streptococcus was reported to have increased in all eight studies. Collectively, these results indicate that several specific types of commensal microbiota coexist in the atherosclerotic plaque and gut or in the blood and gut of patients with CHD.

Table 6. Microbiota populations common to at least two body sites.

Microbiota	Plaque + Fecal	Blood + Fecal
Veillonella	√	
Proteobacteria	√	
Streptococcus	√	
Clostridiales		√

The columns in the middle and on the right indicate the types of microbiota that were found in both the plaque and fecal samples or in the blood and fecal samples of those with coronary heart disease.

4. Discussion

In this study, we compared the bacterial compositions of the microbiota of the blood, gut, and atherosclerotic plaque from 16 relevant studies of patients with CHD. This approach allowed us to generate a relatively comprehensive description of the microbial communities associated with CHD. This comparison of blood, gut, and atherosclerotic plaque samples was necessary to identify members of the normal microbiome that may translocate from one body habitat to another where they may contribute to disease. We specifically identified several common types of commensal microbiota that existed or coexisted in atherosclerotic plaques, blood, and gut that were associated with CHD. However, we did not observe any similarities between the microbiota populations in the blood and plaque, or between the blood, plaque, and gut of the patients assessed by the 16 included studies, which may have been due to the paucity of relevant studies meeting the inclusion criteria. Our findings suggest that specific types of commensal microbiota, such as Streptococcus, Lachnospiraceae, and Clostridiales, may have a stronger predictive value in CHD. Moreover, the atherosclerotic plaque and blood microbiota may, at least in part, be derived from those present in the gut.

In this study, we found that the expression of Streptococcus was increased in the gut but was also present in atherosclerotic plaque samples; this may represent a previously unappreciated core member of the atherosclerotic plaque communities. This organism is known to be implicated in endocarditis [27]; however, the role of Streptococcus in CHD has not yet been reported. Its increased expression in the gut and its presence in atherosclerotic plaques suggests that it may directly affect the pathogenesis of atherosclerosis. Recently, some studies have revealed that the gut microbiome directly affects immune responses that regulate chronic inflammatory diseases, such as atherosclerosis [4,5], and it is becoming clear that microbiota-derived bioactive compounds can signal to distant organs, contributing to the development of cardiovascular disease states [28]. In addition, the molecular mechanism involving the "molecular mimicry" of microbial antigens has also been found to be associated with atherosclerosis [29]. For example, Binder et al. showed that pneumococcal vaccination decreases the formation of atherosclerotic lesions through a molecular mimicry mechanism between Streptococcus pneumoniae and oxidized low-density lipoprotein (LDL) [30], while our previous clinical research revealed that many autoantibodies that differ from those found in chronic autoimmune diseases are associated with atherosclerosis [31]. In parallel with these findings, a recent study reported that autoantibodies produced by B lymphocytes are present in plaques and may cross-react with the outer membrane proteins of bacteria, as well as with a cytoskeletal protein involved in atherogenesis [32]. Moreover, Saita et al. also demonstrated that B cells present in both the coronary and carotid plaques of patients with cardiovascular diseases locally produce antibodies that are capable of reacting in response to antigens of the gut microbiota and that they may cross-react with self-antigens. Furthermore, immunoglobulin G1 (IgG1) is secreted in human coronary atherosclerotic lesions and recognizes the outer membrane proteins of Enterobacteriaceae [33]. These findings demonstrate that in human atherosclerotic plaques, a local cross-reactive immune response may occur, wherein antibodies cross-react with a bacterial antigen and a self-protein. In addition, antibodies and B lymphocytes could play an important role in these disease processes [31,32].

Besides being present in atherosclerotic plaques, Streptococcus expression was also observed to be simultaneously increased in the gut. Recent studies have found that low levels of microbiota can also enter the bloodstream to systemically induce chronic, low-grade inflammation [3,34]. Generally, the intestinal mucosal barrier plays a critical role in preventing the translocation of bacterial components. This barrier is efficient when the microbiome is complex and stable; however, under certain conditions, such as those induced by diets high in fat and cholesterol or in certain diseases, major alterations to the composition of the host microbiota can occur, which have in turn been associated with increased intestinal permeability [35–38]. When the intestinal mucosal barrier becomes compromised, commensal microbes or commensal microbe-derived molecules can readily enter the bloodstream and exert systemic effects, which include the induction of infection or chronic low-grade inflammation and immunoreactivity, affecting multiple immune cell populations; this phenomenon has been found to be prevalent in atherosclerosis [39]. However, the presence of Streptococcus in the blood was not identified in at least two of the relevant studies included in our analysis. Recently, another mechanism has been identified through which bacteria could reach the atherosclerotic plaque, which involves phagocytosis by macrophages at epithelial linings (e.g., of the gut and lung). Upon phagocytosis, macrophages become activated; once they reach the activated endothelium of the atheroma, they leave the bloodstream to enter the atheroma and transform into cholesterol-laden foam cells [40]. In support of this mechanism, patients with cardiovascular disease exhibit a two-fold increase in the number of C. pneumonia-infected peripheral blood mononuclear cells compared with that of controls [11]. Furthermore, the bacteria have been shown to only be present in atheromas and not in healthy aortic tissues in mice [41], and they have been identified in human atherosclerotic plaques [42]. Thus, infected macrophages may specifically target bacteria in atheromas. It remains a possibility that Streptococcus can reach atherosclerotic plaques via the systemic circulation and directly promote local inflammatory cascades or elicit a specific immune response, such as molecular mimicry, thereby indirectly influencing host metabolism and systemic inflammation; however, the specific mechanisms by which Streptococcus regulates the development of atherosclerosis remain unknown and require further investigation.

Study Strengths and Limitations

Although some studies investigating the relationship between commensal microbiota and CHD have been conducted previously [6], our synthetic analysis is the first to investigate the types of commensal microbiota that are commonly associated with CHD. Moreover, our findings revealed several specific types of commensal microbiota that commonly exist or coexist in the atherosclerotic plaque, blood, or feces of patients with CHD. This could be valuable knowledge for future studies investigating this association, as it reveals that the microbiota of the atherosclerotic plaque may, at least in part, be derived from the gut and that these specific types of commensal microbiota may have predictive value for CHD.

A limitation of this study was that only 16 relevant publications met the criteria for inclusion, with only three contributing to a comparison of bacterial populations in the atherosclerotic plaque and with only two studies contributing to that in the blood. This limited our ability to generate a precise descriptive summary of the 'real-world' changes in relative commensal microbiota populations. Furthermore, there were several differences in the methodology of these studies, such as the region of genetic quantification, which could have influenced the results or may even have been significant sources of potential inaccuracy. In addition, the types and proportions of commensal microbiota could also have been influenced by several patient characteristics, such as diet (including regional differences) [43]. The addition of new evidence to the field will significantly reduce the effects of these limitations in future analyses.

Further studies should investigate specific types of commensal microbiota, as well as factors that modulate or inhibit their activity. In addition, more information is required to verify the predictive value and mechanisms of commensal microbiota in CHD patients.

5. Conclusions

In summary, this study revealed key types of bacteria associated with CHD, as well as several types that were simultaneously present in the atherosclerotic plaque, blood, or gut. In addition, the atherosclerotic plaques and blood samples of patients contained numerous bacteria from different phyla. Our findings strongly support the hypothesis that the gut can be a source of atherosclerotic plaque- and blood-associated bacteria. Although our findings are based on the data from a limited number of studies, they clearly suggest that several specific types of commensal microbiota have a predictive value for CHD. More prospective studies are needed to further evaluate this relationship and to identify the mechanisms that drive it.

Author Contributions: Conceptualization, L.C. and T.I.; methodology, H.D. and K.A.; data curation, L.C.; writing—original draft preparation, L.C.; writing—review and editing, L.C.; supervision, K.T. and T.I. All authors have read and agreed to the published version of the manuscript.

Funding: This research was funded by the National Natural Science Foundation of China (grant number 81900388). The funding source had no involvement in the study design, in the collection, analysis, and interpretation of data, in the writing of the report, or in the decision to submit the article for publication.

Conflicts of Interest: The authors declare no conflict of interest.

References

1. Dalen, J.E.; Alpert, J.S.; Goldberg, R.J.; Weinstein, R.S. The epidemic of the 20(th) century: Coronary heart disease. *Am. J. Med.* **2014**, *127*, 807–812. [CrossRef]
2. Finegold, J.A.; Asaria, P.; Francis, D.P. Mortality from ischaemic heart disease by country, region, and age: Statistics from World Health Organisation and United Nations. *Int. J. Cardiol.* **2013**, *168*, 934–945. [CrossRef]
3. Brown, J.M.; Hazen, S.L. The gut microbial endocrine organ: Bacterially derived signals driving cardiometabolic diseases. *Annu. Rev. Med.* **2015**, *66*, 343–359. [CrossRef]
4. Fatkhullina, A.R.; Peshkova, I.O.; Dzutsev, A.; Aghayev, T.; McCulloch, J.A.; Thovarai, V.; Badger, J.H.; Vats, R.; Sundd, P.; Tang, H.-Y. An Interleukin-23-Interleukin-22 Axis Regulates intestinal microbial homeostasis to protect from diet-induced atherosclerosis. *Immunity* **2018**, *49*, 943–957. [CrossRef]
5. Jonsson, A.L.; Backhed, F. Role of gut microbiota in atherosclerosis. *Nat. Rev. Cardiol.* **2017**, *14*, 79–87. [CrossRef]
6. Chen, L.; Ishigami, T.; Doi, H.; Arakawa, K.; Tamura, K. Gut microbiota and atherosclerosis: Role of B cell for atherosclerosis focusing on the gut-immune-B2 cell axis. *J. Mol. Med.* **2020**, *98*, 1235–1244. [CrossRef] [PubMed]
7. Eckburg, P.B.; Bik, E.M.; Bernstein, C.N.; Purdom, E.; Dethlefsen, L.; Sargent, M.; Gill, S.R.; Nelson, K.E.; Relman, D.A. Diversity of the human intestinal microbial flora. *Science* **2005**, *308*, 1635–1638. [CrossRef]
8. Turnbaugh, P.J.; Hamady, M.; Yatsunenko, T.; Cantarel, B.L.; Duncan, A.; Ley, R.E.; Sogin, M.L.; Jones, W.J.; Roe, B.A.; Affourtit, J.P. A core gut microbiome in obese and lean twins. *Nature* **2009**, *457*, 480–484. [CrossRef]
9. Costello, E.K.; Lauber, C.L.; Hamady, M.; Fierer, N.; Gordon, J.I.; Knight, R. Bacterial community variation in human body habitats across space and time. *Science* **2009**, *326*, 1694–1697. [CrossRef] [PubMed]
10. Nasidze, I.; Li, J.; Quinque, D.; Tang, K.; Stoneking, M. Global diversity in the human salivary microbiome. *Genome Res.* **2009**, *19*, 636–643. [CrossRef] [PubMed]
11. Koren, O.; Spor, A.; Felin, J.; Fåk, F.; Stombaugh, J.; Tremaroli, V.; Behre, C.J.; Knight, R.; Fagerberg, B.; Ley, R.E. Human oral, gut, and plaque microbiota in patients with atherosclerosis. *Proc. Natl. Acad. Sci. USA* **2011**, *108* (Suppl. 1), 4592–4598. [CrossRef] [PubMed]
12. Tuomisto, S.; Huhtala, H.; Martiskainen, M.; Goebeler, S.; Lehtimäki, T.; Karhunen, P.J. Age-dependent association of gut bacteria with coronary atherosclerosis: Tampere Sudden Death Study. *PLoS ONE* **2019**, *14*, e0221345. [CrossRef]
13. Liu, H.H.; Chen, X.; Hu, X.M.; Niu, H.T.; Tian, R.; Wang, H.; Pang, H.; Jiang, L.; Qiu, B.; Chen, X. Alterations in the gut microbiome and metabolism with coronary artery disease severity. *Microbiome* **2019**, *7*, 68. [CrossRef] [PubMed]
14. Emoto, T.; Yamashita, T.; Sasaki, N.; Hirota, Y.; Hayashi, T.; So, A.; Kasahara, K.; Yodoi, K.; Matsumoto, T.; Mizoguchi, T. Analysis of Gut Microbiota in Coronary Artery Disease Patients: A Possible Link between Gut Microbiota and Coronary Artery Disease. *J. Atheroscler. Thromb.* **2016**, *23*, 908–921. [CrossRef] [PubMed]

15. Cui, L.; Zhao, T.; Hu, H.; Zhang, W.; Hua, X. Association Study of Gut Flora in Coronary Heart Disease through High-Throughput Sequencing. *BioMed Res. Int.* **2017**, *2017*, 3796359. [CrossRef]
16. Yoshida, N.; Emoto, T.; Yamashita, T.; Watanabe, H.; Hayashi, T.; Tabata, T.; Hoshi, N.; Hatano, N.; Ozawa, G.; Sasaki, N. Bacteroides vulgatus and Bacteroides dorei Reduce Gut Microbial Lipopolysaccharide Production and Inhibit Atherosclerosis. *Circulation* **2018**, *138*, 2486–2498. [CrossRef]
17. Amar, J.; Lelouvier, B.; Servant, F.; Lluch, J.; Burcelin, R.; Bongard, V.; Elbaz, M. Blood Microbiota Modification After Myocardial Infarction Depends Upon Low-Density Lipoprotein Cholesterol Levels. *J. Am. Heart Assoc.* **2019**, *8*, e011797. [CrossRef]
18. Emoto, T.; Yamashita, T.; Kobayashi, T.; Sasaki, N.; Hirota, Y.; Hayashi, T.; So, A.; Kasahara, K.; Yodoi, K.; Matsumoto, T. Characterization of gut microbiota profiles in coronary artery disease patients using data mining analysis of terminal restriction fragment length polymorphism: Gut microbiota could be a diagnostic marker of coronary artery disease. *Heart Vessel.* **2017**, *32*, 39–46. [CrossRef]
19. Toya, T.; Corban, M.T.; Marrietta, E.; Horwath, I.E.; Lerman, L.O.; Murray, J.A.; Lerman, A. Coronary artery disease is associated with an altered gut microbiome composition. *PLoS ONE* **2020**, *15*, e0227147. [CrossRef]
20. Zhu, Q.; Gao, R.; Zhang, Y.; Pan, D.; Zhu, Y.; Zhang, X.; Yang, R.; Jiang, R.; Xu, Y.; Qin, H. Dysbiosis signatures of gut microbiota in coronary artery disease. *Physiol. Genom.* **2018**, *50*, 893–903. [CrossRef] [PubMed]
21. Gao, J.; Yan, K.T.; Wang, J.X.; Dou, J.; Wang, J.; Ren, M.; Ma, J.; Zhang, X.; Liu, Y. Gut microbial taxa as potential predictive biomarkers for acute coronary syndrome and post-STEMI cardiovascular events. *Sci. Rep.* **2020**, *10*, 2639. [CrossRef]
22. Zheng, Y.Y.; Wu, T.T.; Liu, Z.Q.; Li, A.; Guo, Q.Q.; Ma, Y.Y.; Zhang, Z.L.; Xun, Y.L.; Zhang, J.C.; Wang, W.R. Gut Microbiome-Based Diagnostic Model to Predict Coronary Artery Disease. *J. Agric. Food Chem.* **2020**, *68*, 3548–3557. [CrossRef]
23. Alhmoud, T.; Kumar, A.; Lo, C.C.; Al-Sadi, R.; Clegg, S.; Alomari, I.; Zmeilia, T.; Gleasne, C.D.; Mcmurry, K.; Dichosa, A.E.K. Investigating intestinal permeability and gut microbiota roles in acute coronary syndrome patients. *Hum. Microbiome J.* **2019**, *13*, 100059. [CrossRef]
24. Jie, Z.; Xia, H.; Zhong, S.L.; Feng, Q.; Li, S.; Liang, S.; Zhong, H.; Liu, Z.; Gao, Y.; Zhao, H. The gut microbiome in atherosclerotic cardiovascular disease. *Nat. Commun.* **2017**, *8*, 845. [CrossRef]
25. Li, C.W.; Gao, M.; Zhang, W.; Chen, C.Y.; Zhou, F.Y.; Hu, Z.X.; Zeng, C. Zonulin Regulates Intestinal Permeability and Facilitates Enteric Bacteria Permeation in Coronary Artery Disease. *Sci. Rep.* **2016**, *6*, 29142. [CrossRef] [PubMed]
26. Pisano, E.; Severino, A.; Bugli, F.; Pedicino, D.; Sterbini, F.P.; Martini, C. Microbial signature in plaque and gut in acute coronary syndrome: Pathogenetic implications. *Giornale Italiano Cardiol.* **2019**, *20*, 111S–112S.
27. Casalta, J.P.; Fournier, P.E.; Habib, G.; Riberi, A.; Raoult, D. Prosthetic valve endocarditis caused by Pseudomonas luteola. *BMC Infect. Dis.* **2005**, *5*, 82. [CrossRef] [PubMed]
28. Caesar, R.; Reigstad, C.S.; Bäckhed, H.K.; Reinhardt, C.; Ketonen, M.; Lundén, G.Ö.; Cani, P.D.; Bäckhed, F. Gut-derived lipopolysaccharide augments adipose macrophage accumulation but is not essential for impaired glucose or insulin tolerance in mice. *Gut* **2012**, *61*, 1701–1707. [CrossRef] [PubMed]
29. Riley, E.; Dasari, V.; Frishman, W.H.; Sperber, K. Vaccines in Development to Prevent and Treat Atherosclerotic Disease. *Cardiol. Rev.* **2008**, *16*, 288–300. [CrossRef] [PubMed]
30. Binder, C.J.; Horkko, S.; Dewan, A.; Chang, M.-K.; Kieu, E.P.; Goodyear, C.S.; Shaw, P.X.; Palinski, W.; Witztum, J.L.; Silverman, G.J. Pneumococcal vaccination decreases atherosclerotic lesion formation: Molecular mimicry between Streptococcus pneumoniae and oxidized LDL. *Nat. Med.* **2003**, *9*, 736–743. [CrossRef]
31. Ishigami, T.; Abe, K.; Aoki, I.; Minegishi, S.; Ryo, A.; Matsunaga, S.; Matsuoka, K.; Takeda, H.; Sawasaki, T.; Umemura, S. Anti-interleukin-5 and multiple autoantibodies are associated with human atherosclerotic diseases and serum interleukin-5 levels. *FASEB J.* **2013**, *27*, 3437–3445. [CrossRef]
32. Canducci, F.; Saita, D.; Foglieni, C.; Piscopiello, M.R.; Chiesa, R.; Colombo, A.; Cianflone, D.; Maseri, A.; Clementi, M.; Burioni, R. Cross-reacting antibacterial auto-antibodies are produced within coronary atherosclerotic plaques of acute coronary syndrome patients. *PLoS ONE* **2012**, *7*, e42283. [CrossRef] [PubMed]
33. Saita, D.; Ferrarese, R.; Foglieni, C.; Esposito, A.; Canu, T.; Perani, L.; Ceresola, E.R.; Visconti, L.; Burioni, R.; Clementi, M. Adaptive immunity against gut microbiota enhances apoE-mediated immune regulation and reduces atherosclerosis and western-diet-related inflammation. *Sci. Rep.* **2016**, *6*, 29353. [CrossRef] [PubMed]
34. Neves, A.L.; Coelho, J.; Couto, L.; Leite-Moreira, A.; Roncon-Albuquerque, R. Metabolic endotoxemia: A molecular link between obesity and cardiovascular risk. *J. Mol. Endocrinol.* **2013**, *51*, R51–R64. [CrossRef] [PubMed]
35. David, L.A.; Maurice, C.F.; Carmody, R.N.; Gootenberg, D.B.; Button, J.E.; Wolfe, B.E.; Ling, A.V.; Devlin, A.S.; Varma, Y.; Fischbach, M.A. Diet rapidly and reproducibly alters the human gut microbiome. *Nature* **2014**, *505*, 559–563. [CrossRef]
36. Ghosh, S.S.; Bie, J.; Wang, J.; Ghosh, S. Oral Supplementation with Non-Absorbable Antibiotics or Curcumin Attenuates Western Diet-Induced Atherosclerosis and Glucose Intolerance in LDLR−/− Mice—Role of Intestinal Permeability and Macrophage Activation. *PLoS ONE* **2014**, *9*, e108577. [CrossRef] [PubMed]
37. Sato, J.; Kanazawa, A.; Ikeda, F.; Yoshihara, T.; Goto, H.; Abe, H.; Komiya, K.; Kawaguchi, M.; Shimizu, T.; Ogihara, T. Gut Dysbiosis and Detection of "Live Gut Bacteria" in Blood of Japanese Patients with Type 2 Diabetes. *Diabetes Care* **2014**, *37*, 2343–2350. [CrossRef] [PubMed]
38. Zhang, D.; Chen, G.; Manwani, D.; Mortha, A.; Xu, C.; Faith, J.J.; Burk, R.D.; Kunisaki, Y.; Jang, J.E.; Scheiermann, C. Neutrophil ageing is regulated by the microbiome. *Nature* **2015**, *525*, 528–532. [CrossRef]

39. Arakawa, K.; Ishigami, T.; Nakai-Sugiyama, M.; Chen, L.; Doi, H.; Kino, T.; Minegishi, S.; Saigoh-Teranaka, S.; Sasaki-Nakashima, R.; Hibi, K. Lubiprostone as a potential therapeutic agent to improve intestinal permeability and prevent the development of atherosclerosis in apolipoprotein E-deficient mice. *PLoS ONE* **2019**, *14*, e0218096. [CrossRef]
40. Campbell, L.A.; Kuo, C.C. Chlamydia pneumoniae–an infectious risk factor for atherosclerosis? *Nat. Rev. Microbiol.* **2004**, *2*, 23–32. [CrossRef]
41. Moazed, T.C.; Kuo, C.; Grayston, J.T.; Campbell, L.A. Murine models of Chlamydia pneumoniae infection and atherosclerosis. *J. Infect. Dis.* **1997**, *175*, 883–890. [CrossRef] [PubMed]
42. Ott, S.J.; El Mokhtari, N.E.; Musfeldt, M.; Hellmig, S.; Freitag, S.; Rehman, A.; Kühbacher, T.; Nikolaus, S.; Namsolleck, P.; Blaut, M. Detection of diverse bacterial signatures in atherosclerotic lesions of patients with coronary heart disease. *Circulation* **2006**, *113*, 929–937. [CrossRef] [PubMed]
43. Heidenreich, P.A.; Mamic, P. Is Our Diet Turning Our Gut Microbiome Against Us? *J. Am. Coll. Cardiol.* **2020**, *75*, 773–775. [CrossRef] [PubMed]

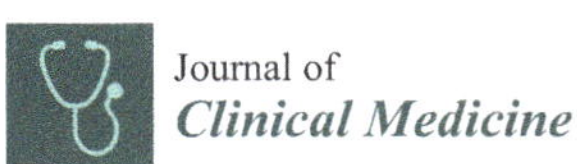
Journal of
Clinical Medicine

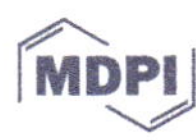

Article

Home-Measured Blood Pressure Is Associated with Handgrip Strength in Patients with Type 2 Diabetes: The KAMOGAWA-HBP Study

Tomonori Kimura, Emi Ushigome *, Yoshitaka Hashimoto, Naoko Nakanishi, Masahide Hamaguchi, Mai Asano, Masahiro Yamazaki and Michiaki Fukui

Department of Endocrinology and Metabolism, Graduate School of Medical Science, Kyoto Prefectural University of Medicine, Kyoto 602-8566, Japan; tomok05@koto.kpu-m.ac.jp (T.K.); y-hashi@koto.kpu-m.ac.jp (Y.H.); naoko-n@koto.kpu-m.ac.jp (N.N.); mhama@koto.kpu-m.ac.jp (M.H.); maias@koto.kpu-m.ac.jp (M.A.); masahiro@koto.kpu-m.ac.jp (M.Y.); michiaki@koto.kpu-m.ac.jp (M.F.)
* Correspondence: emis@koto.kpu-m.ac.jp; Tel.: +81-75-251-5505; Fax: +81-75-252-3721

Abstract: The association between blood pressure measured at home and handgrip strength in patients with diabetes has not been investigated. Therefore, in this study, we aimed to assess this association among patients with type 2 diabetes. In this cross-sectional study, 157 patients with type 2 diabetes underwent muscle tests and morning and evening blood-pressure measurements at home in triplicate for 14 consecutive days throughout the study period. Univariate and multivariate regression analyses were conducted to analyze the relationship between home blood-pressure parameters and handgrip strength. The average age and hemoglobin A1c of the patients were 70.5 years and 7.1%, respectively. Morning diastolic blood pressure of [β (95% confidence interval; CI): 0.20 (0.03, 0.37)] was associated with handgrip strength in men, while morning systolic blood pressure of [−0.09 (−0.15, −0.04)], morning pulse pressure of [−0.14 (−0.21, −0.08)], and evening pulse pressure of [−0.12 (−0.19, −0.04)] were associated with handgrip strength in women. Home-measured blood pressure was associated with handgrip strength. Sex differences were found in the relationship between home blood-pressure parameters and handgrip strength.

Keywords: handgrip strength; home blood pressure; type 2 diabetes

Citation: Kimura, T.; Ushigome, E.; Hashimoto, Y.; Nakanishi, N.; Hamaguchi, M.; Asano, M.; Yamazaki, M.; Fukui, M. Home-Measured Blood Pressure Is Associated with Handgrip Strength in Patients with Type 2 Diabetes: The KAMOGAWA-HBP Study. *J. Clin. Med.* **2021**, *10*, 1913. https://doi.org/10.3390/jcm10091913

Academic Editor: Tomoaki Ishigami

Received: 11 March 2021
Accepted: 26 April 2021
Published: 28 April 2021

1. Introduction

Hypertension is the most common risk factor for cardiovascular diseases (CVDs), and it remains highly prevalent worldwide [1]. Observational data suggest that the treatment of hypertension reduces the risk of diabetic nephropathy and CVD in patients with type 2 diabetes [2]. Home-measured blood pressure (HBP), considered as an important therapeutic parameter, has a strong predictive power for mortality compared with office-measured blood pressure (BP) [3]. Moreover, increased pulse pressure (PP) measured at home is significantly associated with the development of microvascular and macrovascular complications in patients with type 2 diabetes [4]. Patients with type 2 diabetes often suffer from reduced muscle mass and strength [5]. Recent studies have reported that high muscle strength is associated with a lower risk of future CVD events [6]. Moreover, it was reported that increased handgrip strength was associated with lower SBP [7–9] and higher DBP [10]. However, no studies have investigated the relationship between HBP parameters and handgrip strength in patients with diabetes. Thus, we aimed to evaluate this association among patients with type 2 diabetes.

2. Materials and Methods

2.1. Study Design

This study was a cross-sectional study, and baseline data from patients participating in both the type 2 diabetes HBP cohort study (KAMOGAWA-HBP study [3]) and the cohort study on muscle test [11] were used in the present study. Both cohorts included patients who regularly attended the diabetes outpatient clinic at the Kyoto Prefectural University of Medicine Hospital. We evaluated the association of HBP and PP with handgrip strength in patients with type 2 diabetes [11]. All procedures used in this study were approved by the local research ethics committee and were conducted in accordance with the Declaration of Helsinki. Written informed consent was obtained from each patient.

2.2. Patients

In this cross-sectional study, 903 and 274 patients with type 2 diabetes underwent blood-pressure measurement at home and a muscle test, respectively, between 2008 and 2017. We included 164 patients who underwent both HBP measurement and handgrip strength measurement. Among them, 2 and 5 patients were excluded because of insufficient data on HBP and unavailability of handgrip strength data, respectively. The study population finally comprised 157 patients (94 men, 63 women, Figure 1). The diagnosis of type 2 diabetes was based on the criteria published by the American Diabetes Association [12].

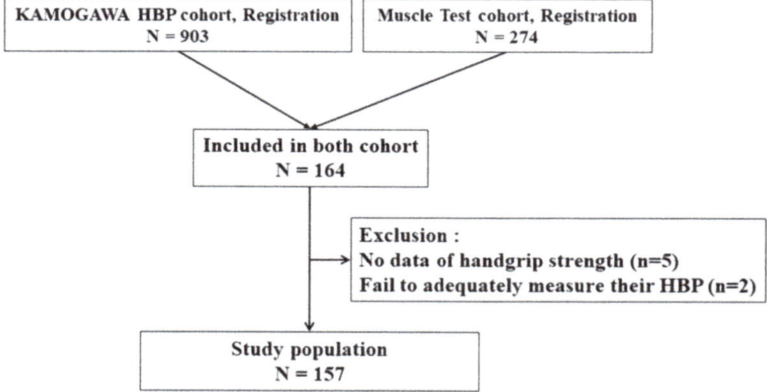

Figure 1. Flow diagram for the KAMOGAWA-HBP cohort.

2.3. BP Measurements

The BP of each patient was measured using the HEM-70801C automated BP monitor (Omron Healthcare Co., Ltd., Kyoto, Japan). Morning and evening BP measurements were performed in triplicate for 14 consecutive days. Morning BP was measured within 1 h of waking, before eating breakfast or taking any drugs, while the patient was seated, and had rested for at least 5 min. Evening BP measurement was performed immediately before going to bed. The cuff was placed over the bare upper arm and was positioned at the heart level [13]. We calculated the mean values of the three morning and evening BP measurements. PP was calculated as systolic BP (SBP) minus diastolic BP (DBP).

2.4. Measurements of Grip Strength

Handgrip strength was measured twice in the outpatient examination room using a dynamometer (Smedley, Takei Scientific Instruments Co., Ltd., Niigata, Japan) with each hand in a standing position with elbows fully extended. The values were checked by the attending physician, and the maximum value among them was used in this study.

2.5. Data Collection

Venous blood was collected after an overnight fast, for biochemical measurements. Hemoglobin A1c (HbA1c) was measured using high-performance liquid chromatography, and results were expressed as a national glycohemoglobin standardization program unit. Body mass index was defined as body weight (kg) divided by the square of the height (m).

Patient information, such as age, smoking status (no smoking/current or past smoking), exercise (without exercise habits/with exercise habits), and antihypertensive medication use (without antihypertensive medication/with antihypertensive medication), was collected using a standardized questionnaire at the time of study entry.

2.6. Statistical Analysis

Statistical analysis was performed using JMP software version 10.0.2 (SAS Institute Inc., Cary, NC, USA). A p value of <0.05 was considered statistically significant. Continuous variables are presented as mean ± standard deviation. Pearson's correlation analysis was used to investigate the relationship between values of handgrip strength measurement and SBP, DBP, and PP. Univariate and multivariate regression analyses were performed to analyze the relationship between HBP and PP, and handgrip strength. β coefficients were calculated to compare the relationship between HBP and PP, and handgrip strength. To adjust the effects of various factors on handgrip strength, the following known risk factors for handgrip strength were considered as covariates: age, smoking status, exercise, BMI, HbA1c, and antihypertensive medication use [14–17]. Missing data were excluded from the statistical analyses.

3. Results

Clinical characteristics of the study participants are presented in Table 1.

Table 1. Clinical characteristics of study participants.

	All	Men	Women	p
N	157	94	63	-
Age (year)	70.5 (8.5)	69.8 (8.9)	71.5 (7.8)	0.201
BMI (kg/m^2)	23.7 (3.8)	24.0 (3.1)	23.2 (4.4)	0.263
Handgrip strength (kg)	27.0 (9.2)	32.4 (7.4)	18.8 (4.1)	<0.0001
Smoking (never/past or current)	52/105	14/80	38/25	<0.0001
Regular exercise (yes/no)	102/53	47/45	55/8	<0.0001
Antihypertensive drug use (yes/no)	88/69	59/35	29/34	0.539
HbA1c (%)	7.1 (0.8)	7.1 (0.8)	7.1 (0.8)	0.572
Average of morning SBP (mmHg)	133.6 (19.9)	133.4 (18.2)	133.8 (22.4)	0.914
Average of morning DBP (mmHg)	75.4 (11.0)	76.8 (10.9)	73.2 (10.8)	0.043
Average of morning PP (mmHg)	58.2 (15.0)	56.6 (13.6)	60.6 (16.7)	0.107
Average of evening SBP (mmHg)	129.2 (17.9)	128.1 (16.5)	130.8 (19.8)	0.342
Average of evening DBP (mmHg)	70.3 (9.8)	70.7 (10.1)	69.7 (9.4)	0.548
Average of evening PP (mmHg)	58.9 (14.0)	57.4 (12.9)	61.1 (15.4)	0.104

For categorical variables, the number is presented. For continuous variables, the average (standard deviation) is presented. HbA1c, hemoglobin A1c; BMI, body mass index; SBP, systolic blood pressure; DBP, diastolic blood pressure; PP, pulse pressure.

The average (standard deviation) age and HbA1c value were 70.5 (8.5) years and 7.1 (0.8)%, respectively. Eighty-eight patients (56.1%) were treated with antihypertensive drugs. The average values of morning SBP, morning DBP, and morning PP were 133.6 (19.9) mmHg, 75.4 (11.0) mmHg, and 58.2 (15.0) mmHg, respectively. The mean handgrip strength value was 32.4 (7.4) kg in men and 18.8 (4.1) kg in women. In the univariate analysis, morning DBP of [β (95% confidence interval; CI): 0.21 (0.08, 0.34)] and evening DBP of [0.19 (0.04, 0.34)] were associated with handgrip strength in men, while morning SBP of [−0.08 (−0.12, −0.03)], morning PP of [−0.13 (−0.19, −0.08)], evening SBP of [−0.07 (−0.12, −0.02)], and evening PP of [−0.13 (−0.19, −0.07)] were associated with handgrip strength in women (Table 2). In the multivariate analysis, morning DBP of [0.20 (0.03, 0.37)] was associated with handgrip strength in men, while morning SBP of [−0.09 (−0.15, −0.04)], morning PP of [−0.14 (−0.21, −0.08)], and evening PP of [−0.12 (−0.19, −0.04)] were associated with handgrip strength in women (Table 2).

Table 2. Unadjusted and adjusted regression analyses on handgrip strength.

	Men		Women	
	Unadjusted	Adjusted †	Unadjusted	Adjusted †
Morning systolic blood pressure	0.04 (−0.05, 0.12)	0.09 (−0.01, 0.19)	−0.08 (−0.12, −0.03)	−0.09 (−0.15, −0.04)
Morning diastolic blood pressure	0.21 (0.08, 0.34)	0.20 (0.03, 0.37)	−0.01 (−0.11, 0.09)	−0.04 (−0.15, 0.08)
Morning pulse pressure	−0.07 (−0.18, 0.04)	0.02 (−0.10, 0.19)	−0.13 (−0.19, −0.08)	−0.14 (−0.21, −0.08)
Evening systolic blood pressure	0.02 (−0.08, 0.11)	0.04 (−0.06, 0.14)	−0.07 (−0.12, −0.02)	−0.06 (−0.12, −0.002)
Evening diastolic blood pressure	0.19 (0.04, 0.34)	0.10 (−0.08, 0.28)	0.04 (−0.07, 0.16)	0.04 (−0.09, 0.17)
Evening pulse pressure	−0.09 (−0.21, 0.03)	0.01 (−0.13, 0.15)	−0.13 (−0.19, −0.07)	−0.12 (−0.19, −0.04)

Data are β coefficients (95% confidence interval). † Adjusted for age, smoking, exercise, body mass index, hemoglobin A1c, and use of antihypertensive medications.

4. Discussion

4.1. Principal Findings

We assessed, for the first time, the association between HBP parameters and handgrip strength among patients with type 2 diabetes. The main findings of this study were the association of HBP parameters with handgrip strength and the sex differences in the relationship between HBP parameters and handgrip strength. Morning DBP was associated with handgrip strength in men, while morning SBP, morning PP, and evening PP were associated with handgrip strength in women.

4.2. Interpretations

In addition to an age-related decrease in activity level and changes in nutrient intake, molecular mechanisms, such as insulin resistance, oxidative stress, chronic inflammation, and changes in sex hormones, have been postulated to contribute to muscle weakness [18]. Type 2 diabetes and hypertension have the same background factors as those mentioned above and are likely to complicate each other. Thus, muscle weakness and BP may be associated in patients with type 2 diabetes. A correlation exists between increased PP and flow-mediated dilatation [19]. The decline in endothelial function is accelerated by aging, hypertension, diabetes mellitus, and dyslipidemia, and it has been shown to affect atherosclerosis development. Higashi, et al. [20] proposed that nitric oxide release may underlie the association between muscle strength and BP. Moreover, age-related loss of nitric oxide synthase in the skeletal muscle was reported to cause reductions in calpain S-nitrosylation, which leads to age-related loss of muscle mass [21].

In this study, the association between HBP and grip strength was stronger in women than in men. This result is consistent with previous reports in which arterial stiffness, measured using cardio-ankle vascular index, was significantly associated with handgrip strength in Japanese non-hypertensive women but not in men [22]. The similarities between the two studies, in which women were older and had higher SBP and lower DBP than men, may have influenced the results. In women, the production levels of estradiol and progesterone declines during menopause [23], and these hormonal changes may also enhance age-related atherosclerosis and muscle weakness [24]. Moreover, a meta-analysis of nearly 10,000 post-menopausal women showed that hormone therapy beneficially affects muscle strength [25]. Estrogen protects skeletal muscle against apoptosis through its effects on heat shock protein and mitochondria [26]. In addition, abnormal inflammatory and satellite cell responses during estrogen deficiency contribute to the loss of muscle strength in women [27].

In the present study, SBP and PP were negatively associated with handgrip strength in women. On the contrary, Taekema et al. [28] found that higher SBP and PP levels were associated with higher handgrip strength in the oldest participants (all 85 years). This is contrary to the results of our study, due to the differences in the patients' backgrounds. The increase in vascular resistance with aging was speculated to require greater pressure as a mechanism to maintain tissue perfusion, to prevent further damage to ischemic peripheral organs such as skeletal muscles [28].

In this study, DBP was positively associated with handgrip strength in men. Lower levels of DBP were reported to be associated with an increased risk of CVD and death [29]. This may reflect an association between lower DBP levels and more serious comorbidities, including arteriosclerotic vascular disease [30]. Moreover, the absolute values of the β coefficient for morning DBP were higher in men. In the present study, the average of morning DBP was higher in men than in women, which might suggest that men are less likely to have advanced atherosclerosis. Therefore, it is possible that the impact of lower DBP on handgrip strength was stronger in men.

This study has several limitations. First, a cross-sectional design was adopted, which did not show the precise determination of the cause–effect relationship between HBP parameters and handgrip strength. Prospective studies are required to evaluate their association. Second, the small sample size could have influenced the results obtained. Therefore, further studies on bigger groups are needed to fully understand the relationship between HBP and handgrip strength in patients with type 2 diabetes. Third, detailed data on the intake of protein and total energy, which might affect muscle strength, were not available. Fourth, there is no quality control of HBP measurements to ensure that the recommendations given to patients are systematically followed. Fifth, this study included patients with a relatively high capacity for self-care, who were able to self-monitor their HBP. Because of this selection bias, the results of this study may not be applicable to all patients with diabetes. Finally, the mechanism underlying the association between HBP parameters and handgrip strength could not be elucidated because of missing data on inflammatory or oxidative stress markers.

5. Conclusions

Our study showed the association between HBP and handgrip strength, particularly in female patients with type 2 diabetes.

Author Contributions: Collection, analysis and interpretation of research data, and manuscript drafting and revision, T.K.; collection, analysis, and interpretation of data, and manuscript revision, E.U., Y.H., N.N., M.H., M.A., M.Y. and M.F. All authors have read and agreed to the published version of the manuscript.

Funding: Emi Ushigome has received grants from the Astellas Foundation for Research on Metabolic Disorders (Grant number: 4024) and the Japanese Study Group for Physiology and Management of Blood Pressure. The Donated Fund Laboratory of Diabetes therapeutics is an endowment department, supported with an unrestricted grant from Ono Pharmaceutical Co., Ltd.

Institutional Review Board Statement: The protocol for this research project has been approved by a suitably constituted Ethics Committee of the institution and it conforms to the provisions of the Declaration of Helsinki. Committee of the institutional review board of the Kyoto Prefectural University of Medicine hospital, approval no. RBMR-E-349 and RBMR-E-466.

Informed Consent Statement: Written informed consent was obtained from all the patients.

Data Availability Statement: All materials are available for use from the corresponding author.

Acknowledgments: The authors would like to thank Naoko Higo, Terumi Kaneko and Machiko Hasegawa at the Kyoto Prefectural University of Medicine for teaching the patients how to measure their BP, and Sayoko Tanaka and Fumie Takenaka at the Kyoto Prefectural University of Medicine for their secretarial assistance.

Conflicts of Interest: Emi Ushigome has received personal fees from Astellas Pharma Inc., Daiichi Sankyo Co., AstraZeneca plc, Ltd., Kowa Pharmaceutical Co., Ltd., Kyowa Hakko Kirin Company Ltd., MSD K.K., Mitsubishi Tanabe Pharma Corp., Novo Nordisk Pharma Ltd., Taisho Toyama Pharmaceutical Co., Ltd., Takeda Pharmaceutical Co., Ltd., Nippon Boehringer Ingelheim Co. and Sumitomo Dainippon Pharma Co., Ltd., outside the submitted work. Yoshitaka Hashimoto has received grants from Asahi Kasei Pharma, personal fees from Daiichi Sankyo Co., Ltd., Mitsubishi Tanabe Pharma Corp., Sanofi K.K. and Novo Nordisk Pharma Ltd., outside the submitted work. Masahide Hamaguchi has received grants from Mitsubishi Tanabe Pharma Corp., Daiichi Sankyo Co.,

Ltd., Asahi Kasei Pharma, Nippon Boehringer Ingelheim Co., Ltd., Takeda Pharmaceutical Company Limited, Astellas Pharma Inc., Sanofi K.K., Sumitomo Dainippon Pharma Co., Ltd., Novo Nordisk Pharma Ltd., Kyowa Kirin Co., Ltd., and Eli Lilly Japan K.K., outside the submitted work. Mai Asano has received personal fees from Abbott Japan Co., Ltd., Novo Nordisk Pharma Ltd., Kowa Pharmaceutical Co., Takeda Pharmaceutical Co., Ltd., AstraZeneca plc, Ltd., and Ono Pharmaceutical Co., Ltd., outside the submitted work. Masahiro Yamazaki reports personal fees from Kowa Company, Ltd., AstraZeneca PLC, MSD K.K., Sumitomo Dainippon Pharma Co., Ltd., Kyowa Hakko Kirin Co., Ltd., Kowa Pharmaceutical Co., Ltd., Daiichi Sankyo Co., Ltd., Takeda Pharmaceutical Company Limited, and Ono Pharma Co., Ltd., outside the submitted work. Michiaki Fukui has received grants from Kissei Pharma Co., Ltd., Daiichi Sankyo Co., Ltd., Takeda Pharma Co., Ltd., Sanofi K.K., Astellas Pharma Inc., MSD K.K., Ltd., Nippon Boehringer Ingelheim Co., Ltd., Kyowa Hakko Kirin Co., Kowa Pharmaceutical Co., Ltd., Mitsubishi Tanabe Pharma Co., Sanwa Kagaku Kenkyusho Co., Ltd. Novo Nordisk Pharma Ltd., Ono Pharma Co., Ltd., Eli Lilly Japan K.K., Taisho Pharma Co., Ltd., Terumo Co., Sumitomo Dainippon Pharma Co., Ltd., Abbott Japan Co., Ltd., Johnson & Johnson K.K. Medical Co., Teijin Pharma Ltd., and Nippon Chemiphar Co., Ltd. and has received personal fees from Nippon Boehringer Ingelheim Co., Ltd., Mitsubishi Tanabe Pharma Corp., Kissei Pharma Co., Sanofi K.K., Takeda Pharma Co., Ltd., Daiichi Sankyo Co., Ltd., MSD K.K., Kyowa Kirin Co., Ltd., Kowa Pharma Co., Ltd., Novo Nordisk Pharma Ltd., Astellas Pharma Inc., Sumitomo Dainippon Pharma Co., Ltd., Ono Pharma Co., Ltd., Eli Lilly Japan K.K., Arkley Inc., Taisho Pharma Co., Ltd., Bayer Yakuhin, Ltd., AstraZeneca K.K., Abbott Japan Co., Ltd., Medtronic Japan Co., Ltd., Sanwa Kagaku Kenkyusho Co., Ltd., Mochida Pharma Co., Ltd., Teijin Pharma Ltd. and Nipro Cor., outside the submitted work.

References

1. Kearney, P.M.; Whelton, M.; Reynolds, K.; Muntner, P.; Whelton, P.K.; He, J. Global burden of hypertension: Analysis of worldwide data. *Lancet* **2005**, *365*, 217–223. [CrossRef]
2. Ismail-Beigi, F.; Craven, T.; Banerji, M.A.; Basile, J.; Calles, J.; Cohen, R.M.; Cuddihy, R.; Cushman, W.C.; Genuth, S.; Grimm, R.; et al. Effect of intensive treatment of hyperglycaemia on microvascular outcomes in type 2 diabetes: An analysis of the accord randomised trial. *Lancet* **2010**, *376*, 419–430. [CrossRef]
3. Ushigome, E.; Oyabu, C.; Tanaka, T.; Hasegawa, G.; Ohnishi, M.; Tsunoda, S.; Ushigome, H.; Yokota, I.; Nakamura, N.; Oda, Y.; et al. Impact of masked hypertension on diabetic nephropathy in patients with type II diabetes: A KAMOGAWA-HBP study. *J. Am. Soc. Hypertens.* **2018**, *12*, 364–371.e1. [CrossRef] [PubMed]
4. Knudsen, S.T.; Poulsen, P.L.; Hansen, K.W.; Ebbehøj, E.; Bek, T.; Mogensen, C.E. Pulse pressure and diurnal blood pressure variation: Association with micro- and macrovascular complications in type 2 diabetes. *Am. J. Hypertens.* **2002**, *15*, 244–250. [CrossRef]
5. Martone, A.M.; Bianchi, L.; Abete, P.; Bellelli, G.; Bo, M.; Cherubini, A.; Corica, F.; Di Bari, M.; Maggio, M.; Manca, G.M.; et al. The incidence of sarcopenia among hospitalized older patients: Results from the Glisten study. *J. Cachexia Sarcopenia Muscle* **2017**, *8*, 907–914. [CrossRef]
6. Timpka, S.; Petersson, I.F.; Zhou, C.; Englund, M. Muscle strength in adolescent men and risk of cardiovascular disease events and mortality in middle age: A prospective cohort study. *BMC Med.* **2014**, *12*, 62. [CrossRef]
7. Hess, N.C.; Carlson, D.J.; Inder, J.D.; Jesulola, E.; McFarlane, J.R.; Smart, N.A. Clinically meaningful blood pressure reductions with low intensity isometric handgrip exercise. A randomized trial. *Physiol. Res.* **2016**, *65*, 461–468. [CrossRef]
8. Carlson, D.J.; Inder, J.; Palanisamy, S.K.; McFarlane, J.R.; Dieberg, G.; Smart, N.A. The efficacy of isometric resistance training utilizing handgrip exercise for blood pressure management: A randomized trial. *Medicine* **2016**, *95*, e5791. [CrossRef]
9. Sayer, A.A.; Syddall, H.E.; Dennison, E.M.; Martin, H.J.; Phillips, D.I.; Cooper, C.; Byrne, C.D. Grip strength and the metabolic syndrome: Findings from the Hertfordshire cohort study. *QJM* **2007**, *100*, 707–713. [CrossRef]
10. Ji, C.; Zheng, L.; Zhang, R.; Wu, Q.; Zhao, Y. Handgrip strength is positively related to blood pressure and hypertension risk: Results from the national health and nutrition examination survey. *Lipids Health Dis.* **2018**, *17*, 86. [CrossRef]
11. Hashimoto, Y.; Kaji, A.; Sakai, R.; Hamaguchi, M.; Okada, H.; Ushigome, E.; Asano, M.; Yamazaki, M.; Fukui, M. Sarcopenia is associated with blood pressure variability in older patients with type 2 diabetes: A cross-sectional study of the KAMOGAWA-DM cohort study. *Geriatr. Gerontol. Int.* **2018**, *18*, 1345–1349. [CrossRef] [PubMed]
12. Expert Committee on the Diagnosis and Classification of Diabetes Mellitus. Report of the expert committee on the diagnosis and classification of diabetes mellitus. *Diabetes Care* **2003**, *26*, 5–20. [CrossRef]
13. Imai, Y.; Otsuka, K.; Kawano, Y.; Shimada, K.; Hayashi, H.; Tochikubo, O.; Miyakawa, M.; Fukiyama, K. Japanese society of hypertension (JSH) guidelines for self-monitoring of blood pressure at home. *Hypertens. Res.* **2003**, *26*, 771–782. [CrossRef] [PubMed]
14. Chilima, D.M.; Ismail, S.J. Nutrition and handgrip strength of older adults in rural Malawi. *Public Health Nutr.* **2001**, *4*, 11–17. [CrossRef]

15. Kallman, D.A.; Plato, C.C.; Tobin, J.D. The role of muscle loss in the age-related decline of grip strength: Cross-sectional and longitudinal perspectives. *J. Gerontol.* **1990**, *45*, 82–88. [CrossRef]
16. Steffl, M.; Bohannon, R.W.; Petr, M.; Kohlikova, E.; Holmerova, I. Relation between cigarette smoking and sarcopenia: Meta-analysis. *Physiol. Res.* **2015**, *64*, 419–426. [CrossRef]
17. Srikanthan, P.; Hevener, A.L.; Karlamangla, A.S. Sarcopenia exacerbates obesity-associated insulin resistance and dysglycemia: Findings from the national health and nutrition examination survey III. *PLoS ONE* **2010**, *5*, e10805. [CrossRef] [PubMed]
18. Kohara, K. Sarcopenic obesity in aging population: Current status and future directions for research. *Endocrine* **2014**, *45*, 15–25. [CrossRef]
19. Chamoit-Clerc, P.; Renaud, J.F.; Safar, M.E. Pulse pressure, aortic reactivity, and endothelium dysfunction in old hypertensive rats. *Hypertension* **2001**, *37*, 313–321. [CrossRef]
20. Higashi, Y.; Sasaki, S.; Kurisu, S.; Yoshimizu, A.; Sasaki, N.; Matsuura, H.; Kajiyama, G.; Oshima, T. Regular aerobic exercise augments endothelium-dependent vascular relaxation in normotensive as well as hypertensive subjects: Role of endothelium-derived nitric oxide. *Circulation* **1999**, *100*, 1194–1202. [CrossRef]
21. Samengo, G.; Avik, A.; Fedor, B.; Whittaker, D.; Myung, K.H.; Wehling-Henricks, M.; Tidball, J.G. Age-related loss of nitric oxide synthase in skeletal muscle causes reductions in calpain S-nitrosylation that increase myofibril degradation and sarcopenia. *Aging Cell* **2012**, *11*, 1036–1045. [CrossRef]
22. Yamanashi, H.; Kulkarni, B.; Edwards, T.; Kinra, S.; Koyamatsu, J.; Nagayoshi, M.; Shimizu, Y.; Maeda, T.; Cox, S.E. Association between atherosclerosis and handgrip strength in non-hypertensive populations in India and Japan. *Geriatr. Gerontol. Int.* **2018**, *18*, 1071–1078. [CrossRef] [PubMed]
23. Baber, R.J.; Panay, N.; Fenton, A.; Baber, R.J.; Panay, N.; Fenton, A.; Pérez López, F.R.; Storch, E.; Villaseca, P.; Llaneza, P. 2016 IMS recommendations on women's midlife health and menopause hormone therapy. *Climacteric* **2016**, *19*, 109–150. [CrossRef]
24. Valenti, G. Adrenopause: An imbalance between dehydroepiandrosterone (DHEA) and cortisol secretion. *J. Endocrinol. Invest.* **2002**, *25*, 29–35. [PubMed]
25. Greising, S.M.; Baltgalvis, K.A.; Lowe, D.A.; Warren, G.L. Hormone therapy and skeletal muscle strength: A meta-analysis. *J. Gerontol. A Biol. Sci. Med. Sci.* **2009**, *64*, 1071–1081. [CrossRef] [PubMed]
26. Lee, C.E.; McArdle, A.; Griffiths, R.D. The role of hormones, cytokines and heat shock proteins during age-related muscle loss. *Clin. Nutr.* **2007**, *26*, 524–534. [CrossRef] [PubMed]
27. Collins, B.C.; Laakkonen, E.K.; Lowe, D.A. Aging of the musculoskeletal system: How the loss of estrogen impacts muscle strength. *Bone* **2019**, *123*, 137–144. [CrossRef]
28. Taekema, D.G.; Maier, A.B.; Westendorp, R.G.J.; de Craen, A.J.M. Higher blood pressure is associated with higher handgrip strength in the oldest old. *Am. J. Hypertens.* **2011**, *24*, 83–89. [CrossRef]
29. Carpenter, M.A.; John, A.; Weir, M.R.; Smith, S.R.; Hunsicker, L.; Kasiske, B.L.; Kusek, J.W.; Bostom, A.; Ivanova, A.; Levey, A.S.; et al. Cardiovascular disease, and death in the folic acid for vascular outcome reduction in transplantation trial. *J. Am. Soc. Nephrol.* **2014**, *25*, 1554–1562. [CrossRef]
30. Franklin, S.S.; Larson, M.G.; Khan, S.A.; Wong, N.D.; Leip, E.P.; Kannel, W.B.; Levy, D. Does the relation of blood pressure to coronary heart disease risk change with aging? The framingham heart study. *Circulation* **2001**, *103*, 1245–1249. [CrossRef]

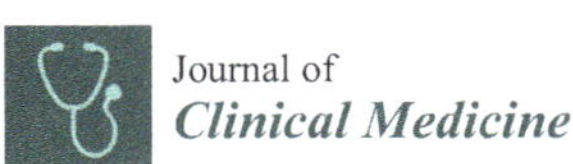
Journal of
Clinical Medicine

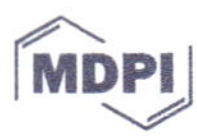

Article

Impact of Isolated High Home Systolic Blood Pressure and Diabetic Nephropathy in Patients with Type 2 Diabetes Mellitus: A 5-Year Prospective Cohort Study

Nobuko Kitagawa [1,†], Noriyuki Kitagawa [1,2,†], Emi Ushigome [1,*], Hidetaka Ushigome [3], Isao Yokota [4], Naoko Nakanishi [1], Masahide Hamaguchi [1], Mai Asano [1], Masahiro Yamazaki [1] and Michiaki Fukui [1]

1 Department of Endocrinology and Metabolism, Graduate School of Medical Science, Kyoto Prefectural University of Medicine, Kyoto 602-8566, Japan; nobuko-s@koto.kpu-m.ac.jp (N.K.); nori-kgw@koto.kpu-m.ac.jp (N.K.); naoko-n@koto.kpu-m.ac.jp (N.N.); mhama@koto.kpu-m.ac.jp (M.H.); maias@koto.kpu-m.ac.jp (M.A.); masahiro@koto.kpu-m.ac.jp (M.Y.); michiaki@koto.kpu-m.ac.jp (M.F.)
2 Department of Endocrinology and Metabolism, Kameoka Municipal Hospital, Kyoto 621-8585, Japan
3 Department of Organ Transplantation and General Surgery, Graduate School of Medical Science, Kyoto Prefectural University of Medicine, Kyoto 602-8566, Japan; ushi@koto.kpu-m.ac.jp
4 Department of Biostatistics, Graduate School of Medicine, Hokkaido University, Hokkaido 060-8638, Japan; yokotai@pop.med.hokudai.ac.jp
* Correspondence: emis@koto.kpu-m.ac.jp; Tel.: +81-75-251-5505
† Address: 465, Kajii cho, Kamigyo-ku, Kyoto-city, Kyoto 602-8566, Japan.

Citation: Kitagawa, N.; Kitagawa, N.; Ushigome, E.; Ushigome, H.; Yokota, I.; Nakanishi, N.; Hamaguchi, M.; Asano, M.; Yamazaki, M.; Fukui, M. Impact of Isolated High Home Systolic Blood Pressure and Diabetic Nephropathy in Patients with Type 2 Diabetes Mellitus: A 5-Year Prospective Cohort Study. *J. Clin. Med.* **2021**, *10*, 1929. https://doi.org/10.3390/jcm10091929

Academic Editor: Tomoaki Ishigami

Received: 16 March 2021
Accepted: 26 April 2021
Published: 29 April 2021

Publisher's Note: MDPI stays neutral with regard to jurisdictional claims in published maps and institutional affiliations.

Abstract: Background: A previous 2-year cohort study has shown that isolated high home systolic blood pressure (IH-HSBP) may increase the risk of diabetic nephropathy, using normal HBP as a reference. However, this association has not been previously assessed in the medium to long term. Methods: This prospective 5-year cohort study of 424 patients, with normal or mildly increased albuminuria, investigated the effect of IH-HSBP on the risk of diabetic nephropathy in patients with type 2 diabetes mellitus. Diabetic nephropathy was defined as an advancement from normal or mildly increased albuminuira to moderate or severely increased albuminuria. Results: Among 424 patients, 75 developed diabetic nephropathy during the study period. The adjusted odds ratio for developing diabetic nephropathy given IH-HSBP was 2.39 (95% confidence interval, 1.15–4.96, $p = 0.02$). The odds ratio for developing nephropathy in patients with IH-HSBP younger than 65 years was higher than that in patients with IH-HSBP older than 65 years. Conclusion: IH-HSBP was associated with an increased risk of diabetic nephropathy among type 2 diabetes mellitus patients with normal or mildly increased albuminuria in the medium to long term. The results support and strengthen previous reports. These findings suggest that IH-HSBP might be a useful marker in disease prognostication.

Keywords: albuminuria; diabetes mellitus; isolated high home systolic blood pressure; diabetic nephropathy

1. Introduction

Home blood pressure (HBP) control is paramount to diabetic nephropathy prevention [1]. Several important factors of HBP, including day-to-day variability [2] or pulse pressure [3], have been reported as relevant to the risk of diabetic nephropathy.

Isolated systolic hypertension (ISH) is diagnosed when systolic blood pressure (SBP) is hypertensive, while diastolic blood pressure (DBP) is normotensive [4]. ISH has been shown to increase the risk of premature mortality in patients with cardiovascular disease; it is a common form of hypertension [5–7].

ISH expressed as HBP (home ISH) has also been shown to affect the risk of diabetic nephropathy. In fact, our group has previously shown that isolated high home systolic blood pressure (IH-HSBP) might be a useful marker in the prognostication of diabetic nephropathy, based on data from a 2-year cohort study [8]. Nevertheless, the follow-up period in that study was relatively short, likely limiting its statistical power. To address this limitation, we performed a follow-up study with patients diagnosed with type 2 diabetes mellitus (DM), aiming to provide a valid assessment of the impact of ISH on the risk of diabetic nephropathy in this patient group over the medium to long term.

2. Design and Methods

We used the same resources in our previous study, which is based on data from the HBP cohort of patients with type 2 diabetes mellitus who had regularly attended the diabetes outpatient clinic at the Kyoto Prefectural University of Medicine Hospital or other general hospitals located in Japan (KAMOGAWA-HBP study) [1].

The present study included patients with type 2 DM; the impact of HBP on the risk of diabetic nephropathy was evaluated. Nephropathy was graded as follows: normal or mild albuminuria, defined as urinary albumin/creatinine ratio (UACR) < 30 mg per gram of creatinine (mg/g Cr); moderately increased albuminuria (microalbuminuria), defined as UACR 30–300 mg/g Cr; or severely increased albuminuria (macroalbuminuria), defined as UACR > 300 mg/g Cr [9–14]. The development of diabetic nephropathy was defined as an advancement from normal or mild albuminuira to moderately or severely increased albuminuria within 5 years. The study protocol was approved by the local Research Ethics Committee, RBMR-E-349; the study adhered to the principles of the Declaration of Helsinki, and informed consent was obtained from all patients prior to enrollment.

2.1. Data Collection

Blood samples for biochemical measurements were taken in the morning. Serum lipid profile (including levels of triglycerides, low-density lipoprotein cholesterol, and high-density lipoprotein cholesterol) and levels of creatinine and hemoglobin A1C (HbA1c), and of other biochemical markers, were assessed by standard laboratory methods. The data collection of urinary samples was performed simultaneously with the beginning of HBP measurements. An immunoturbidimetric assay was used to measure UACR; the mean value of three consecutive urinary measurements was equivalent to UACR. Levels of HbA1c were classified and reported according to the National Glycohemoglobin Standardization Program guidelines, as recommended by the Japan Diabetes Society [15]. Data on patient demographic and clinical characteristics, including sex, age, duration of DM, smoking status, and those who consumed alcohol or antihypertensive medication were collected at the same time as HBP measurements began. To measure brachial–ankle pulse wave velocity (baPWV), the volume plethysmographic method was used, which was also the method utilized in our previous cohort study [16]. Diagnosis of diabetic nephropathy was based on the Diagnostic Nephropathy Study Group criteria [17]. Alcohol drinking status (never, social, or everyday) and smoking status (never, past, or current) were checked by interview. Type 2 DM was diagnosed when a fasting plasma glucose level was more than 126 mg/dl (7.0 mmol/L), or a random plasma glucose was more than 200 mg/dl (11.1 mmol/L), based on the American Diabetes Association criteria [18].

2.2. HBP Measurements

Patients were instructed to measure their BP 3 times each morning and evening for 14 consecutive days, and the 14-day average of the 3 morning and 3 evening mean values were calculated for each. Patients were instructed to measure their morning BP within 1 h of waking up, before breakfast, before taking medication, having sat, and having rested for at least 5 min [19]. Similar instructions applied to evening BP measurements, which were obtained before bedtime. Eating was prohibited for over one hour before measurement before going to bed. Moreover, patients were instructed that the cuff of the measuring device should be placed around the contralateral side of the dominant arm, with its position maintained at the level of the heart. HBP measurements were performed with an automated device—HEM-70801C (Omron Healthcare Co. Ltd., Kyoto, Japan)—which used a digital display to present values of SBP/DBP and heart rate, measured using the cuff-oscillometric method. HEM-70801C uses the same components and BP-determining algorithm as those of another device, HEM-705IT, which was previously validated and satisfied the criteria of the British Hypertension Society protocol [20].

In the Japanese Society of Hypertension Guidelines for the Management of Hypertension (JSH 2019) [21], the target level of HBP control is under 125/75 mmHg in hypertensive patients with DM. Patients were classified into 4 groups based on HBP levels: normal HBP (morning SBP < 125 mmHg and morning DBP < 75 mmHg), isolated high IH-HSBP (morning SBP > 125 mmHg and morning DBP < 75 mmHg), isolated high home DBP (IH-HDBP) (morning SBP < 125 mmHg and morning DBP > 75 mmHg), and high HBP (morning SBP > 125 mmHg and morning DBP > 75 mmHg) [21,22].

2.3. Statistical Analysis

Participant baseline characteristics were reported as median, with interquartile range or count, as suitable. Logistic regression analysis was used to assess the relationship between IH-HSBP, IH-HDBP, and high HBP, and the risk of diabetic nephropathy, with "normal HBP" set as a reference. The following factors were included as covariates in the adjusted models: sex, body mass index (BMI), duration of diabetes, levels of HbA1c, of total cholesterol, of creatinine, and use of antihypertensive medication (Model 2). Separate adjustments were made for the use of renin–angiotensin–aldosterone system inhibitors instead of other antihypertensive medications (Model 3).

In addition, subgroup analyses were performed for age (≥65 years vs. <65 years) and SBP control (≥135 mmHg vs. <135 mmHg). JSH2019 [21] adopted 135/85 mmHg as the diagnostic criterion for hypertension based on HBP. p-values < 0.05 were considered indicative of statistically significant findings. Statistical analyses were performed using JMP version 13.2 software (SAS Institute Inc., Cary, NC, USA).

3. Results

A total of 1372 consecutive patients with type 2 DM, aged 20–90 years, were recruited for this study. In all, 64 and 422 patients were excluded due to insufficient HBP and UACR data, respectively. In addition, there were 148 patients who were newly prescribed angiotensin II receptor blocker (ARB) or angiotensin-converting-enzyme inhibitor (ACE-I), or who stopped using them during follow-up. Another 263 patients who had moderately or severely increased albuminuria were also excluded.

The final sample included 424 patients with normal or mild albuminuria (Figure 1). Among them, during 5-year follow-up period, 74 patients developed moderately increased albuminuria and 1 patient developed severely increased albuminuria.

Patient baseline demographic and clinical characteristics are presented in Tables 1 and 2. Median (interquartile range) age, duration of diabetes, BMI, and levels of total cholesterol and those of HbA1C were 64.0 (59.0–70.0) years, 9.0 (4.8–15.0) years, 23.0 (21.4–25.3) kg/m^2, 191 (170–212) mg/dL, and 6.6% (6.2%–7.3%), respectively. The patients in the IH-HSBP group were older than those in the high HBP group (69.6 vs. 60.6 years, $p < 0.001$). The unadjusted odds ratio (OR) with 95% confidence interval (CI) of developing diabetic nephropathy, given IH-HSBP, IH-HDBP, and high HBP, was 2.68 (1.36–5.30), 0.78 (0.21–2.81), and 1.63 (0.87–3.04), respectively (Table 3), using normal HBP as a reference. In multivariate analyses, adjusted OR (95% CI) of developing diabetic nephropathy, given IH-HSBP, was 2.36% (1.14%–4.89%, $p = 0.02$) in Model 2 and 2.39% (1.15%–4.96%, $p = 0.02$) in Model 3 (Table 3).

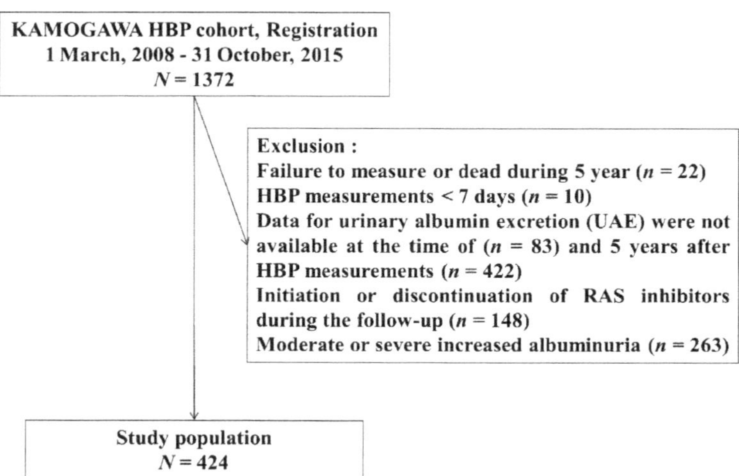

Figure 1. Study flow diagram for the registration of patients.

Table 1. Characteristics of patients.

Sex	
Male	228 (53.8)
Female	196 (46.2)
Age (y)	64.0 (59.0–70.0)
Duration of diabetes (y)	9.0 (4.8–15.0)
Body mass index (kg/m^2)	23.0 (21.4–25.3)
Mean morning systolic blood pressure (mmHg)	128.1 (117.4–138.2)
Mean morning diastolic blood pressure (mmHg)	73.2 (66.5–79.9)
Mean evening systolic blood pressure (mmHg)	123.4 (115.0–133.1)
Mean evening diastolic blood pressure (mmHg)	67.7 (61.9–74.2)
Clinic systolic blood pressure (mmHg)	136.0 (123.0–146.0)
Clinic diastolic blood pressure (mmHg)	76.7 (70.0–80.3)
Hemoglobin A1c (mmol/mol)	52.0 (48.6–59.5)
Total cholesterol (mg/dL)	191 (170–212)
Creatinine (mg/dL)	0.70 (0.58–0.83)
eGFR (ml/min/1.73^2)	75.0 (63.1–89.0)
baPWV	1762 (1501–2002)
Smoking status	
Current smoker	63 (18.1)
Past smoker	109 (31.3)
Alcohol drinking	
everyday	99 (28.6)
social	71 (20.5)
Diabetic complications	
Retinopathy	84 (23.5)
Neuropathy	118 (31.8)
Neuropathy	118 (31.8)
Macrovascular disease	101 (27.0)
Use of antihypertensive medication	192 (45.2)
RAS (−/+)	267/156

For categorical variables, n (%) is presented. For continuous variables, median (interquartile range) is presented. eGFR, estimated glemerular filtration rate; baPWV, brachial–ankle pulse wave velocity; RAS, renin–angiotensin–aldosterone system.

Table 2. Characteristics of patients according to the 4 groups based on HBP levels.

Hypertension Status (n)	Normal HBP Group (152)	Isolated High HSBP Group (83)	Isolated High HDBP Group (30)	High HBP Group (159)
Male/female	74/78	40/43	19/11	95/64
Age (y)	64 (58–70)	69 (63–75)	60 (45–65)	63 (58–70)
Body mass index (kg/m^2)	22.1 (20.9–24.1)	22.5 (21.2–24.7)	23.8 (21.7–26.1)	24.0 (21.8–26.4)
Mean morning systolic blood pressure (mmHg)	115.5 (107.7–119.0	133.3 (128.8–139.6)	120.0 (116.9–122.2)	139.0 (132.2–146.1)
Mean morning diastolic blood pressure (mmHg)	66.3 (62.6–69.0)	69.4 (64.8–72.1)	77.2 (76.4–81.6)	81.6 (77.9–86.7)
Mean evening systolic blood pressure (mmHg)	112.9 (107.6–119.3)	129.6 (123.6–136.3)	118.4 (114.7–123.5)	131.1 (123.7–140.1)
Mean evening diastolic blood pressure (mmHg)	62.9 (58.7–67.2)	63.5 (60.0–67.6)	74.3 (70.9–77.6)	75.1 (70.4–80.6)
Clinic systolic blood pressure (mmHg)	124.1 (114.5–134.8)	141.3 (134.8–151.2)	126.8 (119.0–143.3)	140.7 (130.6–153.0)
Clinic diastolic blood pressure (mmHg)	71.7 (65.8–76.0)	71.7 (65.6–77.7)	82.3 (78.3–92.0)	83.0 (78.7–86.7)
Hemoglobin A1c (%)	6.5 (6.2–7.1)	6.8 (6.2–7.5)	6.4 (6.0–6.8)	6.7 (6.2–7.3)
Total cholesterol (mg/dL)	188.5 (164.8–211.5)	192 (170.5–206)	189 (167–209)	191 (175–216)
Creatinine (mg/dL)	0.67 (0.55–0.80)	0.69 (0.55–0.85)	0.70 (0.62–0.78)	0.70 (0.58–0.83)
eGFR (ml/min/1.73^2)	77.8 (64.0–95.0)	71.1 (58.0–85.0)	84.5 (76.0–96.8)	75.0 (64.3–86.0)
baPWV (cm/sec)	1584 (1411–1858)	1844 (1645–2059)	1491 (1281–2150)	1726 (1509–1995)
Smoking status (never/past/current)	89/42/20	45/16/21	19/7/4	85/42/27
Alcohol drinking (never/social/everyday)	97/34/20	53/9/20	16/8/6	69/35/49
Retinopathy (NDR/SDR/PDR)	120/13/13	52/18/10	24/4/1	124/19/8
Neuropathy (−/+)	111/41	57/25	28/1	120/37
Macrovascular complication (−/+)	131/21	68/15	29/1	139/20
Antihypertensive medication (−/+)	103/49	39/44	22/8	68/91
RAS (−/+)	116/36	43/40	23/7	85/73

HBP, home blood pressure; HSBP, home systolic blood pressure; HDBP, home diastolic blood pressure; eGFR, estimated glemerular filtration rate; baPWV, brachial–ankle pulse wave velocity; NDR, no diabetic retinopathy; SDR, simple diabetic retinopathy; PDR, proliferative diabetic retinopathy; −, without; +, with. For categorical variables, n is presented. For continuous variables, median (interquartile range) is presented.

In subgroup analyses, an adjusted OR (95% CI) for developing nephropathy, given IH-HSBP, was 1.68 (0.66–4.27) among age > 65 years (Table 4); meanwhile, in age < 65 years, an adjusted OR (95% CI) was 3.06% (0.63%–15.0%) (Table 4), using normal HBP as a reference.

In subgroup analysis of SBP control, in patients with equal to or more than 135 mmHg, the adjusted odds ratio (95% CI) of IH-HSBP, using normal HBP as a reference group for the development of diabetic nephropathy, was 5.39% (1.92–18.6%) (Table 5). In patients with <135 mmHg, the adjusted odds ratio (95% CI) of IH-HSBP was 0.71% (0.32–1.35%) (Table 5). The odds of each adjusting factor for the development of diabetic nephropathy are presented in Table 6.

Table 3. Unadjusted and adjusted odds ratios for the development of diabetic nephropathy.

Hypertension Status (n)	Model 1		* Model 2		* Model 3	
	Unadjusted OR (95%CI)	*p* Value	Adjusted OR (95%CI)	*p* Value	Adjusted OR (95%CI)	*p* Value
Normal HBP group (152)	1		1		1	
Isolated high HSBP group (83)	2.68 (1.36–5.30)	0.004	2.36 (1.14–4.89)	0.020	2.39 (1.15–4.96)	0.019
Isolated high HDBP group (30)	0.78 (0.21–2.81)	0.701	0.54 (0.12–2.53)	0.438	0.54 (0.12–52.5)	0.434
High HBP group (159)	1.63 (0.87–3.04)	0.126	1.57 (0.79–3.12)	0.193	1.60 (0.81–3.17)	0.173

HBP, home blood pressure; HSBP, home systolic blood pressure; normal HBP (morning SBP < 125 mmHg and morning DBP < 75 mmHg); isolated high HSBP (morning SBP > 125 mmHg and morning DBP < 75 mmHg); isolated high HDBP (morning SBP < 125 mmHg and morning DBP > 75 mmHg); and high HBP (morning SBP > 125 mmHg and morning DBP > 75 mmHg). * Model 2: Odds ratios were adjusted for sex, age, duration of diabetes mellitus, body mass index, hemoglobin A1C, total cholesterol, creatinine, and the use of antihypertensive medications. * Model 3: Odds ratios were adjusted for variables in Model 2 and additional adjustment for the use of renin–angiotensin system inhibitors instead of the use of antihypertensive medications.

Table 4. Unadjusted and adjusted odds ratios for the development of diabetic nephropathy in patients equal to or more than 65 years old and less than 65 years old.

Hypertension Status	Model 1		* Model 2		* Model 3	
	Unadjusted OR (95%CI)	*p* Value	Adjusted OR (95%CI)	*p* Value	Adjusted OR (95%CI)	*p* Value
		≥65 years old				
Normal HBP group	1		1		1	
Isolated high HSBP group	1.90 (0.85–4.23)	0.116	1.70 (0.67–4.33)	0.263	1.68 (0.66–4.27)	0.275
		<65 years old				
Normal HBP group	1		1		1	
Isolated high HSBP group	3.08 (0.76–12.5)	0.116	3.07 (0.62–15.1)	0.167	3.06 (0.63–15.0)	0.167

HBP, home blood pressure; HSBP, home systolic blood pressure; * Model 2: Odds ratios were adjusted for sex, age, duration of diabetes mellitus, body mass index, hemoglobin A1C, total cholesterol, creatinine, and the use of antihypertensive medications. * Model 3: Odds ratios were adjusted for variables in Model 2 and additional adjustment for the use of renin–angiotensin system inhibitors instead of the use of antihypertensive medications.

Table 5. Unadjusted and adjusted odds ratios for the development of diabetic nephropathy in patients according to systolic blood pressure.

Hypertension Status	Model 1		* Model 2		* Model 3	
	Unadjusted OR (95%CI)	*p* Value	Adjusted OR (95%CI)	*p* Value	Adjusted OR (95%CI)	*p* Value
		≥135 mmHg				
Normal HBP group	1		1		1	
Isolated high HSBP group	4.21 (1.73–12.6)	0.0009	5.59 (2.02–19.1)	0.0005	5.39 (1.92–18.6)	0.0008
		<135 mmHg				
Normal HBP group	1		1		1	
Isolated high HSBP group	1.31 (0.63–2.52)	0.452	0.75 (0.33–1.57)	0.449	0.71 (0.32–1.35)	0.384

HBP, home blood pressure; HSBP, home systolic blood pressure; * Model 2: Odds ratios were adjusted for sex, age, duration of diabetes mellitus, body mass index, hemoglobin A1C, total cholesterol, creatinine, and the use of antihypertensive medications. * Model 3: Odds ratios were adjusted for variables in Model 2 and additional adjustment for the use of renin–angiotensin system inhibitors instead of use of antihypertensive medications.

Table 6. The odds of each adjusting factor for the development of diabetic nephropathy according to systolic blood pressure.

	SBP Control ≥ 135 mmHg	SBP Control < 135 mmHg
Sex	0.86 (0.36–1.98)	0.69 (0.36–1.29)
Duration of diabetes	0.99 (0.95–1.04)	0.98 (0.95–1.01)
Body mass index	1.08 (0.97–1.22)	0.93 (0.86–1.01)
Hemoglobin A1c	1.12 (0.73–1.80)	0.73 (0.52–1.03)
Total cholesterol	1.00 (0.99–1.02)	0.99 (0.98–1.003)
Creatinine	1.13 (0.51–6.26)	0.74 (0.13–4.56)
Use of antihypertensive medication	0.90 (0.38–2.06)	0.69 (0.37–1.32)
Use of RAS	1.00 (0.43–2.29)	0.78 (0.40–1.56)

SBP, systolic blood pressure; RAS, renin–angiotensin–aldosterone system.

4. Discussion

In the present study, IH-HSBP was associated with an increased risk of transition to moderate or severe albuminuria in patients with type 2 DM during a 5-year follow-up period.

The results are in line with the previous 2-year cohort study [8]. The mechanism likely to account for the association between IH-HSBP and diabetic nephropathy risk has been described elsewhere [23–29]. Increased arterial stiffness has been associated with the development of ISH [30]. Further arterial aging might result in additional increase of IH-HSBP, which is a risk factor for target organ dysfunction [31] and diabetic nephropathy [32]. The association between proteinuria and high BP is strictly related to very high risk of cardiovascular disease in type 2 diabetes [33,34]. In advanced type 2 diabetic nephropathy, appropriate management is of great importance [35]. So, we should adequately man-age home SBP. In HBP management, especially, we should clarify the association be-tween albuminuria and isolated high HSBP.

In the present study, IH-HSBP was associated with an increased risk of diabetic nephropathy; however, high HBP was not. The patients in the IH-HSBP group were older than those in the high HBP group. When arterial stiffness was compared between the IH-HSBP and High-HBP groups using baPWV measurements, there appeared to be higher arterial stiffness among patients in the IH-HSBP group than in those in the High-HBP group (Table S1) [16,36]. Arterial aging in IH-HSBP may be associated with increased odds for the development of diabetic nephropathy. Similarly, the isolated high HDBP group was not associated with an increased risk of diabetic nephropathy development. Those in the isolated HDBP group were younger, had a short duration of diabetes, lower baPWV, and also lower HSBP than the isolated high HSBP group (Table S2). For these reasons, only the isolated HSBP was associated with an increased risk of diabetic nephropathy development in this study.

The effect of IH-HSBP on the development of diabetic nephropathy, defined using estimated glomerular filtration rate (eGFR), is very important. Then, we analyzed the association between IH-HSBP and the development of diabetic nephropathy, defined using eGFR, and found that there was no relationship between them. We examined the association between changes in eGFR and the factors which were associated with IH-HSBP, including duration of diabetes or baPWV, and found no association. We assume that development of diabetic nephropathy, defined using ACR but not eGFR, was associated with pathophysiology of IH-HSBP in this study, although the precise mechanism is not unclear. Moreover, in this study, the mean (standard deviation) change in eGFR over 5 years was -0.37 (7.92) mL/min/1.73^2, which might be too small to properly analyze the development of diabetic nephropathy.

Initiation or discontinuation of anti-diabetic medications such as sodium glucose co-transporter (SGLT2) inhibitors may affect intra-glomerular pressure and the progression of diabetic nephropathy. However, SGLT2 inhibitors were not used at the start or during the initial 2-year follow-up period of this study. Among 424 patients with type 2 DM in the present cohort, 24 patients were newly prescribed SGLT2 inhibitors during the study period. Nevertheless, use of SGLT2 inhibitors did not affect the risk of diabetic nephropathy associated with IH-HSBP. Most present study patients were prescribed these agents for less than one year, which might have reduced their impact on outcomes of interest. Further studies are needed to examine this effect.

ISH among young-to-middle-aged Japanese people is associated with premature mortality due to cardiovascular disease [37]. In the present study, age-stratified subgroup analysis revealed that the adjusted OR was higher among patients aged <65 years than in those aged ≥65 years. These findings were consistent with those of our previous study [8], in that the association between IH-HSBP and diabetic nephropathy was weakened in patients ≥ 65. Among the patients with IH-HSBP ≥ 65, the progression of diabetic nephropathy was observed in 9.4% (2-year) and 9.5% (5-year). The progression of diabetic nephropathy did not increase over 3 years among the patients with IH-HSBP ≥ 65. Therefore, the association between IH-HSBP and diabetic nephropathy was weakened in patients aged ≥65. Meanwhile, subgroup analyses stratified by SBP status revealed that IH-HSBP increased the risk of diabetic nephropathy only in patients with SBP ≥ 135 mmHg. Patients with IH-HSBP may be at a lower risk if their SBP measurements meet the hypertension diagnostic criteria of less than 135 mmHg [21]. It should be noted that patients in this group were older and more likely to take antihypertensive medications than patients with SBP < 135 mmHg (Table S3). Patients with SBP ≥ 135 mmHg had remarkable ISH, which would be associated with arterial damage and diabetic nephropathy.

To the best of our knowledge, this is the first study to evaluate the impact of IH-HSBP on the risk of diabetic nephropathy in patients with type 2 DM over the medium to long term. The results support and strengthen previous reports. In addition, the risk of younger patients with ISH was elucidated through the 5-year follow-up period.

Nevertheless, this study has several limitations, which should be considered when interpreting its findings. First, we did not have data on salt intake, protein intake, or levels of exercise, which would be associated with the development of diabetic nephropathy [27,38–41]. In this regard, we could not clearly identify the prognostic significance of HBP for the development of diabetic nephropathy, even in a longer study. Second, only Japanese men and women were included in the study population. Therefore, these findings might not be generalized to other ethnic groups. Third, only single baseline measurements of BP were performed. This may be potential bias. However, the association of target organ damage was confirmed by BP at baseline or during follow-up [21]. Single BP assessments would be reliable when the addition of subsequent values does not significantly alter the results. Fourth, another important issue is the ultrasound findings on kidneys in the baseline, particularly the size of kidneys, which should be hypertrophic or enlarged before a moderately increased albuminuria development. However, these were not the ultrasound findings on kidneys. Fifth, the risk of ISH, defined by home BP on developing albuminuria in diabetic patients, was similar after the follow-up period and was prolonged for 3 years. The results were essentially similar to previous findings, and thus could not add new information for clinical science. We should at least prolong the follow-up period up to 10 years or more. Finally, a non-albuminuric phenotype has for years been reported in diabetic kidney disease (DKD) of type 2 DM [42]. Therefore, many patients with type 2 DM, despite being normoalbuminuric if they have a GRF of <60 mil/min/1.73m^2, still have DKD. In the present study, we did not include patients with a GFR of <60 mil/min/1.73m^2. Thus, we were not able to evaluate the decline in renal function in the definition of DKD in this study. Further studies will be conducted in the future.

5. Conclusions

In conclusion, IH-HSBP in patients with type 2 diabetes mellitus was a prognostic factor for the development of diabetic nephropathy in a prospective 5-year cohort study.

Supplementary Materials: The following are available online at https://www.mdpi.com/article/10.3390/jcm10091929/s1, Table S1: The comparison of arterial stiffness among patients with isolated high HSBP or High-HBP, Table S2: The comparison of the patients with isolated high HSBP or isolated high HDBP, Table S3: The comparison of patients according to systolic blood pressure.

Author Contributions: N.K. (Nobuko Kitagawa) or N.K. (Noriyuki Kitagawa) designed the study, performed data analyses, and reviewed/edited the manuscript; E.U. designed the study, contributed to the collection of research data, performed data analyses, drafted the manuscript, and was the main study physician responsible for the KAMOGAWA-HBP study in Kyoto Prefectural University of Medicine, Graduate School of Medical Science; H.U., N.N. and M.H. designed the study protocol, reviewed data reports, and reviewed the study manuscript; I.Y. supervised data analysis, contributed to manuscript preparation, contributed to discussion, and reviewed/edited the manuscript; M.A. and M.Y. designed the study protocol, reviewed data reports, and reviewed the study manuscript; M.F. designed the protocol, performed data analyses, drafted the manuscript, and was the principal investigator of the Kyoto Prefectural University of Medicine, Graduate School of Medical Science, and lead principal investigator for the study. All authors reviewed and provided edits and comments on manuscript drafts. E.U. is the guarantor of this work and, as such, had full access to all the data in the study and takes responsibility for the integrity of the data and the accuracy of the data analysis. All authors have read and agreed to the published version of the manuscript.

Funding: EU received grant support from the Japanese Study Group for Physiology and Management of Blood Pressure, and the Astellas Foundation for Research on Metabolic Disorders (grant number: 4024).

Institutional Review Board Statement: The study design was approved by the appropriate ethics review board. The ethics committee of Kyoto Prefectural University of Medicine approved the study, and the study was conducted in accordance with Declaration of Helsinki.

Informed Consent Statement: All study participants provided informed consent.

Data Availability Statement: Data are available upon reasonable request to the corresponding author.

Acknowledgments: We thank Naoko Higo R.N., Machiko Hasegawa R.N., and Terumi Kaneko R.N. of the Kyoto Prefectural University of Medicine for teaching patients how to measure their blood pressure, and Sayoko Horibe, Hiroko Kawamura, and Aiko Aida, also of the Kyoto Prefectural University of Medicine, for their secretarial assistance. We thank Editage for English language editing.

Conflicts of Interest: N.K., N.K., E.U., H.U., N.N., M.H., M.A., M.Y., and M.F. have received grant and research support from AstraZeneca plc, Astellas Pharma Inc., Bristol-Myers Squibb K.K., Daiichi Sankyo Co., Ltd., Eli Lilly Japan K.K., Kyowa Hakko Kirin Company Ltd., Kowa Pharmaceutical Co., Ltd., Kissei Pharmaceutical Co., Ltd., MSD K.K., Mitsubishi Tanabe Pharma Corp., Novo Nordisk Pharma Ltd., Nippon Chemiphar Company Ltd., Sanwa Kagaku Kenkyusho Co., Ltd., Sanofi K.K., Taisho Toyama Pharmaceutical Co., Ltd., Takeda Pharmaceutical Co., Ltd., and TERUMO Co. I.Y. has received grants from Japan Society for the Promotion of Science KAKENHI, and Health, Labour and Welfare Policy Research Grants, speaker fees from Chugai Pharmaceutical Co, AstraZeneca plt, Japan Tabacco Pharamaceutical Division, and Nippon Shinyaku Co. The remaining authors have nothing to declare. The sponsors were not involved in the study design; in the collection, analysis, interpretation of data; nor in the writing of this manuscript; nor in the decision to submit the article for publication. The authors, their immediate families, and any research foundations with which they are affiliated have not received any financial payments or other benefits from any commercial entity related to the subject of this article. The authors declare that, although they are affiliated with a department that is supported financially by a pharmaceutical company, the authors received no current funding for this study, and department affiliation does not alter their adherence to all journal policies on sharing data and materials.

References

1. Ushigome, E.; Oyabu, C.; Tanaka, T.; Hasegawa, G.; Ohnishi, M.; Tsunoda, S.; Ushigome, H.; Yokota, I.; Nakamura, N.; Oda, Y.; et al. Impact of masked hypertension on diabetic nephropathy in patients with type II diabetes: A KAMOGAWA-HBP study. *J. Am. Soc. Hypertens.* **2018**, *12*, 364–371. [CrossRef] [PubMed]
2. Ushigome, E.; Matsumoto, S.; Oyabu, C.; Kitagawa, N.; Tanaka, T.; Hasegawa, G.; Ohnishi, M.; Tsunoda, S.; Ushigome, H.; Yokota, I.; et al. Prognostic significance of day-by-day variability of home blood pressure on progression to macroalbuminuria in patients with diabetes. *J. Hypertens.* **2018**, *36*, 1068–1075. [CrossRef] [PubMed]

3. Kitagawa, N.; Ushigome, E.; Matsumoto, S.; Oyabu, C.; Ushigome, H.; Yokota, I.; Asano, M.; Tanaka, M.; Yamazaki, M.; Fukui, M. Prognostic significance of home pulse pressure for progression of diabetic nephropathy: KAMOGAWA-HBP Study. *Hypertens. Res.* **2018**, *41*, 363–371. [CrossRef] [PubMed]
4. Bulpitt, C.J.; Fletcher, A.E.; Thijs, L.; Steassen, J.A.; Antikainen, R.; Davidson, C.; Fagard, R.; Gil-Extremera, B.; Jääskivi, M.; O'Brien, E.; et al. Symptoms reported by elderly patients with isolated systolic hypertension: Baseline data from the SYST-EUR trial. Systolic Hypertension in Europe. *Age Ageing* **1999**, *28*, 15–22. [CrossRef] [PubMed]
5. Lakatta, E.G. Mechanism of hypertension in the elderly. *J. Am. Geriatr. Soc.* **1989**, *37*, 780–790. [CrossRef]
6. Messerli, F.H.; Ventura, H.; Aristimuno, G.G.; Suarez, D.H.; Dreslinski, G.R.; Frohlich, E.D. Arterial compliance in systolic hypertension. *Clin. Exp. Hypertens.* **1982**, *4*, 1037–1044. [CrossRef]
7. Hozawa, A.; Ohkubo, T.; Nagai, K.; Kikuya, M.; Matubara, M.; Tsuji, I.; Ito, S.; Satoh, H.; Hisamichi, S.; Imai, Y. Prognosis of isolatedsystolic and isolated diastolic hypertension as assessed by self-measurement of blood pressure at home: The Ohasamastudy. *Arch. Intern. Med.* **2000**, *160*, 3301–3306. [CrossRef]
8. Kitagawa, N.; Ushigome, E.; Tanaka, T.; Hasegawa, G.; Nakamura, N.; Ohnishi, M.; Tsunoda, S.; Ushigome, H.; Yokota, I.; Kitagawa, N.; et al. Isolated high home systolic blood pressure in patients with type 2 diabetes is a prognostic factor for the development of diabetic nephropathy: KAMOGAWA-HBP Study. *Diabetes Res. Clin. Pract.* **2019**, *158*, 107920. [CrossRef]
9. Gerstein, H.C.; Mann, J.; Yi, Q.; Zinman, B.; Dinneen, S.F.; Hoogwerf, B.; Hallé, J.P.; Young, J.; Rashkow, A.; Joyce, C.; et al. Hope Study Investigators. Albuminuria and risk of cardiovascular events, death, and heart failure in diabetic and nondiabetic individuals. *JAMA* **2001**, *286*, 421–426. [CrossRef]
10. Kramer, H.; Jacobs, D.R.; Bild, D.; Post, W.; Saad, M.F.; Detrano, R.; Tracy, R.; Cooper, R.; Liu, K. Urine albumin excretion and subclinical cardiovascular disease: The multi-ethnic study of atherosclerosis. *Hypertension* **2005**, *46*, 38–43. [CrossRef]
11. Krolewski, A.S.; Niewczas, M.A.; Skupien, J.; Gohda, T.; Smiles, A.; Eckfeldt, J.H.; Doria, A.; Warram, J.H. Early progressive renal decline precedes the onset of microalbuminuria and its progression to macroalbuminuria. *Diabetes Care* **2014**, *37*, 226–234. [CrossRef]
12. Ushigome, E.; Fukui, M.; Sakabe, K.; Tanaka, M.; Inada, S.; Omoto, A.; Tanaka, T.; Fukuda, W.; Atsuta, H.; Ohnishi, M.; et al. Uncontrolled home blood pressure in the morning is associated with nephropathy in Japanese type 2 diabetes. *Heart Vessels* **2011**, *26*, 609–615. [CrossRef]
13. Nakade, Y.; Toyama, T.; Furuichi, K.; Kitajima, S.; Miyajima, Y.; Fukamachi, M.; Sagara, A.; Shinozaki, Y.; Hara, A.; Shimizu, M.; et al. Impact of kidney function and urinary protein excretion on intima–media thickness in Japanese patients with type 2 diabetes. *Clin. Exp. Nephrol.* **2015**, *19*, 909–917. [CrossRef] [PubMed]
14. Levey, A.S.; Eckardt, K.U.; Dorman, N.M.; Christiansen, S.L.; Cheung, M.; Jadoul, M.; Winkelmayer, W.C. Nomenclature for kidney function and disease-executive summary and glossary from a Kidney Disease: Improving Global Outcomes (KDIGO) consensus conference. *Eur. Heart J.* **2020**, *41*, 4592–4598. [CrossRef] [PubMed]
15. Kashiwagi, A.; Kasuga, M.; Araki, E.; Oka, Y.; Hanafusa, T.; Ito, H.; Tominaga, M.; Oikawa, S.; Noda, M.; Kawamura, T.; et al. Committee on the Standardization of Diabetes Mellitus-Related Laboratory Testing of Japan Diabetes Society. International clinical harmonization of glycated hemoglobin in Japan: From Japan Diabetes Society to National Glycohemoglobin Standardization Program values. *J. Diabetes Investig.* **2012**, *3*, 39–40. [PubMed]
16. Kitagawa, N.; Ushigome, E.; Matsumoto, S.; Oyabu, C.; Ushigome, H.; Yokota, I.; Asano, M.; Tanaka, M.; Yamazaki, M.; Fukui, M. Threshold value of home pulse pressure predicting arterial stiffness in patients with type 2 diabetes: KAMOGAWA-HBP study. *J. Clin. Hypertens.* **2018**, *20*, 472–477. [CrossRef]
17. Wada, T.; Haneda, M.; Furuichi, K.; Babazono, T.; Yokoyama, H.; Iseki, K.; Araki, S.; Ninomiya, T.; Hara, S.; Suzuki, Y.; et al. Research Group of Diabetic Nephropathy, Ministry of Health, Labour, and Welfare of Japan. Clinical impact of albuminuria and glomerular filtration rate on renal and cardiovascular events, and all-cause mortality in Japanese patients with type 2 diabetes. *Clin. Exp. Nephrol.* **2014**, *18*, 621–622. [CrossRef]
18. Expert Committee on the Diagnosis and Classification of Diabetes Mellitus. Report of the Expert Committee on the Diagnosis and Classification of Diabetes Mellitus. *Diabetes Care* **2002**, *25*, S5–S20. [CrossRef]
19. Imai, Y.; Otsuka, K.; Kawano, Y.; Shimada, K.; Hayashi, H.; Tochikubo, O.; Miyakawa, M.; Fukiyama, K.; Japan Society of Hypertension. Japanese Society of Hypertension (JSH) guidelines for self-monitoring of blood pressure at home. *Hypertens. Res.* **2003**, *26*, 771–782. [CrossRef]
20. Coleman, A.; Fraaman, P.; Steel, S.; Shennan, A. Validation of the Omron 705IT (HEM-759-E) oscillometric blood pressure monitoring device according to the British Hypertension Society protocol. *Blood Press. Monit.* **2006**, *11*, 27–32. [CrossRef] [PubMed]
21. Umemura, S.; Arima, H.; Arima, S.; Asayama, K.; Dohi, Y.; Hirooka, Y.; Horio, T.; Hoshide, S.; Ikeda, S.; Ishimitsu, T.; et al. The Japanese Society of Hypertension Guidelines for the Management of Hypertension (JSH 2019). *Hypertens. Res.* **2019**, *42*, 1235–1481. [CrossRef]
22. Kai, H. Blood pressure management in patients with type 2 diabetes mellitus. *Hypertens. Res.* **2017**, *40*, 721–729. [CrossRef]
23. Franklin, S.S.; Gustin, W., IV.; Wong, N.D.; Larson, M.G.; Weber, M.A.; Kannel, W.B.; Levy, D. Hemodynamic patterns of age-related changes in blood pressure. Framingham Heart Study. *Circulation* **1997**, *96*, 308–315. [CrossRef] [PubMed]
24. Safar, M.E. Arterial aging-hemodynamic changes and therapeutic options. *Nat. Rev. Cardiol.* **2010**, *7*, 442–449. [CrossRef] [PubMed]

25. Mitchell, G.F.; Conlin, P.R.; Dunlap, M.E.; Lacourrvciere, Y.; Arnold, J.M.O.; Ogilvie, R.I.; Neutel, J.; Izzo, J.L., Jr.; Pfeffer, M.A. Aortic diameter, wall stiffness, and wave reflection in systolic hypertension. *Hypertension* **2008**, *51*, 105–111. [CrossRef] [PubMed]
26. Messerli, F.H.; Frohlich, E.D.; Suarez, D.H.; Dreslinski, G.R.; Dunn, F.G.; Cole, F.E. Borderline hypertension: Relationship between age, hemodynamics, and circulating catecholamines. *Circulation* **1981**, *64*, 760–764. [CrossRef] [PubMed]
27. Julius, S.; Pascual, A.V.; London, R. Role of parasympathetic inhibition in the hyperkinetic type borderline hypertension. *Circulation* **1971**, *44*, 413–418. [CrossRef] [PubMed]
28. Ekundayo, O.J.; Allman, R.M.; Sanders, P.W.; Aban, I.; Love, T.E.; Arnett, D.; Ahmed, A. Isolated systolic hypertension and incident heart failure in older adults: A propensity-matched study. *Hypertension* **2009**, *53*, 458–465. [CrossRef]
29. D'Sell, D.R.; Monnier, V.M. Molecular basis of arterial stiffening: Role of glycation—A mini-review. *Gerontology* **2012**, *58*, 227–237.
30. Kamoi, K.; Miyakoshi, M.; Soda, S.; Kaneko, S.; Nakagawa, O. Usefulness of home blood pressure measurement in the morning in type 2 diabetic patients. *Diabetes Care* **2002**, *25*, 2218–2223. [CrossRef]
31. Tomiyama, H.; Shiina, K.; Nakano, H.; Iwasaki, Y.; Matsumoto, C.; Fujii, M.; Chikamori, T.; Yamashina, A. Arterial stiffness and pressure wave reflection in the development of isolated diastolic hypertension. *J. Hypertens.* **2020**, *38*, 2000–2007. [CrossRef] [PubMed]
32. Ushigome, E.; Hamaguchi, M.; Matsumoto, S.; Oyabu, C.; Omoto, A.; Tanaka, T.; Fukuda, W.; Hasegawa, G.; Mogami, S.; Ohnishi, M.; et al. Optimal home SBP targets for preventing the progression of diabetic nephropathy in patients with type 2 diabetes mellitus. *J. Hypertens.* **2015**, *33*, 1853–1859, discussion 1859. [CrossRef] [PubMed]
33. Minutolo, R.; Gabbai, F.B.; Provenzano, M.; Chiodini, P.; Borrelli, S.; Garofalo, C.; Sasso, F.C.; Santoro, D.; Bellizzi, V.; Conte, G.; et al. Cardiorenal prognosis by residual proteinuria level in diabetic chronic kidney disease: Pooled analysis of four cohort studies. *Nephrol. Dial. Transplant.* **2018**, *33*, 1942–1949. [CrossRef] [PubMed]
34. Sasso, F.C.; Nicola, L.D.; Carbonara, O.; Nasti, R.; Minutolo, R.; Salvatore, T.; Conte, G.; Torella, R. Cardiovascular risk factors and disease management in type 2 diabetic patients with diabetic nephropathy. *Diabetes Care* **2006**, *29*, 498–503. [CrossRef]
35. Minutolo, R.; Sasso, F.C.; Chiodini, P.; Cianciaruso, B.; Carbonara, O.; Zamboli, P.; Tirino, G.; Pota, A.; Torella, R.; Conte, G.; et al. Management of cardiovascular risk factors in advanced type 2 diabetic nephropathy: A comparative analysis in nephrology, diabetology and primary care settings. *J. Hypertens.* **2006**, *24*, 1655–1661. [CrossRef]
36. Ninomiya, T.; Kojima, I.; Doi, Y.; Fukuhara, M.; Hirakawa, Y.; Hata, J.; Kitazono, T.; Kiyohara, Y. Brachial-ankle pulse wave velocity predicts the development of cardiovascular disease in a general Japanese population: The Hisayama study. *J. Hypertens.* **2013**, *31*, 477–483. [CrossRef] [PubMed]
37. Hiramatsu, T.; Miura, K.; Ohkubo, T.; Kadota, A.; Kondo, K.; Kita, Y.; Hayakawa, T.; Kanda, H.; Okamura, T.; Okayama, A.; et al. NIPPON DATA80 Research Group. Isolated systolic hypertension and 29-year cardiovascular mortality risk in Japanese adults aged 30–49 years. *J. Hypertens.* **2020**, *38*, 2230–2236. [CrossRef] [PubMed]
38. Ha, S.K. Dietary salt intake and hypertension Electrolyte. *Blood Press.* **2014**, *12*, 7–18. [CrossRef]
39. Machnik, A.; Neuhofer, W.; Jantsch, J.; Dahlmann, A.; Tammela, T.; Machura, K.; Park, J.K.; Beck, F.X.; Müller, D.N.; Derer, W.; et al. Macrophages regulate salt-dependent volume and blood pressure through a vascular endothelial growth factor-C-dependent buffering mechanism. *Nat. Med.* **2009**, *15*, 545–552. [CrossRef]
40. Zhu, H.G.; Jiang, Z.S.; Gong, P.Y.; Zhang, D.M.; Zou, Z.W.; Zhang, Q.; Ma, H.M.; Guo, Z.G.; Zhao, J.Y.; Dong, J.J.; et al. Efficacy of low-protein diet for diabetic nephropathy: A systematic review of randomized controlled trials. *Lipids Health Dis.* **2018**, *17*, 141. [CrossRef]
41. Zhao, W.; Katzmarzyk, P.T.; Horswell, R.; Wang, Y.; Li, W.; Johnson, J.; Heymsfield, S.B.; Cefalu, W.T.; Ryan, D.H.; Hu, G. Aggressive blood pressure control increases coronary heart disease risk among diabetic patients. *Diabetes Care* **2013**, *36*, 3287–3296. [CrossRef] [PubMed]
42. Penno, G.; Solini, A.; Orsi, E.; Bonora, E.; Fondelli, C.; Trevisan, R.; Vedovato, M.; Cavalot, F.; Lamacchia, O.; Scardapane, M.; et al. Non-albuminuric renal impairment is a strong predictor of mortality in individuals with type 2 diabetes: The Renal In-sufficiency And Cardiovascular Events (RIACE) Italian multicentre study. *Diabetologia* **2018**, *61*, 2277–2289. [CrossRef] [PubMed]

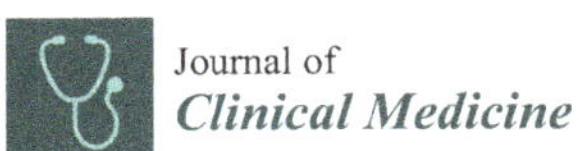
Journal of
Clinical Medicine

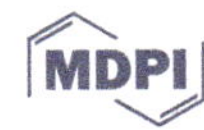

Article

Associations between High-Density Lipoprotein Functionality and Major Adverse Cardiovascular Events in Patients Who Have Undergone Coronary Computed Tomography Angiography

Hiroko Inoue [1], Yuhei Shiga [2,*], Kenji Norimatsu [1,2], Kohei Tashiro [2], Makito Futami [1,2], Yasunori Suematsu [2], Makoto Sugihara [2], Hiroaki Nishikawa [1], Yousuke Katsuda [1] and Shin-ichiro Miura [1,2,*]

1 Department of Cardiology, Fukuoka University Nishijin Hospital, Fukuoka 814-8522, Japan; hiroco61@fukuoka-u.ac.jp (H.I.); kenjimm020010@yahoo.co.jp (K.N.); makito8718@yahoo.co.jp (M.F.); hiroaki@fukuoka-u.ac.jp (H.N.); katsuda@fukuoka-u.ac.jp (Y.K.)
2 Department of Cardiology, Fukuoka University School of Medicine, Fukuoka 814-0180, Japan; kohei.t1027@gmail.com (K.T.); ysuematsu@fukuoka-u.ac.jp (Y.S.); msma93@adm.fukuoka-u.ac.jp (M.S.)
* Correspondence: yuheis@fukuoka-u.ac.jp (Y.S.); miuras@cis.fukuoka-u.ac.jp (S.-i.M.); Tel.: +81-92-801-1011 (Y.S. & S.-i.M.)

Citation: Inoue, H.; Shiga, Y.; Norimatsu, K.; Tashiro, K.; Futami, M.; Suematsu, Y.; Sugihara, M.; Nishikawa, H.; Katsuda, Y.; Miura, S.-i. Associations between High-Density Lipoprotein Functionality and Major Adverse Cardiovascular Events in Patients Who Have Undergone Coronary Computed Tomography Angiography. *J. Clin. Med.* **2021**, *10*, 2431. https://doi.org/10.3390/jcm10112431

Academic Editor: Sandro Gelsomino

Received: 25 April 2021
Accepted: 26 May 2021
Published: 30 May 2021

Publisher's Note: MDPI stays neutral with regard to jurisdictional claims in published maps and institutional affiliations.

Abstract: The present study aimed to investigate the associations between high-density lipoprotein (HDL) functionality and major adverse cardiovascular events (MACE) in patients who have undergone coronary computed tomography angiography (CCTA). We performed a prospective cohort study and enrolled 151 patients who underwent CCTA and had a follow-up of up to 5 years. We measured cholesterol efflux capacity (CEC), caspase-3/7 activity and monocyte chemoattractant protein-1 (MCP-1) secretion as bioassays of HDL functionality. The patients were divided into MACE(−) (n = 138) and MACE(+) (n = 13) groups. While there was no significant difference in %CEC, caspase-3/7 activity or MCP-1 secretion between the MACE(−) and MACE(+) groups, total CEC and HDL cholesterol (HDL-C) in the MACE(+) group were significantly lower than those in the MACE(−) group. Total CEC was correlated with HDL-C. A receiver-operating characteristic curve analysis showed that there was no significant difference between the areas under the curves for total CEC and HDL-C. In conclusion, total CEC in addition to HDL-C, but not %CEC, was associated with the presence of MACE. On the other hand, HDL functionality with regard to anti-inflammatory and anti-apoptosis effects was not associated with MACE.

Keywords: high-density lipoprotein; cholesterol efflux capacity; major adverse cardiovascular events

1. Introduction

In patients who are treated for atherosclerotic cardiovascular disease (ASCVD), there is a possibility of some residual risks even when the low-density lipoprotein cholesterol (LDL-C) level has been significantly reduced [1,2]. Such residual risks include high levels of the triglyceride (TG), a low level of high-density lipoprotein cholesterol (HDL-C) and other uncontrolled risk factors [1–6]. A recent study in a Japanese cohort indicated that extremely high HDL-C (≥90 mg/dL) had an adverse effect on ASCVD mortality [7]. HDL mainly enhances reverse cholesterol transport, such as the cholesterol efflux capacity (CEC), as well as having anti-oxidative, anti-inflammatory and anti-apoptosis functions [8–10]. Recently, it has been considered that both HDL quality and HDL quantity are important for preventing CVD. Prospective studies revealed that CEC was inversely correlated with the incidence of CV events [11]. We also reported that the restenosis rates after coronary stent implantation were associated with CEC [12]. Thus, HDL functionality is a critical residual risk factor for ASCVD.

Coronary computed tomography angiography (CCTA) has become more widely available in many general hospitals and enables the accurate non-invasive assessment of coronary artery stenosis for screening of coronary artery disease (CAD). In our previous cross-sectional study, high levels of HDL-C at the time of CCTA were associated with a reduced presence and severity of CAD [13]. In addition, total CEC and HDL-C were associated with the presence of CAD, while %CEC was not [14]. However, that study did not analyze the associations between various HDL functionalities, including CEC and the prognosis. Therefore, we determined the associations in this study.

2. Materials and Methods

In our previous study, 204 consecutive subjects who underwent CCTA for screening of CAD and were either clinically suspected to have CAD or had at least one cardiovascular risk factor were enrolled, and CEC was measured [14]. In this study, we excluded 53 of those patients due to the absence of follow-up (n = 8) and an insufficient volume of blood samples for further analysis of HDL functionality (n = 45), and finally analyzed HDL functionality in 151 patients.

We followed the patients for up to 5 years (average, 3.7 ± 0.7 years) and divided them into those with ((+) group, n = 13) and without ((−) group, n = 138) a major adverse cardiovascular event (MACE), where MACE was defined as all-cause deaths, acute myocardial infarction, coronary revascularization and ischemic stroke as a composite primary endpoint. When the patients had significant coronary stenosis as assessed by CCTA and received coronary intervention immediately after CCTA, the intervention was not included in MACE as coronary revascularization. We measured HDL functionality including CEC, caspase 3/7 activity associated with apoptosis and the secretion of monocyte chemotactic protein-1 (MCP-1) associated with inflammation. The protocol in this study was approved by the ethics committee of the Fukuoka University Hospital (# 09-10-02). All subjects gave their written informed consent to participate.

2.1. Evaluation of Coronary Stenosis Using CCTA

We assessed coronary stenosis using CCTA [13,14]. All patients were scanned by 64-multidetector row CT on an Aquilion 64 (TOSHIBA, Tokyo, Japan). The region of interest was placed within the ascending aorta. The scan was started when the CT density reached 100 Hounsfield Units higher than the baseline density. The scan was performed between the tracheal bifurcation and the diaphragm. All segments were evaluated according to the 15-segment American Heart Association coronary artery model. Fifteen segments of coronary arteries were evaluated. CAD was defined as any narrowing of the normal contrast-enhanced lumen to more than 50% in at least one major coronary artery that could be identified in multi-planar reconstructions or cross-sectional images. The number of significantly stenosed coronary vessels (0, 1, 2 and 3VD) was determined. In addition, the atherosclerotic severity of coronary artery disease was assessed in terms of the Gensini score.

2.2. Evaluation of CAD Risk Factors and Left Ventricular Ejection Fraction (LVEF)

Age, gender, body mass index (BMI), systolic blood pressure (SBP), diastolic BP (DBP), smoking status (current vs. nonsmoker), family history (myocardial infarction (MI), angina pectoris or sudden death) and chronic kidney disease (CKD) were collected as risk factors for CAD. Data of serum levels of LDL-C, HDL-C, triglycerides (TG), hemoglobin A1c (HbA1c) and fasting blood glucose (FBG) were also collected. LVEF was assessed by transthoracic echocardiography. BMI was calculated as weight (kg)/height (m^2). BP was determined as the mean of two measurements obtained in an office setting by the conventional cuff method using a mercury sphygmomanometer after at least 5 min of rest. The presence of dyslipidemia (DL), hypertension (HTN), diabetes mellitus (DM) and use of medication were obtained from medical records. Patients who had SBP $\geq$ 140 mmHg and/or DBP $\geq$ 90 mmHg at present or who were taking antihypertensive treatment were considered to have HTN. Patients with LDL-C ≥ 140 mg/dL, TG ≥ 150 mg/dL and/or HDL-C < 40 mg/dL or who were taking lipid-lowering treatment were considered to have DL. Patients with FBG ≥ 126 mg/dL, HbA1c ≥6.5% or who were receiving a glucose-lowering drug were considered to have DM. We calculated the estimated glomerular filtration rate (eGFR) from the data of serum creatinine, age, body size and gender. We defined CKD as when eGFR was less than 60 mL per minute per 1.73 m^2 body surface area.

2.3. Measurement of HDL CEC

We examined HDL CEC with an ex vivo system that used J774 macrophages and HDL isolated from plasma of the study patients by ultracentrifugation [14]. Briefly, J774 macrophages were cultured and radiolabeled with 2 µCi/mL of ^{3}H-cholesterol for 24 h. The day after labeling, the cells were washed and incubated with 8-Br-cAMP to upregulate ATP-binding cassette A1 transporter. Efflux medium containing isolated HDL (15 µg) was added for 4 h. Radiolabeled cholesterol counts were analyzed for the cell compartment and media. Percentage (%) of CEC was calculated as follows: (radioactivity in the medium/total radioactivity (radioactivity in medium + cells extracted with NaOH/NaCl)) × 100-CEC in sample-free medium. Total CEC was also calculated as the percentage of cholesterol efflux capacity/100 × HDL-C level.

2.4. Measurement of Secretion of Monocyte Chemotactic Protein 1 (MCP-1)

We evaluated the HDL-induced secretion of MCP-1 with an ex vivo system using human coronary endothelial cells (HCECs, Clonetics, San Diego, CA, USA) [15] and apo-B-depleted plasma from the study participants as samples. HCECs were cultured and grown in media. In the experiments, HCECs were washed with medium. The cells were incubated with 5 µg/mL of samples under the same conditions for 24 h. After 24 h, the secretion of MCP-1 in the medium from HCECs was measured by a Human CCL2/MCP-1 Quantikine ELISA Kit (R & D Systems, Minneapolis, MN, USA). The relative secretion of MCP-1 in each sample was calculated by the ratio of the secretion in each sample to the secretion in standard HDL (EMD Millipore Corp., Billerica, MA, USA). The relative total secretion of MCP-1 was also calculated as the relative secretion of the MCP-1/100 × HDL-C level.

2.5. Measurement of Caspase 3/7 Activity

We analyzed the HDL-suppressed caspase 3/7 activity with an ex vivo system that used the H9C2 cell line of embryonic rat cardiomyoblasts (ATCC®, CRL-1446™, Manassas, VA, USA) and apo-B-depleted plasma from the study participants as samples. We used cardiomyoblasts to analyze anti-apoptosis by HDL because HDL may prevent the progression of cardiac dysfunction related to apoptosis. H9C2 cells were cultured and grown in media. In the experiments, H9C2 cells were grown under serum-free conditions for 2 h. After 2 h, the cells were incubated with 5 µg/mL of samples for an additional 6 h. The caspase 3/7 activities in the H9C2 cells were measured by the Caspase-Glo® 3/7Assay System (Promega Corp., Madison, WI, USA). Relative caspase 3/7 activity in each sample was calculated by the ratio of the activity in each sample to the activity in standard HDL. Relative total caspase 3/7 activity was also calculated as the relative caspase 3/7 activity/100 × HDL-C level.

2.6. Statistical Analysis

The statistical analysis was performed using IBM SPSS statistics software, version 22 (SPSS Inc., Chicago, IL, USA) and EZR, which is used in R (The R Foundation for Statistical Computing, Vienna, Austria). More precisely, it is a modified version of R Commander designed to add statistical functions frequently used in biostatistics [16]. Continuous variables are shown as mean ± standard deviation. Continuous and categorical variables were compared between the groups by the *t* test and a Chi-square analysis, respectively. We performed a Wilcoxon rank-sum test when continuous variables did not show a normal distribution expressed as a median value and interquartile range.

The Spearman rank correlation coefficient was used to evaluate associations between the groups. A receiver-operating characteristic (ROC) curve analysis was used to determine the cut-off of the total CEC or HDL-C to distinguish between with and without MACE at the highest possible sensitivity and specificity levels. Area under the curve (AUC) values were compared between total CEC and HDL-C by a Chi-square analysis. A value of $p < 0.05$ was considered significant.

3. Results

3.1. Patient Characteristics in All Patients and in the MACE(+) and MACE(−) Groups

Table 1 shows the patient characteristics in all patients and in the MACE(+) and MACE(−) groups. The mean age was 65 (58–71) years and BMI was 23 ± 3 kg/m^2 in all patients. The frequencies of HTN, DL and DM in all patients were 78%, 71% and 23%, respectively. The MACE(+) group showed a higher level of %smoking and a lower level of HDL-C than the MACE(−) group. There were no significant differences in other factors, including %CAD, the number of VD, Gensini score, left ventricular ejection fraction (LVEF), %CKD, eGFR and medications between the MACE(+) and MACE(−) groups.

Table 1. Patient characteristics in all patients, the MACE(+) group and the MACE(−) group.

	All Patients (*n* = 151)	MACE(+) Group (*n* = 13)	MACE(−) Group (*n* = 138)
Age (years)	65 (58–71)	67 (58–70)	64 (58–71)
Male (%)	62	62	57
BMI (kg/m^2)	23 ± 3	23 ± 4	23 ± 3
Smoking (%)	39	62 *	34
HTN (%)	78	77	71
SBP (mmHg)	134 (123–146)	136 (123–146)	133 (123–146)
DBP (mmHg)	76 ± 12	79 ± 19	76 ± 11
DL (%)	71	77	64
LDL-C (mg/dL)	108 ± 28	94 ± 28	109 ± 28
HDL-C (mg/dL)	50 (43–61)	46 (33–50) *	51 (44–62)
TG (mg/dL)	114 (79–159)	113 (76–187)	114 (79–156)
DM (%)	23	23	21
HbA1c (%)	5.6 (5.3–6.2)	5.8 (5.4–6.6)	5.6 (5.3–6.2)
FBG (mg/dL)	101 (93–114)	101 (93–124)	101 (93–114)
CKD (%)	5	8	6
eGFR (mL/min/1.73 m^2)	66 ± 14	67 ± 10	68 ± 14
LVEF (%)	68 ± 9	67 ± 12	68 ± 5
CAD (%)	48	61	47
The number of VD	0.92 ± 1.10	1.38 ± 1.32	0.88 ± 1.07
Gensini score	12 ± 15	16 ± 15	11 ± 14
Medications			
ARB/ACE-I (%)	44	46	41
CCB (%)	35	31	33
β-blocker (%)	17	0	17
Diuretic (%)	13	15	12
Statin (%)	34	46	35
EPA (%)	2	8	2
Insulin (%)	10	8	6
Sulfonylurea (%)	13	23	12
Biguanide (%)	10	23	9
DPP4-I (%)	10	15	9

MACE: major adverse cardiovascular events, *BMI:* body mass index, *HTN:* hypertension, *SBP:* systolic blood pressure, *DBP:* diastolic BP, *DL:* dyslipidemia, *LDL-C:* low-density lipoprotein cholesterol, *HDL-C:* high-density lipoprotein cholesterol, *TG:* triglyceride, *DM:* diabetes mellitus, *HbA1c* hemoglobin A1c, *FBG:* fasting blood glucose, *CKD: chronic kidney disease*, *eGFR:* estimated glomerular filtration rate, *LVEF:* left ventricular ejection fraction, *CAD:* coronary artery disease, *the number of VD:* the number of significant stenosed coronary vessels, *ARB/ACE-I:* angiotensin II receptor blocker/angiotensin converting enzyme inhibitor, *CCB:* calcium channel blocker, *EPA:* eicosapentaenoic acid, *DPP4-I:* dipeptidyl peptidase-4-inhibitor. * $p < 0.05$ vs. MACE(−) group.

3.2. %CEC, Total CEC and HDL-C in the MACE(+) and MACE(−) Groups

As shown in Figure 1A–C, the MACE(+) group showed significantly lower total CEC ($p = 0.030$) and HDL-C levels ($p = 0.014$) than the MACE(−) group, while there was no difference in %CEC between the groups.

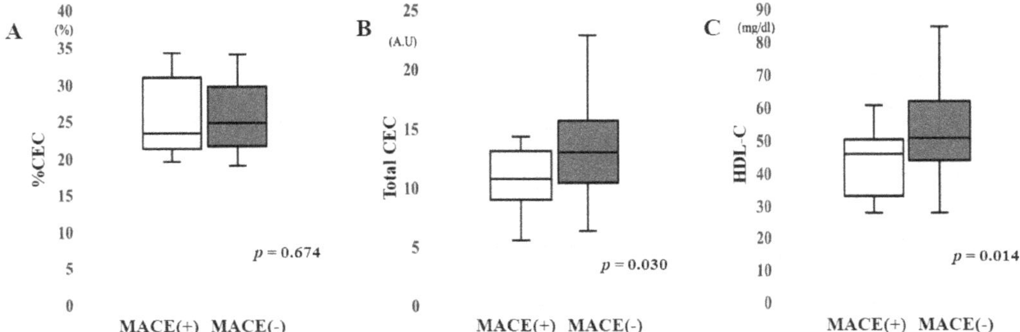

Figure 1. (**A**) %CEC, (**B**) total CEC and (**C**) HDL-C in the MACE(+) and MACE(−) groups. *A.U*: arbitrary unit.

3.3. Relative Caspase 3/7 Activity, Relative Total Caspase 3/7 Activity, Relative Secretion of MCP-1 and Relative Total Secretion of MCP-1 in the MACE(+) and MACE(−) Groups

Figure 2 shows caspase 3/7 activity and the secretion of MCP-1. There were no differences in relative caspase 3/7 activity ($p = 0.819$), relative total caspase 3/7 activity ($p = 0.745$), the relative secretion of MCP-1 ($p = 0.235$) or relative total secretion of MCP-1 ($p = 0.307$) between the groups.

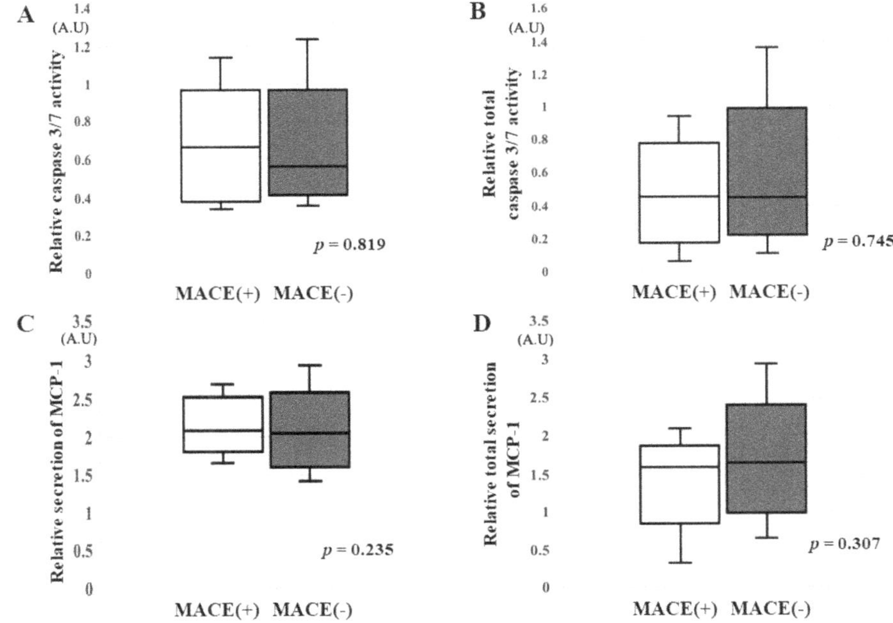

Figure 2. (**A**) Relative caspase 3/7 activity, (**B**) relative total caspase 3/7 activity, (**C**) relative secretion of MCP-1 and (**D**) relative total secretion of MCP-1 in the MACE(+) and MACE(−) groups. *A.U*: arbitrary unit.

3.4. Correlations between %CEC, Total CEC and HDL-C in All Patients

Total CEC was positively correlated with HDL-C in all patients ($r = 0.793$, $p < 0.001$), whereas %CEC showed no correlation ($r = 0.024$, $p = 0.769$) (Figure 3A,B).

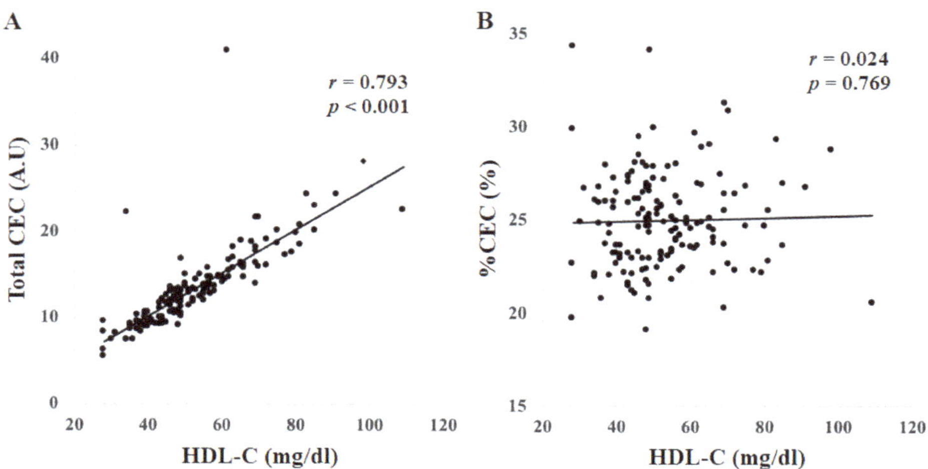

Figure 3. Correlations between (**A**) %CEC, (**B**) total CEC and HDL-C in all patients. *A.U*: arbitrary unit.

3.5. Cut-Off Values of Total CEC or HDL-C Levels for the Diagnosis of MACE in All Patients

A ROC curve analysis showed that the AUC for total CEC and HDL-C were 0.682 and 0.696, respectively, in all patients (Figure 4A,B). The cut-off levels of total CEC and HDL-C that gave the greatest sensitivity and specificity for the presence of CAD were 12.4 (sensitivity 0.572, specificity 0.692) and 47 mg/dL (sensitivity 0.659, specificity 0.692), respectively. There was no significant difference between the AUC for total CEC and HDL-C ($p = 0.656$), which indicated that these two factors contributed to MACE to a similar extent.

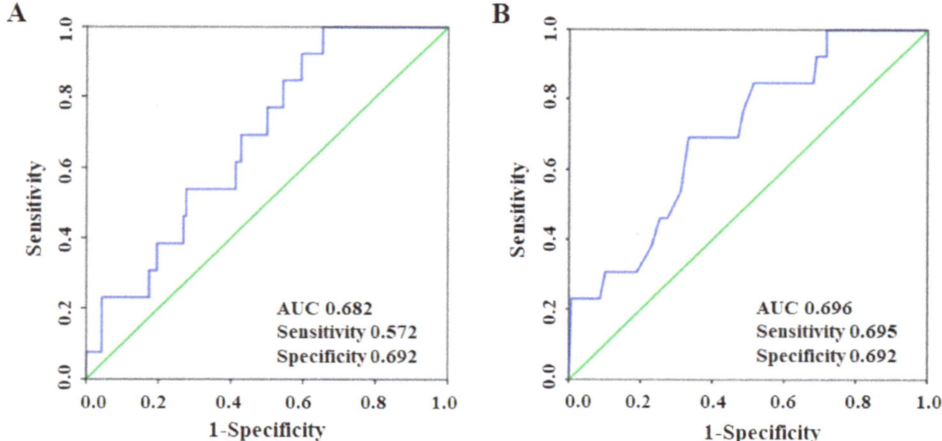

Figure 4. Cut-off values of (**A**) total CEC or (**B**) HDL-C levels for the diagnosis of MACE in all patients.

4. Discussion

In this study, we hypothesized that HDL functionality, CEC in particular, was associated with MACE. The main finding was that total CEC and HDL-C in the MACE(+) group were significantly lower than those in the MACE(−) group. In addition, total CEC was correlated with HDL-C. These two factors contributed to MACE to a similar extent. On the other hand, HDL functionality with regard to anti-inflammatory and anti-apoptosis effects was not associated with MACE.

We showed that total CEC and HDL-C in the MACE(+) group were significantly lower than those in the MACE(−) group. We measured %CEC using isolated HDL by ultracentrifugation to eliminate the effects of other lipoproteins as much as possible, since several studies have reported that other lipoproteins might influence cholesterol efflux capacity [17,18]. By this method, we could estimate the efflux capacity for a fixed amount of isolated HDL. This reflects the effect of the per unit capacity of HDL, but not total CEC in the bloodstream. Therefore, %CEC was normalized to total CEC in blood by the HDL-C concentration. Although we used HDL without the effects of other lipoproteins to measure pure CEC, %CEC values alone could not predict the occurrence of MACE. The involvement of other lipoproteins, other than Apo-AI, was also considered. Since the MACE (+) group had significantly lower HDL levels and the total CEC, which is the cholesterol uptake rate multiplied by the HDL-C value, was associated with MACE, the HDL-C value itself was at least related to MACE. In addition, since the correlation coefficient between HDL-C and total CEC was 0.793, which is a relatively strong correlation, it may be possible to predict MACE from the HDL-C value without measuring total CEC. However, the HDL-C value is 20–30% of the weight of HDL, and it is not clear whether the HDL-C value alone directly reflects the functionality of HDL itself. In any case, these results show that both HDL quality and quantity are important. In this study, the cut-off levels of total CEC and HDL-C for the presence of MACE according to a ROC curve analysis were 12.4 and 47 mg/dL, respectively. To the best of our knowledge, only our previous report has addressed the cut-off levels of the total CEC for the diagnosis of CAD [14]. In that study, the total CEC in the presence of CAD was 12.2, which is similar to the value observed here. Next, the cut-off level of HDL-C for the presence of MACE was 47 mg/dL, which is neither high nor low compared to values in the literature [6,19]. The cut-off level of HDL-C for the diagnosis of CAD was 48 mg/dL [14], which is similar to the cut-off for the presence of MACE. In addition, after adjusting for demographics, co-morbidities, lipid profile, statin use and date of procedure, our model demonstrated a U-shaped association between HDL-C and overall mortality, with HDL-C levels of 30–50 mg/dL associated with the most favorable outcomes, and HDL-C levels <30 mg/dL or >50 mg/dL associated with worse outcomes [20]. Decreased HDL-C levels were associated with a significantly increased risk of CV events in women (<49 mg/dL in women) but not in men (<42 mg/dL in men) [21]. According to the Japan Atherosclerosis Society Guidelines for Prevention of Atherosclerotic Cardiovascular Diseases 2017, serum HDL-C levels should be maintained ≥40 mg/dL for the primary and secondary prevention of CVD [6]. Thus, the cut-off level of HDL-C at 47 mg/dL, while relatively low, seems to be reasonable. On the other hand, higher levels of HDL-C have not been found to be associated with atheroprotection [7,22–24]. In NIPPON DATA90, high HDL-C (60–79 mg/dL) was associated with a significantly reduced risk of CAD, whereas very high HDL-C (≥80 mg/dL) was not [24]. Recently, extremely high levels of HDL-C (≥90 mg/dL) were significantly associated with an increased risk of ASCVD mortality, an increased risk of CAD and ischemic stroke in a pooled analysis of Japanese cohorts (EPOCH-JAPAN) [7]. In any case, our results suggest that when patients show a total CEC less than around 12.4 and/or HDL-C less than around 47 mg/dL at the time of CCTA, they might develop MACE in the future.

HDL functionality with regard to anti-inflammation and anti-apoptosis was not associated with MACE in this study. Many studies have shown that vascular inflammation is associated with adverse events and C-reactive protein is a critical biomarker of CVD [25–30]. HDL mainly acts as a scavenger, removing deposited cholesterol from macrophages. It also provides anti-inflammation and anti-apoptosis effects. Inflammation and apoptosis are associated with not only HDL function, but also with many other inflammation factors (MCP-1 [30], interleukin-6 and -8 [31], etc.) and apoptosis factors (tumor necrosis factor-a, B-cell lymphoma 2 [32], etc.). Thus, anti-inflammation and anti-apoptosis by HDL were not associated with MACE.

This study has several important limitations. First, although the sample size was relatively small, which limited our ability to determine significance, such as in the ROC analysis, including the cut-off levels of total CEC and HDL-C, which may be affected by gender-specific differences, we found that total CEC clearly had a significant correlation with MACE. Second, the population was only selected from Japan and the findings may not be applicable to other populations. Third, the CEC assay itself has several limitations because cell-based assays are labor-intensive. We did not analyze the anti-oxidative function of HDL. Fourth, we divided patients according to the presence of MACE and the duration of follow-up was only up to five years. A large-scale survey with a longer follow-up and further analysis will be needed.

5. Conclusions

Total CEC was correlated with HDL-C. Total CEC in addition to HDL-C, but not %CEC, was associated with the presence of MACE. These two factors contributed to MACE to a similar extent. On the other hand, HDL functionality with regard to anti-inflammatory and anti-apoptosis effects was not associated with MACE.

Author Contributions: Conceptualization, S.-i.M.; Data curation, Y.S. (Yuhei Shiga), K.T. and M.F.; Formal analysis, H.I. and Y.S. (Yuhei Shiga); Investigation, H.I., K.N., K.T. and M.F.; Methodology, Y.S. (Yuhei Shiga); Project administration, S.-i.M.; Resources, K.N. and K.T.; Supervision, H.N., Y.K. and S.-i.M.; Validation, H.I., Y.S. (Yuhei Shiga) and K.N.; Visualization, M.S., H.N. and Y.K.; Writing—original draft, H.I.; Writing—review and editing, Y.S. (Yasunori Suematsu) and S.-i.M. All authors have read and agreed to the published version of the manuscript.

Funding: This study has not received funding.

Institutional Review Board Statement: The study was conducted according to the guidelines of the Declaration of Helsinki and approved by the ethics committee of Fukuoka University Hospital.

Informed Consent Statement: Written informed consent was obtained from all subjects involved in the study.

Data Availability Statement: The data that support the findings of this study are available from the corresponding author upon reasonable request.

Conflicts of Interest: The authors declare that there is no conflict of interest.

References

1. Barter, P.; Gotto, A.M.; LaRosa, J.C.; Maroni, J.; Szarek, M.; Grundy, S.M.; Kastelein, J.J.P.; Bittner, V.; Fruchart, J.-C. HDL Cholesterol, Very Low Levels of LDL Cholesterol, and Cardiovascular Events. *N. Engl. J. Med.* **2007**, *357*, 1301–1310. [CrossRef] [PubMed]
2. O'Keefe, J.H.; Cordain, L.; Harris, W.H.; Moe, R.M.; Vogel, R. Optimal low-density lipoprotein is 50 to 70 mg/dL: Lower is better and physiologically normal. *J. Am. Coll. Cardiol.* **2004**, *43*, 2142–2146. [CrossRef]
3. Ogita, M.; Miyauchi, K.; Miyazaki, T.; Naito, R.; Konishi, H.; Tsuboi, S.; Dohi, T.; Kasai, T.; Yokoyama, T.; Okazaki, S.; et al. Low high-density lipoprotein cholesterol is a residual risk factor associated with long-term clinical outcomes in diabetic patients with stable coronary artery disease who achieve optimal control of low-density lipoprotein cholesterol. *Heart Vessel.* **2013**, *29*, 35–41. [CrossRef] [PubMed]
4. Gordon, T.; Castelli, W.P.; Hjortland, M.C.; Kannel, W.B.; Dawber, T.R. High density lipoprotein as a protective factor against coronary heart disease. *Am. J. Med.* **1977**, *62*, 707–714. [CrossRef]
5. The AIM-HIGH Investigators Niacin in Patients with Low HDL Cholesterol Levels Receiving Intensive Statin Therapy. *N. Engl. J. Med.* **2011**, *365*, 2255–2267. [CrossRef] [PubMed]
6. Kinoshita, M.; Yokote, K.; Arai, H.; Iida, M.; Ishigaki, Y.; Ishibashi, S.; Umemoto, S.; Egusa, G.; Ohmura, H.; Okamura, T.; et al. Japan Atherosclerosis Society (JAS) Guidelines for Prevention of Atherosclerotic Cardiovascular Diseases 2017. *J. Atheroscler. Thromb.* **2018**, *25*, 846–984. [CrossRef]

7. Hirata, A.; Sugiyama, D.; Watanabe, M.; Tamakoshi, A.; Iso, H.; Kotani, K.; Kiyama, M.; Yamada, M.; Ishikawa, S.; Murakami, Y.; et al. Association of extremely high levels of high-density lipoprotein cholesterol with cardiovascular mortality in a pooled analysis of 9 cohort studies including 43,407 individuals: The EPOCH–JAPAN study. *J. Clin. Lipidol.* **2018**, *12*, 674–684.e5. [CrossRef]
8. Dimmeler, S.; Haendeler, J.; Zeiher, A.M. Regulation of endothelial cell apoptosis in atherothrombosis. *Curr. Opin. Lipidol.* **2002**, *13*, 531–536. [CrossRef]
9. Farbstein, D.; Levy, A.P. HDL dysfunction in diabetes: Causes and possible treatments. *Expert Rev. Cardiovasc. Ther.* **2012**, *10*, 353–361. [CrossRef]
10. Khera, A.V.; Cuchel, M.; De La Llera-Moya, M.; Rodrigues, A.; Burke, M.F.; Jafri, K.; French, B.C.; Phillips, J.A.; Mucksavage, M.L.; Wilensky, R.L.; et al. Cholesterol Efflux Capacity, High-Density Lipoprotein Function, and Atherosclerosis. *N. Engl. J. Med.* **2011**, *364*, 127–135. [CrossRef]
11. Rohatgi, A.; Khera, A.; Berry, J.D.; Givens, E.G.; Ayers, C.R.; Wedin, K.E.; Neeland, I.J.; Yuhanna, I.S.; Rader, D.R.; De Lemos, J.A.; et al. HDL Cholesterol Efflux Capacity and Incident Cardiovascular Events. *N. Engl. J. Med.* **2014**, *371*, 2383–2393. [CrossRef]
12. Imaizumi, S.; Miura, S.; Takata, K.; Takamiya, Y.; Kuwano, T.; Sugihara, M.; Ike, A.; Iwata, A.; Nishikawa, H.; Saku, K. Association between cholesterol efflux capacity and coronary restenosis after successful stent implantation. *Heart Vessel.* **2015**, *31*, 1257–1265. [CrossRef]
13. Tashiro, K.; Inoue, H.; Shiga, Y.; Tsukihashi, Y.; Imaizumi, T.; Norimatsu, K.; Idemoto, Y.; Kuwano, T.; Sugihara, M.; Nishikawa, H.; et al. Associations Between High Levels of High-Density Lipoprotein Cholesterol and the Presence and Severity of Coronary Artery Disease in Patients Who Have Undergone Coronary Computed Tomography Angiography. *J. Clin. Med. Res.* **2020**, *12*, 734–739. [CrossRef]
14. Norimatsu, K.; Kuwano, T.; Miura, S.; Shimizu, T.; Shiga, Y.; Suematsu, Y.; Miyase, Y.; Adachi, S.; Nakamura, A.; Imaizumi, S.; et al. Significance of the percentage of cholesterol efflux capacity and total cholesterol efflux capacity in patients with or without coronary artery disease. *Heart Vessel.* **2016**, *32*, 30–38. [CrossRef] [PubMed]
15. Miura, S.; Suematsu, Y.; Matsuo, Y.; Imaizumi, S.; Yahiro, E.; Uehara, Y.; Saku, K. Induction of endothelial tube for-mation and anti-inflammation by newly developed apolipoprotein A-I mimetic peptide. *IJC Metab. Endocr.* **2014**, *5*, 70–72. [CrossRef]
16. Kanda, Y. Investigation of the freely available easy-to-use software 'EZR' for medical statistics. *Bone Marrow Transplant.* **2012**, *48*, 452–458. [CrossRef] [PubMed]
17. Chan, D.C.; Hoang, A.; Barrett, P.H.R.; Wong, A.T.Y.; Nestel, P.J.; Sviridov, D.; Watts, G.F. Apolipoprotein B-100 and ApoA-II Kinetics as Determinants of Cellular Cholesterol Efflux. *J. Clin. Endocrinol. Metab.* **2012**, *97*, E1658–E1666. [CrossRef]
18. Melchior, J.T.; Street, S.E.; Andraski, A.B.; Furtado, J.D.; Sacks, F.M.; Shute, R.L.; Greve, E.I.; Swertfeger, D.; Li, H.; Shah, A.S.; et al. Apolipoprotein A-II alters the proteome of human lipoproteins and enhances cholesterol efflux from ABCA1. *J. Lipid Res.* **2017**, *58*, 1374–1385. [CrossRef] [PubMed]
19. Castelli, W.P.; Garrison, R.J.; Wilson, P.W.F.; Abbott, R.D.; Kalousdian, S.; Kannel, W.B. Incidence of Coronary Heart Disease and Lipoprotein Cholesterol Levels. *JAMA* **1986**, *256*, 2835–2838. [CrossRef]
20. Kaur, M.; Ahuja, K.R.; Khubber, S.; Zhou, L.; Verma, B.R.; Meenakshisundaram, C.; Gad, M.M.; Saad, A.; Dhaliwal, K.; Isogai, T.; et al. Effect of High-Density Lipoprotein Cholesterol Levels on Overall Survival and Major Adverse Cardiovascular and Cerebrovascular Events. *Am. J. Cardiol.* **2021**, *146*, 8–14. [CrossRef]
21. Li, Y.-H.; Taiwanese Secondary Prevention for Patients with AtheRosCLErotic Disease (T-SPARCLE) Registry Investigators; Tseng, W.-K.; Yin, W.-H.; Lin, F.-J.; Wu, Y.-W.; Hsieh, I.-C.; Lin, T.-H.; Sheu, W.H.-H.; Yeh, H.-I.; et al. Prognostic effect of high-density lipoprotein cholesterol level in patients with atherosclerotic cardiovascular disease under statin treatment. *Sci. Rep.* **2020**, *10*, 21835. [CrossRef] [PubMed]
22. Di Angelantonio, E.; Sarwar, N.; Perry, P.; Kaptoge, S.; Ray, K.K.; Thompson, A.; Wood, A.M.; Lewington, S.; Sattar, N.; Packard, C.J.; et al. Major lipids, apolipoproteins, and risk of vascular disease. *JAMA J. Am. Med. Assoc.* **2009**, *302*, 1993–2000. [CrossRef]
23. Haase, C.L.; Tybjaerg-Hansen, A.; Grande, P.; Frikke-Schmidt, R. Genetically Elevated Apolipoprotein A-I, High-Density Lipoprotein Cholesterol Levels, and Risk of Ischemic Heart Disease. *J. Clin. Endocrinol. Metab.* **2010**, *95*, E500–E510. [CrossRef]
24. Hirata, A.; Okamura, T.; Sugiyama, D.; Kuwabara, K.; Kadota, A.; Fujiyoshi, A.; Miura, K.; Okuda, N.; Ohkubo, T.; Okayama, A.; et al. The Relationship between Very High Levels of Serum High-Density Lipoprotein Cholesterol and Cause-Specific Mortality in a 20-Year Follow-Up Study of Japanese General Population. *J. Atheroscler. Thromb.* **2016**, *23*, 800–809. [CrossRef]
25. Madsen, C.M.; Varbo, A.; Nordestgaard, B.G. Extreme high high-density lipoprotein cholesterol is paradoxically associated with high mortality in men and women: Two prospective cohort studies. *Eur. Heart J.* **2017**, *38*, 2478–2486. [CrossRef]
26. Retterstol, L.; Eikvar, L.; Bohn, M.; Bakken, A.; Erikssen, J.; Berg, K. C-reactive protein predicts death in patients with previous premature myocardial infarction—A 10 year follow-up study. *Atherosclerosis* **2002**, *160*, 433–440. [CrossRef]
27. Chew, D.P.; Bhatt, D.L.; Robbins, M.A.; Penn, M.S.; Schneider, J.P.; Lauer, M.; Topol, E.J.; Ellis, S.G. Incremental Prognostic Value of Elevated Baseline C-Reactive Protein Among Established Markers of Risk in Percutaneous Coronary Intervention. *Circulation* **2001**, *104*, 992–997. [CrossRef]

28. Nissen, S.E.; Tuzcu, E.M.; Schoenhagen, P.; Crowe, T.; Sasiela, W.J.; Tsai, J.; Orazem, J.; Magorien, R.D.; O'Shaughnessy, C.; Ganz, P. Statin Therapy, LDL Cholesterol, C-Reactive Protein, and Coronary Artery Disease. *N. Engl. J. Med.* **2005**, *352*, 29–38. [CrossRef]
29. Gallacher, J.E. C-reactive protein concentration and risk of coronary heart disease, stroke, and mortality: An individual participant meta-analysis. *Lancet* **2010**, *375*, 132–140. [CrossRef]
30. Wang, Q.; Ren, J.; Morgan, S.; Liu, Z.; Dou, C.; Liu, B. Monocyte Chemoattractant Protein-1 (MCP-1) Regulates Macrophage Cytotoxicity in Abdominal Aortic Aneurysm. *PLoS ONE* **2014**, *9*, e92053. [CrossRef]
31. Kristono, G.A.; Holley, A.S.; Hally, K.E.; Brunton-O'Sullivan, M.M.; Shi, B.; Harding, S.A.; Larsen, P.D. An IL-6-IL-8 score derived from principal component analysis is predictive of adverse outcome in acute myocardial infarction. *Cytokine X* **2020**, *2*, 100037. [CrossRef] [PubMed]
32. Dong, Y.; Chen, H.; Gao, J.; Liu, Y.; Li, J.; Wang, J. Molecular machinery and interplay of apoptosis and autophagy in coronary heart disease. *J. Mol. Cell. Cardiol.* **2019**, *136*, 27–41. [CrossRef] [PubMed]

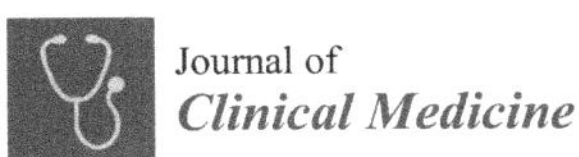

Journal of
Clinical Medicine

MDPI

Article

Increased Plasma Levels of Myosin Heavy Chain 11 Is Associated with Atherosclerosis

Lisa Takahashi [1,2], Tomoaki Ishigami [3], Hirofumi Tomiyama [1], Yuko Kato [2], Hiroyuki Kikuchi [4], Koichiro Tasaki [5], Jun Yamashita [1], Shigeru Inoue [4], Masataka Taguri [6], Toshitaka Nagao [5], Taishiro Chikamori [1], Yoshihiro Ishikawa [7] and Utako Yokoyama [2,7,*]

1 Department of Cardiology, Tokyo Medical University, 6-7-1 Nishi-shinjuku, Shinjuku-ku, Tokyo 160-0023, Japan; lisataka@tokyo-med.ac.jp (L.T.); tomiyama@tokyo-med.ac.jp (H.T.); jyamashi@tokyo-med.ac.jp (J.Y.); chikamd@tokyo-med.ac.jp (T.C.)
2 Department of Physiology, Tokyo Medical University, 6-6-1 Shinjuku, Shinjuku-ku, Tokyo 160-8402, Japan; yukato@tokyo-med.ac.jp
3 Department of Cardio-Renal Medicine and Medical Science, Yokohama City University, 3-9 Fukuura, Yokohama 236-0004, Japan; tommmish@hotmail.com
4 Department of Preventive Medicine and Public Health, Tokyo Medical University, 6-6-1 Shinjuku, Shinjuku-ku, Tokyo 160-8402, Japan; kikuchih@tokyo-med.ac.jp (H.K.); inoue@tokyo-med.ac.jp (S.I.)
5 Department of Pathology, Tokyo Medical University, 6-7-1 Nishi-shinjuku, Shinjuku-ku, Tokyo 160-0023, Japan; k-tasaki@tokyo-med.ac.jp (K.T.); nagao-t@tokyo-med.ac.jp (T.N.)
6 Department of Data Science, Yokohama City University, 22-2 Seto, Kanazawa-ku, Yokohama 236-0027, Japan; masataka.taguri@gmail.com
7 Cardiovascular Research Institute, Yokohama City University, 3-9 Fukuura, Kanazawa-ku, Yokohama 236-0004, Japan; yishikaw@yokohama-cu.ac.jp
* Correspondence: uyokoyam@tokyo-med.ac.jp; Tel.: +81-03-351-6141

Citation: Takahashi, L.; Ishigami, T.; Tomiyama, H.; Kato, Y.; Kikuchi, H.; Tasaki, K.; Yamashita, J.; Inoue, S.; Taguri, M.; Nagao, T.; et al. Increased Plasma Levels of Myosin Heavy Chain 11 Is Associated with Atherosclerosis. *J. Clin. Med.* **2021**, *10*, 3155. https://doi.org/10.3390/jcm10143155

Academic Editor: Emmanuel Androulakis

Received: 10 June 2021
Accepted: 14 July 2021
Published: 16 July 2021

Publisher's Note: MDPI stays neutral with regard to jurisdictional claims in published maps and institutional affiliations.

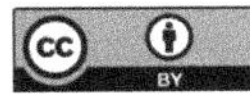

Abstract: Many studies have revealed numerous potential biomarkers for atherosclerosis, but tissue-specific biomarkers are still needed. Recent lineage-tracing studies revealed that smooth muscle cells (SMCs) contribute substantially to plaque formation, and the loss of SMCs causes plaque vulnerability. We investigated the association of SMC-specific myosin heavy chain 11 (myosin-11) with atherosclerosis. Forty-five patients with atherosclerosis and 34 control subjects were recruited into our study. In the atherosclerosis patients, 35 patients had either coronary artery disease (CAD) or peripheral artery disease (PAD), and 10 had both CAD and PAD. Coronary arteries isolated from five patients were subjected to histological study. Circulating myosin-11 levels were higher in the CAD or PAD group than in controls. The area under the receiver operating characteristic curve of myosin-11 was 0.954. Circulating myosin-11 levels in the CAD and PAD group were higher than in the CAD or PAD group, while high-sensitivity C-reactive protein concentrations did not differ between these groups. Multinomial logistic regression analyses showed a significant association of myosin-11 levels with the presence of multiple atherosclerotic regions. Myosin-11 was expressed in the medial layer of human atherosclerotic lesions where apoptosis elevated. Circulating myosin-11 levels may be useful for detecting spatial expansion of atherosclerotic regions.

Keywords: atherosclerosis; immunohistochemistry; biomarkers; smooth muscle cells; myosin heavy chain

1. Introduction

Atherosclerosis is the main pathological process underlying myocardial infarction, heart failure, peripheral artery disease (PAD), stroke, and cerebral infarction, and it has been the leading cause of morbidity and mortality globally [1]. Atherosclerotic plaque formation develops over long periods with chronic inflammation based on complex processes, including the oxidation of accumulated cholesterol-carrying low-density lipoprotein (LDL), immune cell infiltration, production of inflammatory mediators, endothelial dysfunctions, and vascular smooth muscle cell (VSMC) proliferation and migration [2,3]. Plaque instability, in which the activation of proteases for extracellular matrices and the loss of VSMCs are involved, increases the risk of cardiovascular events [4]. Because these pathological changes in the vascular wall are mostly asymptomatic, the detection of atherosclerotic lesions by serological biomarkers before critical clinical features emerge has been extensively investigated [5–9].

In atherosclerotic plaques, differentiated VSMCs that are derived from the tunica media undergo phenotypic switching to proliferative synthetic cells that produce extracellular matrices (ECMs) and contribute to plaque stabilization [10]. In vulnerable plaques, previous studies indicated a high proportion of infiltrated monocytes/macrophages and extracellular lipids rather than VSMCs [4]. Thus, VSMCs have been thought to play relatively minor roles in the progression to rupture-prone atherosclerosis [1,4,10]. Over the past decade, however, studies that used fate-mapping and lineage-tracing revealed that VSMCs account for up to 70% of all plaque cells in murine models of atherosclerosis and that VSMCs contribute to multiple plaque cell phenotypes, i.e., macrophage-like cells, foam cells, osteochondrogenic cells, and mesenchymal stem cells alongside ECM-producing α-smooth muscle actin (αSMA)-positive cells [11–15], which highlight the importance of VSMCs. Thus, VSMCs are a major cell type in plaque formation and play a greater role in atherosclerosis than previously recognized [1].

Loss of VSMCs through cell death, including apoptosis and secondary necrosis, was shown to occur during the progression of atherosclerosis [16,17]. In studies using animal models, relatively acute VSMC apoptosis induced features of plaque vulnerability, such as fibrous cap thinning [18], and chronic apoptosis of VSMCs accelerated plaque growth necrotic core enlargement, plaque calcification, medial expansion and degeneration, elastin breaks, and failure of outward remodeling [19]. In humans, a decrease in the VSMC cell number was correlated with plaque instability [4]. On the basis of these findings, we hypothesized that SMC-specific proteins leak into the circulation from dying cells with the development and spread of atherosclerotic regions.

Some of myosin superfamily members were expressed in a cell-type-specific manner [20] and were reported to be increased in the blood of patients with several diseases, including autoimmune diseases [21], myocardial cell damages [22,23], and skeletal muscle injuries [24]. Myosin heavy chain 11 (myosin-11) is exclusively enriched in VSMCs [25]. A recent report demonstrated that patients with a non-ruptured abdominal aortic aneurysm (AAA), in which VSMCs undergo apoptosis, had significantly higher levels of circulating myosin-11 than normal controls, and its levels were correlated with the maximum aortic diameter [26]. These data indicated that circulating myosin-11 levels are associated with the loss of VSMCs in the vascular wall. We investigated the association of plasma levels of myosin-11 and atherosclerosis to identify a new tissue-specific serological biomarker for atherosclerosis.

2. Materials and Methods

2.1. Study Subjects

Forty-five patients with atherosclerosis were recruited from June in 2013 to January in 2015 at Yokohama City University Hospital. Atherosclerosis patients consisted of two groups: 35 patients with either coronary artery disease (CAD) or PAD (the CAD or PAD group) and 10 patients with both CAD and PAD (the CAD + PAD group). Plasma samples were taken within 1 week before the patients received percutaneous coronary artery intervention or endovascular treatment. Plasma samples from 34 control subjects were collected from age- and sex-ratio-matched healthy volunteers at Maebashi Hirosegawa Clinic who did not have a history of CAD, PAD, cerebrovascular disease, aortic aneurysm, diabetes mellitus, or renal insufficiency. Medical interviews were performed when the subjects were recruited into this study, and their systolic and diastolic blood pressure and body mass index (BMI) were recorded at that time. Plasma samples were stored at −80 °C until analysis. The proximal segments of the left coronary arteries from five patients

(2–5 segments per patient) were collected at autopsies in 2020 at Tokyo Medical University Hospital. Tissues were fixed in 4% paraformaldehyde for histological analysis.

2.2. Clinical and Biochemical Analysis

Plasma levels of myosin-11 were quantified in a specific sandwich enzyme-linked immunosorbent assay (ELISA) (Cusabio Biotech, College Park, MD, USA) in accordance with the manufacturer's instructions. Although the information on antibody-binding sites was not disclosed by the company, the ELISA was reacted to human recombinant coiled-coil domain of myosin-11 (data not shown). High-sensitivity C-reactive protein (hsCRP) was measured by SRL, Inc. (Tokyo, Japan).

2.3. Tissue Staining and Immunohistochemistry

Paraffin-embedded blocks containing the coronary artery tissues were cut into 4 μm–thick sections. Elastica van Gieson staining and Masson's trichrome staining were performed for morphological analysis. We used anti-CD68 (1:200 dilution, M0876, Dako, Carpinteria, CA, USA) to detect macrophages in immunohistochemical staining.

The 5′ and 3′ end of *Myh11* (myosin-11 gene) are alternatively spliced to generate COOH-terminal isoforms (SM1 and SM2) and NH_2-terminal isoforms (SM-A and SM-B) [27]. Among all combinations of the four isoforms (SM1A, SM1B, SM2A, and SM2B) identified in humans [28], the artery expressed exclusively SM1A and SM2A [27]. We, therefore, used anti-SM1 (1:500 dilution, 7600, Yamasa, Chuo-ku, Tokyo, Japan), and anti-SM2 (1:200 dilution, 7601, Yamasa, Chuo-ku, Tokyo, Japan) antibodies to detect myosin-11 isoforms. Biotinylated horse anti-mouse IgG (Vectastain Elite ABC IgG kit, Vector Labs, Burlingame, CA, USA) was used as a secondary antibody. Negative staining of immunohistochemistry was confirmed by the omission of primary antibodies. TdT-mediated dUTP Nick End Labeling (TUNEL) (G7130, Promega Corporation, Madison, WI, USA) was performed to evaluate apoptotic cells.

2.4. Statistical Analysis

In Table 1, the data that are shown as values were statistically analyzed by using the Kruskal-Wallis test, and the data shown as ratios were analyzed by using the chi-square test. Both of these tests were followed by Fisher's least significant difference post hoc test, the Mann-Whitney U-test, or Fisher's exact test, as appropriate. In Table 2, the data that are shown as values were statistically analyzed by using the Mann-Whitney U-test, and the data shown as ratios were analyzed by Fisher's exact test. The data in Figure 1a,b and Figure 2a,b were statistically analyzed by using the Kruskal-Wallis test, followed by Fisher's least-significant-difference post hoc test and the Mann-Whitney U-test. The Mann-Whitney U-test was used in Figure 1c,d. Spearman's correlation analysis was used in Figure 1e. Data were analyzed by using Prism software (version 5.0; GraphPad, San Diego, CA, USA). Receiver-operating characteristic (ROC) analysis was performed by using a binary analysis of factors to evaluate the diagnostic performance. Multinomial logistic regression analyses were used to assess the difference of hsCRP (Model 1) and myosin-11 (Model 2) values within the three groups, after adjusting the Brinkman index (per 100), hypertension (dichotomous), and dyslipidemia status (dichotomous). Before the analysis, both myosin-11 and hsCRP values were transformed into the standardized score (z-score) for comparability. ROC analysis was examined by using SPSS (version 26; IBM Corp., Armonk, NY, USA), and multinomial logistic regression analyses were performed by using Stata (version 15; Stata Corp., College Station, TX, USA). The p-values < 0.05 were considered to be statistically significant.

Table 1. Clinical baseline characteristics of patients with atherosclerosis and controls.

Variables	A	B	C	*p*-Value			
	Controls (*n* = 34)	**CAD or PAD (*n* = 35)**	**CAD + PAD (*n* = 10)**	**A vs. B vs. C**	**A vs. B**	**A vs. C**	**B vs. C**
Age, years	71.2 ± 3.7	69.9 ± 7.4	72 ± 8.5	0.348			
Male gender, *n* (%)	28 (82.4)	30 (85.7)	8 (80.0)	0.923			
Body mass index	23.3 ± 1.2	22.8 ± 3.2	21.7 ± 3.0	0.383			
Systolic BP, mmHg	132 ± 12	131 ± 19	138 ± 22	0.477			
Diastolic BP, mmHg	80 ± 8	66 ± 14	71 ± 13	<0.001 *	<0.001 *	0.047 *	0.262
HDL-cholesterol, mg/dL	58 ± 16	52 ± 14	44 ± 12	0.042 *	0.073	0.024 *	0.262
LDL-cholesterol, mg/dL	118 ± 19	83 ± 23	96 ± 27	<0.001 *	<0.001*	0.018 *	0.105
Triglyceride, mg/dL	101 ± 43	118 ± 67	125 ± 68	0.575			
HbA1c, %	5.5 ± 0.4	6.3 ± 0.9	6.0 ± 0.7	<0.001 *	<0.001 *	0.047 *	0.358
Creatinine, mg/dL	0.7 ± 0.2	3.8 ± 4.7	6.6 ± 5.8	<0.001 *	<0.001 *	<0.001 *	0.25
eGFR, mL/min/1.73 m^2	78 ± 17	45 ± 32	30 ± 33	<0.001 *	<0.001*	<0.001 *	0.198
Hemodialysis, *n* (%)	0 (0)	11 (31.4)	6 (60.0)	<0.001 *	<0.001 *	<0.001 *	0.179
Hypertension, *n* (%)	15 (44.1)	28 (80.0)	9 (90.0)	0.001 *	0.002 *	0.013 *	0.661
Dyslipidemia, *n* (%)	14 (41.2)	28 (80.0)	6 (60.0)	0.004 *	0.001 *	0.472	0.228
Brinkman index	356 ± 423	710 ± 511	948 ± 681	0.006 *	0.008 *	0.014 *	0.286
Diabetes mellitus, *n* (%)	0 (0)	19 (54.3)	6 (60.0)	<0.001 *	<0.001 *	<0.001 *	>0.999
Statins, *n* (%)	1 (2.9)	28 (80.0)	3 (30.0)	<0.001 *	<0.001 *	0.032 *	0.005 *
ACE inhibitor or ARB, *n* (%)	4 (11.8)	20 (57.1)	7 (70.0)	<0.001 *	<0.001 *	0.001*	0.716
β-blocker, *n* (%)	2 (5.9)	21 (60.0)	3 (30.0)	<0.001 *	<0.001 *	0.069	0.151
Acetylsalicylic acid, *n* (%)	0 (0)	30 (85.7)	9 (90.0)	<0.001 *	<0.001 *	<0.001 *	>0.999

Continuous variables are shown as the mean ± SD and categorical variables are expressed as the number (%). * $p < 0.05$; n, number of subjects; CAD, coronary artery disease; PAD, peripheral artery disease; BP, blood pressure; HDL, high-density lipoprotein; LDL, low-density lipoprotein; Hb, hemoglobin; eGFR, estimated glomerular filtration rate; ACE, angiotensin-converting enzyme; ARB, angiotensin receptor blocker; SD, standard deviation.

Table 2. Clinical baseline characteristics of patients with CAD or PAD.

Variables	A	B	*p*-Value
	CAD (*n* = 24)	**PAD (*n* = 11)**	**A vs. B**
Age, years	70 ± 8.2	70 ± 5.3	0.587
Male gender, *n* (%)	21 (87.5)	9 (81.8)	0.656
Body mass index	22.4 ± 2.9	23.8 ± 3.6	0.238
Systolic BP, mmHg	127 ± 19	139 ± 17	0.085
Diastolic BP, mmHg	65 ± 12	67 ± 18	0.687
HDL-cholesterol, mg/dL	50 ± 12	56 ± 17	0.494
LDL-cholesterol, mg/dL	86 ± 22	78 ± 26	0.163
Triglyceride, mg/dL	113 ± 67	126 ± 69	0.472
HbA1c, %	6.3 ± 0.9	6.5 ± 0.8	0.18
Creatinine, mg/dL	2.7 ± 4.0	6.1 ± 5.7	0.252
eGFR, mL/min/1.73 m^2	49 ± 28	37 ± 39	0.43
Hemodialysis, *n* (%)	6 (25.0)	5 (45.5)	0.115
Hypertension, *n* (%)	19 (79.2)	9 (81.8)	0.856
Dyslipidemia, *n* (%)	20 (83.3)	8 (72.7)	0.466
Brinkman index	724 ± 561	679 ± 402	0.847
Diabetes mellitus, *n* (%)	10 (41.7)	9 (81.8)	0.027 *
Statins, *n* (%)	20 (83.3)	8 (72.7)	0.466
ACE inhibitor or ARB, *n* (%)	16 (66.7)	4 (36.4)	0.093
β-blocker, *n* (%)	16 (66.7)	5 (45.5)	0.234
Acetylsalicylic acid, *n* (%)	24 (100)	6 (54.5)	<0.001 *

Continuous variables are shown as the mean ± SD, and categorical variables are expressed as the number (%). * $p < 0.05$; *n*, number of subjects; CAD, coronary artery disease; PAD, peripheral artery disease; BP, blood pressure; HDL, high-density lipoprotein; LDL, low-density lipoprotein; Hb, hemoglobin; eGFR, estimated glomerular filtration rate; ACE, angiotensin-converting enzyme; ARB, angiotensin receptor blocker; SD, standard deviation.

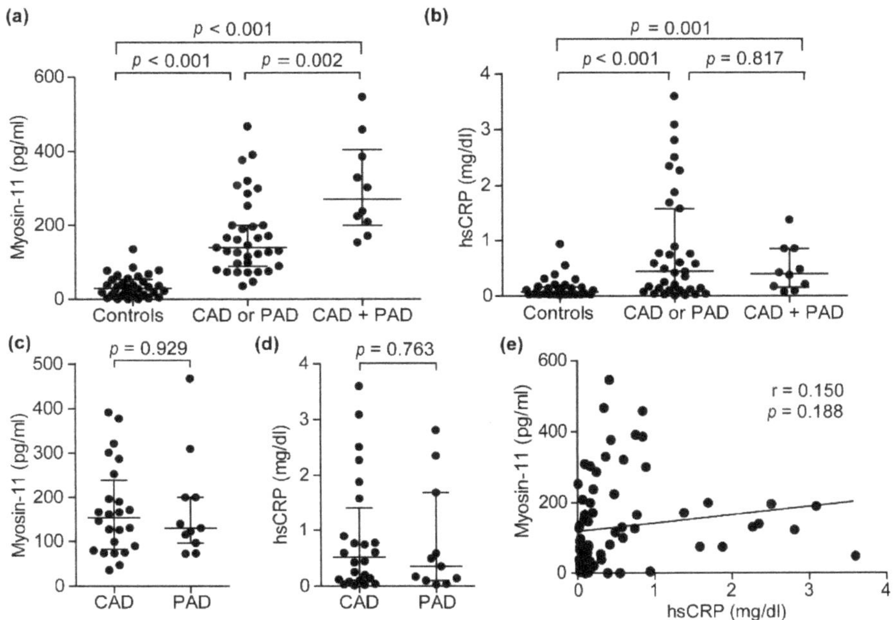

Figure 1. Plasma myosin-11 (myosin heavy chain 11) levels in patients with atherosclerosis. (**a**,**b**) Myosin-11 and hsCRP (high-sensitivity C-reactive protein) concentrations in plasma samples of control subjects (Controls, $n = 34$), patients with CAD (coronary artery disease) or PAD (peripheral artery disease) (CAD or PAD, $n = 35$), and patients with both CAD and PAD (CAD + PAD, $n = 11$). Data are shown as the median with interquartile ranges. (**c**,**d**) Myosin-11 and hsCRP concentrations in plasma samples from CAD ($n = 24$) and PAD ($n = 11$) patients. Data are shown as the median with interquartile ranges. (**e**) Correlation between plasma concentrations of myosin-11 and hsCRP in all patients and controls ($n = 80$).

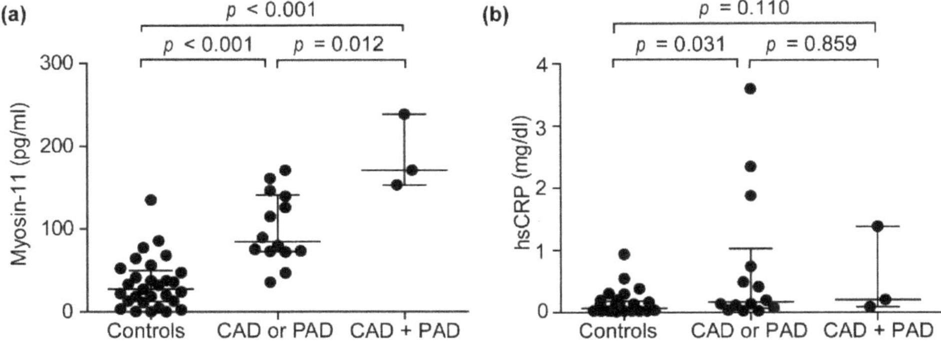

Figure 2. Plasma myosin-11 (myosin heavy chain 11) levels in subjects without renal insufficiency. (**a**,**b**) Myosin-11 and hsCRP (high-sensitivity C-reactive protein) concentrations in plasma samples of control subjects (Controls, $n = 29$), patients with CAD (coronary artery disease) or PAD (peripheral artery disease) (CAD or PAD, $n = 14$), and patients with both CAD and PAD (CAD + PAD, $n = 3$). Data are shown as the median with interquartile ranges.

3. Results

3.1. Characteristics of Patients with Atherosclerosis

Clinical baseline characteristics of patients with atherosclerosis (n = 45) and control subjects (n = 34) are shown in Table 1. Patients with atherosclerosis were divided into two groups: the CAD or PAD group (n = 35), in which patients had either CAD or PAD, and the CAD + PAD group (n = 10), in which patients had both CAD and PAD. There were no significant differences in age, frequencies of male gender, or BMI between the three groups. Both the CAD or PAD group and the CAD + PAD group had a higher frequency of hypertension, dyslipidemia, smokers, renal dysfunction, and diabetes mellitus than the control group, and there were no differences in the frequencies of these populations between the CAD or PAD and the CAD + PAD groups. Use of statins, angiotensin-converting enzyme (ACE) inhibitors, angiotensin receptor blockers (ARBs), β-blockers, and acetylsalicylic acid was also more common among patients with atherosclerosis compared to control subjects. With the exception of statins, there were no differences in the usage of these medications between the CAD or PAD and the CAD + PAD groups.

3.2. Myosin-11 Plasma Levels Were Upregulated in Patients with Atherosclerosis

We measured plasma myosin-11 concentrations in patients with atherosclerosis patients and control subjects using an ELISA that was specific for myosin-11. Plasma myosin-11 levels were higher in the CAD or PAD group (median (25th–75th percentiles): 139.2 (89.3–200.0) pg/mL) and the CAD + PAD group (median (25th–75th percentiles): 252.1 (208.6–386.3) pg/mL) than in control subjects (median (25th–75th percentiles): 30.0 (13.1–53.6) pg/mL) (Figure 1a). In addition, myosin-11 levels were significantly higher in the CAD + PAD group than in the CAD or PAD group (Figure 1a). In this sample set, we analyzed the plasma concentrations of hsCRP, which is the most extensively studied potential biomarker for atherosclerosis [29,30]. Moreover, hsCRP plasma levels were significantly higher in the CAD or PAD group (median (25th–75th percentiles): 0.44 (0.10–1.58) pg/mL) than in control subjects (median (25th–75th percentiles): 0.07 (0.03–0.16) pg/mL) (Figure 1b), while there was no difference in hsCRP between the CAD or PAD group and the CAD + PAD group (median (25th–75th percentiles): 0.42 (0.17–0.85) pg/mL) (Figure 1b).

3.3. Circulating Myosin-11 Levels in Patients with CAD or PAD

Next, we examined whether there was a difference in circulating myosin-11 levels between patients with CAD and PAD. The patient information is shown in Table 2. There were no differences in patient characteristics between CAD and PAD patients except for the frequencies of diabetes mellitus and usage of acetylsalicylic acid. Plasma levels of myosin-11 were similar between CAD patients (median (25th–75th percentiles: 153.5 (82.2–238.8 pg/mL) and PAD patients (median (25th–75th percentiles): 129.7 (96.1–200.0) pg/mL) (Figure 1c). Similar to myosin-11, there was no difference in hsCRP between CAD (median (25th–75th percentiles): 0.52 (0.11–1.41] pg/mL) and PAD (median (25th–75th percentiles): 0.35 (0.10–1.69) pg/mL) patients (Figure 1e). There was no positive association of plasma myosin-11 levels with hsCRP (Figure 1e).

3.4. Circulating Myosin-11 Levels and Clinical Parameters

We analyzed the values of myosin-11 or hsCRP together with traditional clinical risk factors. We performed multinomial logistic regression analyses by using hypertension, dyslipidemia, and the Brinkman index as risk factors. Because we recruited control subjects from among individuals who did not have a history of diabetes mellitus or renal insufficiencies, we did not include these factors in this analysis. The significant association between increased circulating myosin-11 levels and the presence of either CAD or PAD compared to control subjects persisted after adjustment for the risk factors (Table 3, Model 1). Similarly, hsCRP levels had a significant association with the presence of either CAD or PAD (Model 2). When we set the CAD or PAD group as a reference, the significant association between circulating myoin-11 levels and the presence of multiple regions of atherosclerosis (CAD and PAD) (Table 3, Model 1) remained after the adjustment. However, traditional risk factors, i.e., smoking history, hypertension, and dyslipidemia, and plasma levels of hsCRP were not associated with the presence of both CAD and PAD (Models 1 and 2).

Table 3. Association between standardized score of myosin-11/hsCRP and atherosclerosis.

	Controls			CAD or PAD	CAD + PAD		
	AOR	95%CI	*p*-Value	(Reference)	AOR	95%CI	*p*-Value
Model 1							
Myosin-11 [1]	0.01	0.01–0.03	0.002 *	(1.00)	4.10	1.43–11.69	0.008 *
Brinkman index [2]	0.71	0.49–1.03	0.065	(1.00)	1.07	0.92–1.24	0.070
Hypertension	0.03	0.01–0.90	0.044 *	(1.00)	8.76	0.24–323.81	0.598
Dyslipidemia	0.12	0.01–3.52	0.219	(1.00)	0.31	0.05–1.91	0.276
Model 2							
hsCRP [1]	0.02	0.01–0.37	0.008 *	(1.00)	0.58	0.23–1.42	0.232
Brinkman index [2]	0.92	0.80–1.05	0.208	(1.00)	1.10	0.96–1.26	0.183
Hypertension	0.20	0.05–0.85	0.029 *	(1.00)	2.12	0.21–21.37	0.523
Dyslipidemia	0.17	0.04–0.72	0.016 *	(1.00)	0.29	0.05–1.49	0.136

* $p < 0.05$. [1] Values were transformed into a standardized score (z-score) before this analysis. [2] The AORs (adjusted odds ratio) were calculated using a per-100 change to the index. Myosin-11, myosin heavy chain 11; hsCRP, high-sensitivity C-reactive protein; CAD, coronary artery disease; PAD, peripheral artery disease; AOR, adjusted odds ratio; 95%CI, 95% confidence interval.

3.5. The Effects of Renal Function on Circulating Myosin-11 Levels

Although the differences in creatinine levels and estimated glomerular filtration rate (eGFR) between the CAD or PAD group and the CAD + PAD group did not reach significance, atherosclerosis patients had a higher frequency of renal insufficiency. We subsequently investigated the plasma levels of myosin-11 in atherosclerosis patients and control subjects who did not have a renal insufficiency, which was defined by less than 60 mL/min/1.73 m^2 of eGFR. In accordance with the results that are presented in Figure 1, plasma myosin-11 levels were significantly higher in the CAD or PAD group (median (25th–75th percentiles): 84.6 (72.77–140.9) pg/mL) and the CAD + PAD group (median (25th–75th percentiles): 170.9 (152.8–238.0) pg/mL) than in control subjects (median (25th–75th percentiles): 27.5 (12.3–50.1) pg/mL) (Figure 2a). Circulating myosin-11 levels were also higher in the CAD + PAD group than in the CAD or PAD group (Figure 2a). In this dataset, plasma levels of hsCRP were significantly higher in the CAD or PAD group (median (25th–75th percentiles): 0.17 (0.07–1.03) pg/mL) than in control subjects (median (25th–75th percentiles): 0.07 (0.03–0.19) pg/mL) (Figure 2b), while hsCRP levels did not differ between the CAD or PAD group and the CAD + PAD group (median (25th–75th percentiles): 0.21 (0.09–1.38) pg/mL) (Figure 2b).

3.6. Efficacy of Myosin-11 for Diagnosis

We evaluated the diagnostic value using ROC analysis of myosin-11 to detect the presence of either CAD or PAD. The area under the curve (AUC) of myosin-11 was 0.954 (95% confidence interval [CI]: 0.909–0.998, $p < 0.001$), with a specificity of 88% at a sensitivity of 90% (Figure 3a), and the positive predictive value, negative predictive value, accuracy, and cutoff value were 89%, 91%, 90%, and 72.5 pg/mL, respectively. The AUC of hsCRP was 0.771 (95% CI: 0.657–0.884, $p < 0.001$), with a specificity of 29% at a sensitivity of 90%, and the positive predictive value, negative predictive value, and accuracy were 56%, 71%, and 59%, respectively. The AUC of myosin-11 was significantly greater than that of hsCRP ($p < 0.025$) (Figure 3a).

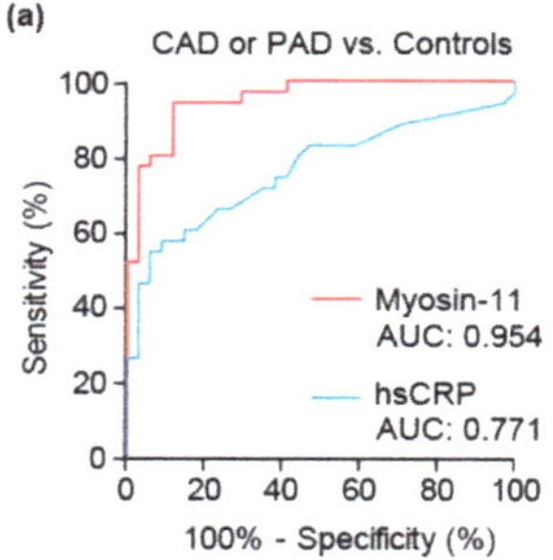

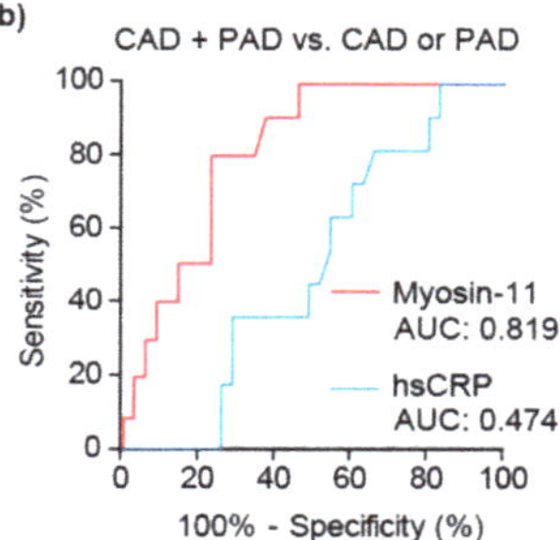

Figure 3. ROC (receiver-operating characteristic) analysis of myosin-11 (myosin heavy chain 11) and hsCRP (high-sensitivity C-reactive protein). (**a**) ROC curves of myosin-11 and hsCRP in patients with CAD (coronary artery disease) or PAD (peripheral artery disease) and control subjects. (**b**) Receiver-operating characteristic curves of myosin-11 and hsCRP in patients with CAD + PAD and CAD or PAD. AUC: the area under the curve.

To further investigate the efficacy of myosin-11 to detect the presence of multiple regions of atherosclerosis, we compared circulating myosin-11 levels between the CAD or PAD group and the CAD + PAD group. The AUC of myosin-11 was 0.814 (95% CI: 0.691–0.938, $p = 0.002$), with a specificity of 63% at a sensitivity of 91% (Figure 3b), and the positive predictive value, negative predictive value, accuracy, and cutoff value were 43%, 96%, 70%, and 168.4 pg/mL, respectively. The AUC of hsCRP was 0.522 (95% CI: 0.339–0.705, $p = 0.827$), with a specificity of 20% at a sensitivity of 91%. The positive predictive value, negative predictive value, and accuracy were 26%, 88%, and 37%, respectively. The AUC of myosin-11 was significantly greater than that of hsCRP ($p = 0.007$) (Figure 3b). These results suggest that circulating myosin-11 levels were increased in patients with atherosclerosis, and its levels may reflect the spatial expansion of atherosclerotic regions.

3.7. Expression of Myosin-11 Isoforms in the Coronary Arteries

Finally, we investigated myosin-11 expression and apoptosis during atherosclerosis progression in humans. The patient information is shown in Table 4.

Table 4. Patient characteristics for histological analyses.

	Age	Gender	Diagnosis	Hypertension	Dyslipidemia	Diabetes Mellitus	Smoking History	Atherosclerosis Lesions
Patient 1	48	M	HCC	−	−	−	−	Type II, III
Patient 2	66	M	Liver cirrhosis	−	−	−	+	Type II, III
Patient 3	71	M	Lung cancer	+	−	+	+	Type III, IV, V
Patient 4	72	M	HCC	−	−	−	+	Type II, III
Patient 5	88	F	CHF	+	−	−	+	Type III, IV, V

HCC, hepatocellular carcinoma; CHF, chronic heart failure.

Proximal regions in human left coronary arteries were evaluated based on the American Heart Association (AHA)-recommended classification of atherosclerotic lesions [31]. Expression of SM1 and SM2 was greatly decreased for both in the intimal layer in Type II through Type V lesions, except in the shoulder region of atheromatous plaque in Type IV lesion and in intraplaque neovasculatures in Type V lesion defined as those in which major parts of the fibromuscular cap represent replacement of tissue disrupted by accumulated lipid and hematoma or organized thrombotic deposits (Figure 4). These findings were consistent with a previous report [28]. Expression of both SM1 and SM2 was gradually decreased in the medial layer as atherosclerosis progressed, while both expression levels were relatively maintained in the medial layer compared to that in the intimal layer (Figure 4).

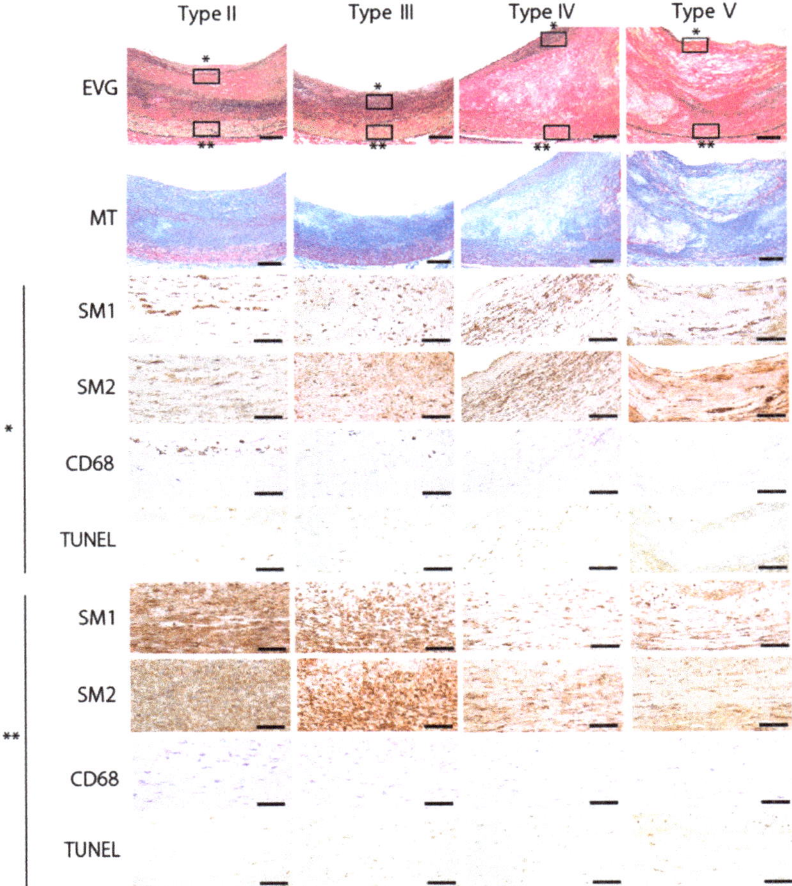

Figure 4. Histological analysis of human coronary arteries. Representative images of EVG (Elastica van Gieson staining), MT (Masson's trichrome staining), and immunohistochemistry for CD68 (a marker of macrophages), SM1 and SM2 (myosin heavy chain 11 isoforms), and TUNEL (TdT-mediated dUTP Nick End Labeling) stain in Type II (patient 4), Type III (patient 1), Type IV (patient 3), and Type V (patient 3) atherosclerotic lesions. * Magnified images of black boxes in the intimal layer. ** Magnified images of black boxes in the medial layer. Scale bars for EVG and MT: 200 μm. Scale bars for immunohistochemistry and TUNEL stain: 50 μm.

TUNEL-positive apoptotic cells were present in the intimal layer in Type II lesion and more advanced atherosclerotic lesions where macrophages were accumulated, as reported previously [32]. In the medial layer, apoptosis was increased in Types III, IV, and V lesions, in which moderate expression of both SM1 and SM2 proteins was observed (Figure 4). These apoptotic cells seemed originate from SMCs, because CD68-positive cells were rarely seen in these areas.

4. Discussion

During the past decade, the importance of VSMCs in atherosclerosis pathology has been re-evaluated [1]. Considerable efforts to identify subjects who are at a higher risk for cardiovascular events have been made, and numerous biomarkers were proposed [5,9]. The associated pathological processes are complex, and proteins related to lipid, inflammation, oxidative stress, coagulation, neurohumoral activity, and myocardial damage have been shown to be associated with the presence of atherosclerosis and vulnerability of atherosclerotic plaques [33]. Although recent studies identified micro-RNA enriched in VSMCs as a potential biomarker for atherosclerosis [5,34], vascular-tissue-specific circulating biomarkers are not currently available. In the present study, we focused on the VSMC-enriched protein myosin-11 and demonstrated increased plasma levels of myosin-11 in patients with CAD or PAD compared to control subjects. Plasma myosin-11 levels did not differ between patients with CAD and PAD, and circulating myosin-11 levels were higher in the CAD + PAD group than in the CAD or PAD group, suggesting that a higher level of circulating myosin-11 is associated with the presence of multiple atherosclerotic regions.

Pathological intimal thickening, which is the first stage of atherosclerosis, progresses to fibroatheromas, which are characterized by the formation of a fibrous cap and a necrotic core [1]. Differentiated mature contractile VSMCs express contractile genes, such as αSMA and myosin-11 [35], and VSMCs in the early stage fibrous cap, which protects against plaque rupture, also express αSMA and myosin-11 [36]. Recent lineage-tracing studies involving the use of *Myh11* (myosin-11 gene)-CreERT2 have demonstrated that VSMC-derived cells contributed substantially to the generation of a plaque core that is composed of αSMA-positive cells, macrophage-like cells, osteochondrogenic cells, and mesenchymal stem-cell-like cells [1,11,13–15]. Most αSMA-positive cells within the fibrous cap are positive for the VSMC-lineage label [37–39]. In the late stage of atherosclerosis, apoptosis is a hallmark of advanced atherosclerotic regions in humans [40]. It was reported that VSMC uptake of oxidized LDL and VSMC-derived foam cell formation seemed to induce VSMC apoptosis [17]. Induction of VSMC apoptosis using SM22α-hDTR/ApoE−/− mice induced fibrous cap thinning, necrotic core enlargement, plaque calcification, and medial degeneration, indicating that VSMC apoptosis accelerates atherosclerosis progression [19]. These data suggest that VSMCs proliferate during the early stage of atherosclerosis, and their loss in the arteries promotes plaque instability. Because myosin-11 is the component of smooth muscle myosin that is a major cytoskeletal/contractile protein of VSMCs and is theoretically not secreted from cells, increased circulating myosin-11 levels were thought to reflect dying VSMCs. In the present study, we measured plasma concentrations of myosin-11 in patients with advanced atherosclerosis in the coronary and peripheral arteries, so we do not know how early a stage of atherosclerosis we could possibly detect. The histology data in the present study demonstrated that expression the of both SM1 and SM2 was greatly decreased in the intimal layer, as reported previously [28], but were relatively maintained in the medial layer of advanced atherosclerotic lesions of human coronary arteries. Apoptosis in VSMCs seemed to be elevated in the medial layer of Type III lesions. Although the immunohistochemistry did not demonstrate that apoptotic SMCs in the medial layer are the source of circulating myosin-11, myosin-11 derived from VSMCs in Type III, as well as in Types IV and V, lesions may possibly affect circulating myosin-11 levels. Further study investigating the association of circulating myosin-11 levels with circulating apoptosis markers, such as cytokeratin-18 M30 antigen [41] and nucleosomes [42], at an asymptomatic early stage in atherosclerosis patients would clarify the timing at which circulating myosin-11 is elevated during atherosclerosis progression.

In a previous study, we conducted a secretome-based analysis of human AAA tissues and found that myosin-11 was abundantly detected in the supernatants of an organ culture of advanced AAA tissues [26]. In addition to the supernatants, circulating myosin-11 levels were increased in patients with AAA, and its levels were correlated with maximum aortic diameter [26]. It is widely recognized that aortic aneurysms that are localized at the abdominal region develop based on atherosclerotic pathological remodeling, and an advanced aneurysmal wall exhibits VSMC apoptosis and medial degeneration [43,44]. Another line of study also demonstrated that circulating myosin-11 levels were significantly increased in the blood immediately after aortic dissection occurred [45,46]. Together with the present study, these findings support the concept that elevated circulating myosin-11 levels seem to reflect the degree of VSMC loss.

An increasing amount of proteomic evidence has identified several circulating protein markers for atherosclerosis [9]. Although contractile genes are downregulated when VSMCs undergo phenotypic switching during atherosclerosis progression [47], VSMC-related cytoskeleton and contracting proteins were identified in tissue extracts and secretome analyses of human atherosclerotic samples, such as carotid or coronary plaques [9]. To the best of our knowledge, however, molecular signatures of circulating myosin-11 in blood derived from patients with atherosclerosis remain uncertain.

VSMCs in the tunica media arise from local progenitor cells, and multiple distinct cell lineages are distributed across the arterial tree [48]. Coronary arteries are derived from pro-epicardium (lateral plate mesoderm) [49]. The infrarenal abdominal aorta and its distal peripheral arteries are derived from the splanchnic mesoderm [50]. A study using liquid chromatography/tandem mass spectrometric analysis (LC–MS/MS) analyses of the human AAA tunica media that is located in infra-renal regions demonstrated that the number of segments in a coiled-coil domain was larger than that of a motor domain in human AAA tissue secretion [26]. Because the infrarenal abdominal aorta and the peripheral arteries share a similar cell lineage, a coiled-coil domain of myosin-11 may be elevated in the blood of PAD patients. The present study, however, did not reveal molecular signatures of myosin-11 detected in the blood of CAD and PAD, because the ELISA used in this study could detect both fragments of myosin-11 containing a coiled-coil domain and full-length myosin-11. Identification of circulating myosin-11 by using mass spectrometric analysis and Western blotting in patients with atherosclerosis of each region, i.e., the coronary and peripheral arteries, would clarify whether myosin-11 in the blood is fragmented or full-length, and provide further information for atherosclerosis pathologies and developing a detection system.

There are several limitations to the present study. The present work was conducted by using a small number of samples, all with advanced atherosclerosis, and therefore, it lacks clinical background variety. Myosin-11 is abundantly expressed in arterial smooth muscle cells, but it is also found in the bladder, intestine, stomach, and uterus [27]. It is theoretically possible that circulating myosin-11 levels are elevated in patients with diseases of these organs. In addition to AAA and dissection of the aorta, circulating myosin-11 levels can be elevated in other vascular diseases, such as aortitis. The effect of gender on circulating myosin-11 levels remains unknown, because the number of female patients in this study was too small for statistical analysis.

The present study involved a higher frequency of renal insufficiency in atherosclerosis patients. A previous study reported that renal function did not increase circulating myosin-11 levels [46], and an analysis involving subjects without renal insufficiency in the present study demonstrated a similar tendency as that seen in the results using all subjects (Figure 2a,b). However, the effect of renal function on circulating myosin-11 levels should be considered, and the clearance of circulating myosin-11 needs to be examined in future studies. Because the progression of atherosclerosis consists of multiple pathological molecular processes, it is unlikely that a single molecule could be used to detect relatively early phase asymptomatic atherosclerosis and to monitor plaque vulnerability.

5. Conclusions

In conclusion, together with other biomarkers, circulating levels of myosin-11, which seem to reflect VSMC loss or damage, may help to detect the presence of atherosclerosis and spatial expansion in atherosclerosis regions.

Author Contributions: Conceptualization, U.Y.; methodology, U.Y.; validation, T.I., H.T., T.C., and Y.I.; formal analysis, L.T., H.K., and S.I.; investigation, L.T., T.I., Y.K., K.T., and U.Y.; resources, T.I., K.T., and T.N.; data curation, L.T., Y.K., H.K., S.I., M.T., and U.Y.; writing—original draft preparation, L.T., Y.K., and U.Y.; writing—review and editing, L.T., Y.K., and U.Y.; visualization, L.T., Y.K., and U.Y.; supervision, H.T., J.Y., T.C., and Y.I.; project administration, U.Y.; funding acquisition, L.T., Y.I., and U.Y. All authors have read and agreed to the published version of the manuscript.

Funding: This work was supported by AMED (U Yokoyama and Y Ishikawa, JP21ek0210117) and was also partially supported by JSPS (L Takahashi, JP20K16533; U Yokoyama, JP20H03650; JP20K21638), and Kitsuen Research Foundation (Y Ishikawa, 1971000014).

Institutional Review Board Statement: The study protocols were approved by the Research Ethics Committee of Yokohama City University Hospital (approval number: B170800045) and Tokyo Medical University (approval number: T2020-0423). The studies were conducted in accordance with the principles outlined in the Declaration of Helsinki.

Informed Consent Statement: Written informed consent was obtained from all the subjects after they received a full explanation of the study of Yokohama City University Hospital. Histological analyses of coronary artery tissues were performed after the public announcement of the study protocol at Tokyo Medical University Hospital.

Data Availability Statement: The data presented in this study are available on request from the corresponding author. The data are not publicly available due to privacy.

Acknowledgments: The authors are grateful to Yuka Sawada and Fumiko Kato for their technical assistance.

Conflicts of Interest: Jun Yamashita and Lisa Takahashi are affiliated with an endowed department sponsored by Abbott Vascular Japan Co., Ltd. However, Abbott Vascular Japan had no role in the study design; in the collection, analysis, and interpretation of data; in the writing of the report; and in the decision to submit the article for publication. The other authors declare no conflict of interest.

References

1. Basatemur, G.L.; Jørgensen, H.F.; Clarke, M.C.H.; Bennett, M.R.; Mallat, Z. Vascular smooth muscle cells in atherosclerosis. *Nat. Rev. Cardiol.* **2019**, *16*, 727–744. [CrossRef]
2. Libby, P.; Buring, J.E.; Badimon, L.; Hansson, G.K.; Deanfield, J.; Bittencourt, M.S.; Tokgözoğlu, L.; Lewis, E.F. Atherosclerosis. *Nat. Rev. Dis. Primers* **2019**, *5*, 56. [CrossRef]
3. Gisterå, A.; Hansson, G.K. The immunology of atherosclerosis. *Nat. Rev. Nephrol.* **2017**, *13*, 368–380. [CrossRef]
4. Davies, M.J.; Richardson, P.D.; Woolf, N.; Katz, D.R.; Mann, J. Risk of thrombosis in human atherosclerotic plaques: Role of extracellular lipid, macrophage, and smooth muscle cell content. *Heart* **1993**, *69*, 377–381. [CrossRef]
5. Hoefer, I.E.; Steffens, S.; Ala-Korpela, M.; Back, M.; Badimon, L.; Bochaton-Piallat, M.L.; Boulanger, C.M.; Caligiuri, G.; Dimmeler, S.; Egido, J.; et al. Novel methodologies for biomarker discovery in atherosclerosis. *Eur. Heart J.* **2015**, *36*, 2635–2642. [CrossRef] [PubMed]
6. da Silva, P.M.; Duarte, J.S.; von Hafe, P.; Gil, V.; de Oliveira, J.N.; de Sousa, G. Standardization of laboratory and lipid profile evaluation: A call for action with a special focus in 2016 ESC/EAS dyslipidaemia guidelines—Full report. *Atheroscler. Suppl.* **2018**, *31*, e1–e12. [CrossRef] [PubMed]
7. Shah, P.K. Biomarkers of plaque instability. *Curr. Cardiol. Rep.* **2014**, *16*, 547. [CrossRef] [PubMed]
8. Viswanathan, V.; Jamthikar, A.D.; Gupta, D.; Shanu, N.; Puvvula, A.; Khanna, N.N.; Saba, L.; Omerzum, T.; Viskovic, K.; Mavrogeni, S.; et al. Low-cost preventive screening using carotid ultrasound in patients with diabetes. *Front. Biosci.* **2020**, *25*, 1132–1171.
9. Eslava-Alcon, S.; Extremera-García, M.J.; González-Rovira, A.; Rosal-Vela, A.; Rojas-Torres, M.; Beltran-Camacho, L.; Sanchez-Gomar, I.; Jiménez-Palomares, M.; Alonso-Piñero, J.A.; Conejero, R.; et al. Molecular signatures of atherosclerotic plaques: An up-dated panel of protein related markers. *J. Proteom.* **2020**, *221*, 103757. [CrossRef]
10. Schwartz, S.M.; Virmani, R.; Rosenfeld, M.E. The good smooth muscle cells in atherosclerosis. *Curr. Atheroscler. Rep.* **2000**, *2*, 422–429. [CrossRef]
11. Shankman, L.S.; Gomez, D.; Cherepanova, O.A.; Salmon, M.; Alencar, G.F.; Haskins, R.M.; Swiatlowska, P.; Newman, A.A.; Greene, E.S.; Straub, A.C.; et al. KLF4-dependent phenotypic modulation of smooth muscle cells has a key role in atherosclerotic plaque pathogenesis. *Nat. Med.* **2015**, *21*, 628–637. [CrossRef]
12. Feil, S.; Fehrenbacher, B.; Lukowski, R.; Essmann, F.; Schulze-Osthoff, K.; Schaller, M.; Feil, R. Transdifferentiation of vascular smooth muscle cells to macrophage-like cells during atherogenesis. *Circ. Res.* **2014**, *115*, 662–667. [CrossRef]

13. Chappell, J.; Harman, J.L.; Narasimhan, V.M.; Yu, H.; Foote, K.; Simons, B.D.; Bennett, M.R.; Jorgensen, H.F. Extensive Proliferation of a Subset of Differentiated, yet Plastic, Medial Vascular Smooth Muscle Cells Contributes to Neointimal Formation in Mouse Injury and Atherosclerosis Models. *Circ. Res.* **2016**, *119*, 1313–1323. [CrossRef]
14. Jacobsen, K.; Lund, M.B.; Shim, J.; Gunnersen, S.; Fuchtbauer, E.M.; Kjolby, M.; Carramolino, L.; Bentzon, J.F. Diverse cellular architecture of atherosclerotic plaque derives from clonal expansion of a few medial SMCs. *JCI Insight* **2017**, *2*. [CrossRef] [PubMed]
15. Dobnikar, L.; Taylor, A.L.; Chappell, J.; Oldach, P.; Harman, J.L.; Oerton, E.; Dzierzak, E.; Bennett, M.R.; Spivakov, M.; Jorgensen, H.F. Disease-relevant transcriptional signatures identified in individual smooth muscle cells from healthy mouse vessels. *Nat. Commun.* **2018**, *9*, 4567. [CrossRef]
16. Kockx, M.M.; De Meyer, G.R.; Muhring, J.; Jacob, W.; Bult, H.; Herman, A.G. Apoptosis and related proteins in different stages of human atherosclerotic plaques. *Circulation* **1998**, *97*, 2307–2315. [CrossRef] [PubMed]
17. Okura, Y.; Brink, M.; Itabe, H.; Scheidegger, K.J.; Kalangos, A.; Delafontaine, P. Oxidized low-density lipoprotein is associated with apoptosis of vascular smooth muscle cells in human atherosclerotic plaques. *Circulation* **2000**, *102*, 2680–2686. [CrossRef] [PubMed]
18. Clarke, M.C.; Figg, N.; Maguire, J.J.; Davenport, A.P.; Goddard, M.; Littlewood, T.D.; Bennett, M.R. Apoptosis of vascular smooth muscle cells induces features of plaque vulnerability in atherosclerosis. *Nat. Med.* **2006**, *12*, 1075–1080. [CrossRef] [PubMed]
19. Clarke, M.C.; Littlewood, T.D.; Figg, N.; Maguire, J.J.; Davenport, A.P.; Goddard, M.; Bennett, M.R. Chronic apoptosis of vascular smooth muscle cells accelerates atherosclerosis and promotes calcification and medial degeneration. *Circ. Res.* **2008**, *102*, 1529–1538. [CrossRef]
20. Hartman, M.A.; Spudich, J.A. The myosin superfamily at a glance. *J. Cell Sci.* **2012**, *125*, 1627–1632. [CrossRef]
21. Myronovkij, S.; Negrych, N.; Nehrych, T.; Redowicz, M.J.; Souchelnytskyi, S.; Stoika, R.; Kit, Y. Identification of a 48 kDa form of unconventional myosin 1c in blood serum of patients with autoimmune diseases. *Biochem. Biophys. Rep.* **2016**, *5*, 175–179. [CrossRef]
22. Seguin, J.R.; Saussine, M.; Ferriere, M.; Leger, J.J.; Leger, J.; Larue, C.; Calzolari, C.; Grolleau, R.; Chaptal, P.A. Myosin: A highly sensitive indicator of myocardial necrosis after cardiac operations. *J. Thorac. Cardiovasc. Surg.* **1989**, *98*, 397–401. [CrossRef]
23. Astorri, E.; Fiorina, P.; Gavaruzzi, G.; Contini, G.A.; Fesani, F. Perioperative myocardial cell damage assessed by immunoradiometric assay of beta-myosin heavy chain serum levels in patients undergoing coronary bypass surgery. *Int. J. Cardiol.* **1996**, *55*, 157–162. [CrossRef]
24. Onuoha, G.N.; Alpar, E.K.; Laprade, M.; Rama, D.; Pau, B. Levels of myosin heavy chain fragment in patients with tissue damage. *Arch. Med Res.* **2001**, *32*, 27–29. [CrossRef]
25. Nagai, R.; Kuro-o, M.; Babij, P.; Periasamy, M. Identification of two types of smooth muscle myosin heavy chain isoforms by cDNA cloning and immunoblot analysis. *J. Biol. Chem.* **1989**, *264*, 9734–9737. [CrossRef]
26. Yokoyama, U.; Arakawa, N.; Ishiwata, R.; Yasuda, S.; Minami, T.; Goda, M.; Uchida, K.; Suzuki, S.; Matsumoto, M.; Koizumi, N.; et al. Proteomic analysis of aortic smooth muscle cell secretions reveals an association of myosin heavy chain 11 with abdominal aortic aneurysm. *Am. J. Physiol. Heart Circ. Physiol.* **2018**, *315*, H1012–H1018. [CrossRef]
27. Koenig, W.; Khuseyinova, N. Biomarkers of atherosclerotic plaque instability and rupture. *Arterioscler. Thromb. Vasc. Biol.* **2007**, *27*, 15–26. [CrossRef]
28. Emerging Risk Factors, C.; Kaptoge, S.; Di Angelantonio, E.; Pennells, L.; Wood, A.M.; White, I.R.; Gao, P.; Walker, M.; Thompson, A.; Sarwar, N.; et al. C-reactive protein, fibrinogen, and cardiovascular disease prediction. *N. Engl. J. Med.* **2012**, *367*, 1310–1320. [CrossRef] [PubMed]
29. Leguillette, R.; Gil, F.R.; Zitouni, N.; Lajoie-Kadoch, S.; Sobieszek, A.; Lauzon, A.M. (+)Insert smooth muscle myosin heavy chain (SM-B) isoform expression in human tissues. *Am. J. Physiol. Cell Physiol.* **2005**, *289*, C1277–C1285. [CrossRef]
30. Stary, H.C. Natural history and histological classification of atherosclerotic lesions: An update. *Arterioscler. Thromb. Vasc. Biol.* **2000**, *20*, 1177–1178. [CrossRef]
31. Aikawa, M.; Sivam, P.N.; Kuro-o, M.; Kimura, K.; Nakahara, K.; Takewaki, S.; Ueda, M.; Yamaguchi, H.; Yazaki, Y.; Periasamy, M.; et al. Human smooth muscle myosin heavy chain isoforms as molecular markers for vascular development and atherosclerosis. *Circ. Res.* **1993**, *73*, 1000–1012. [CrossRef] [PubMed]
32. Lutgens, E.; de Muinck, E.D.; Kitslaar, P.J.; Tordoir, J.H.; Wellens, H.J.; Daemen, M.J. Biphasic pattern of cell turnover characterizes the progression from fatty streaks to ruptured human atherosclerotic plaques. *Cardiovasc. Res.* **1999**, *41*, 473–479. [CrossRef]
33. Blankenberg, S.; Zeller, T.; Saarela, O.; Havulinna, A.S.; Kee, F.; Tunstall-Pedoe, H.; Kuulasmaa, K.; Yarnell, J.; Schnabel, R.B.; Wild, P.S.; et al. Contribution of 30 biomarkers to 10-year cardiovascular risk estimation in 2 population cohorts: The MONICA, risk, genetics, archiving, and monograph (MORGAM) biomarker project. *Circulation* **2010**, *121*, 2388–2397. [CrossRef]
34. Churov, A.; Summerhill, V.; Grechko, A.; Orekhova, V.; Orekhov, A. MicroRNAs as Potential Biomarkers in Atherosclerosis. *Int. J. Mol. Sci.* **2019**, *20*, 5547. [CrossRef]
35. Owens, G.K.; Kumar, M.S.; Wamhoff, B.R. Molecular regulation of vascular smooth muscle cell differentiation in development and disease. *Physiol. Rev.* **2004**, *84*, 767–801. [CrossRef]
36. Misra, A.; Feng, Z.; Chandran, R.R.; Kabir, I.; Rotllan, N.; Aryal, B.; Sheikh, A.Q.; Ding, L.; Qin, L.; Fernandez-Hernando, C.; et al. Integrin beta3 regulates clonality and fate of smooth muscle-derived atherosclerotic plaque cells. *Nat. Commun.* **2018**, *9*, 2073. [CrossRef]

37. Bentzon, J.F.; Sondergaard, C.S.; Kassem, M.; Falk, E. Smooth muscle cells healing atherosclerotic plaque disruptions are of local, not blood, origin in apolipoprotein E knockout mice. *Circulation* **2007**, *116*, 2053–2061. [CrossRef]
38. Bentzon, J.F.; Weile, C.; Sondergaard, C.S.; Hindkjaer, J.; Kassem, M.; Falk, E. Smooth muscle cells in atherosclerosis originate from the local vessel wall and not circulating progenitor cells in ApoE knockout mice. *Arterioscler. Thromb. Vasc. Biol.* **2006**, *26*, 2696–2702. [CrossRef]
39. Yu, H.; Stoneman, V.; Clarke, M.; Figg, N.; Xin, H.B.; Kotlikoff, M.; Littlewood, T.; Bennett, M. Bone marrow-derived smooth muscle-like cells are infrequent in advanced primary atherosclerotic plaques but promote atherosclerosis. *Arterioscler. Thromb. Vasc. Biol.* **2011**, *31*, 1291–1299. [CrossRef]
40. van der Wal, A.C.; Becker, A.E.; van der Loos, C.M.; Das, P.K. Site of intimal rupture or erosion of thrombosed coronary atherosclerotic plaques is characterized by an inflammatory process irrespective of the dominant plaque morphology. *Circulation* **1994**, *89*, 36–44. [CrossRef]
41. Krysko, D.V.; Vanden Berghe, T.; D'Herde, K.; Vandenabeele, P. Apoptosis and necrosis: Detection, discrimination and phagocytosis. *Methods* **2008**, *44*, 205–221. [CrossRef] [PubMed]
42. Holdenrieder, S.; Nagel, D.; Schalhorn, A.; Heinemann, V.; Wilkowski, R.; von Pawel, J.; Raith, H.; Feldmann, K.; Kremer, A.E.; Müller, S.; et al. Clinical relevance of circulating nucleosomes in cancer. *Ann. N. Y. Acad. Sci.* **2008**, *1137*, 180–189. [CrossRef]
43. Golledge, J. Abdominal aortic aneurysm: Update on pathogenesis and medical treatments. *Nat. Rev. Cardiol.* **2019**, *16*, 225–242. [CrossRef] [PubMed]
44. Yoshimura, K.; Morikage, N.; Nishino-Fujimoto, S.; Furutani, A.; Shirasawa, B.; Hamano, K. Current Status and Perspectives on Pharmacologic Therapy for Abdominal Aortic Aneurysm. *Curr. Drug Targets* **2018**, *19*, 1265–1275. [CrossRef]
45. Suzuki, T.; Katoh, H.; Watanabe, M.; Kurabayashi, M.; Hiramori, K.; Hori, S.; Nobuyoshi, M.; Tanaka, H.; Kodama, K.; Sato, H.; et al. Novel biochemical diagnostic method for aortic dissection. Results of a prospective study using an immunoassay of smooth muscle myosin heavy chain. *Circulation* **1996**, *93*, 1244–1249. [CrossRef]
46. Katoh, H.; Suzuki, T.; Hiroi, Y.; Ohtaki, E.; Suzuki, S.; Yazaki, Y.; Nagai, R. Diagnosis of aortic dissection by immunoassay for circulating smooth muscle myosin. *Lancet* **1995**, *345*, 191–192. [CrossRef]
47. Rensen, S.S.; Doevendans, P.A.; van Eys, G.J. Regulation and characteristics of vascular smooth muscle cell phenotypic diversity. *Neth. Heart J.* **2007**, *15*, 100–108. [CrossRef]
48. Bentzon, J.F.; Majesky, M.W. Lineage tracking of origin and fate of smooth muscle cells in atherosclerosis. *Cardiovasc. Res.* **2018**, *114*, 492–500. [CrossRef]
49. Mikawa, T.; Gourdie, R.G. Pericardial mesoderm generates a population of coronary smooth muscle cells migrating into the heart along with ingrowth of the epicardial organ. *Dev. Biol.* **1996**, *174*, 221–232. [CrossRef]
50. Wasteson, P.; Johansson, B.R.; Jukkola, T.; Breuer, S.; Akyurek, L.M.; Partanen, J.; Lindahl, P. Developmental origin of smooth muscle cells in the descending aorta in mice. *Development* **2008**, *135*, 1823–1832. [CrossRef] [PubMed]

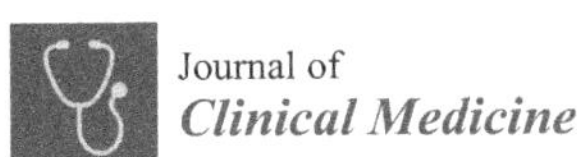
Journal of
Clinical Medicine
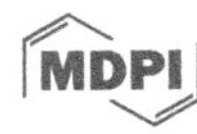

Article

Direct Oral Anticoagulant Therapy for Isolated Distal Deep Vein Thrombosis Associated with Cancer in Routine Clinical Practice

Yutaka Ogino [1], Tomoaki Ishigami [2,*], Ryosuke Sato [1], Hidefumi Nakahashi [1], Yugo Minamimoto [1], Yuichiro Kimura [1], Kozo Okada [1], Yasushi Matsuzawa [1], Noriaki Iwahashi [1], Kiyoshi Hibi [1], Masami Kosuge [1], Toshiaki Ebina [1], Toshiyuki Ishikawa [2], Kouichi Tamura [2] and Kazuo Kimura [1]

1 Department of Cardiology, Yokohama City University Medical Center, Yokohama 232-0024, Japan; ogino-you@hotmail.co.jp (Y.O.); r_satou@yokohama-cu.ac.jp (R.S.); t146060t@yokohama-cu.ac.jp (H.N.); yugo@yokohama-cu.ac.jp (Y.M.); y_kimura@yokohama-cu.ac.jp (Y.K.); kokada2@yokohama-cu.ac.jp (K.O.); matsu@yokohama-cu.ac.jp (Y.M.); niwahash@urahp.yokohama-cu.ac.jp (N.I.); hibikiyo@urahp.yokohama-cu.ac.jp (K.H.); masami-kosuge@pop06.odn.ne.jp (M.K.); tebina@yokohama-cu.ac.jp (T.E.); c_kimura@yokohama-cu.ac.jp (K.K.)
2 Department of Cardiology, Yokohama City University Hospital, Yokohama 236-0004, Japan; tishika@yokohama-cu.ac.jp (T.I.); tamukou@med.yokohama-cu.ac.jp (K.T.)
* Correspondence: tommmish@hotmail.com

Abstract: Background: The efficacy and bleeding complications of direct oral anticoagulant (DOAC) therapy for isolated distal deep vein thrombosis (IDDVT) associated with cancer in routine clinical practice remain unclear. Moreover, prior studies on prolonged therapy for IDDVT are limited. Methods: This retrospective study enrolled 1641 consecutive patients with acute venous thromboembolism (VTE) who had received oral anticoagulant therapy, including warfarin or DOAC, between April 2014 and September 2018 in our institutions. In these patients, 200 patients with cancer-associated IDDVT were evaluated. Results: Mean follow-up period was 780 ± 593 days. Major bleeding and VTE recurrence were observed in 22 (11.0%) and 11 (5.5%) patients, respectively. In multivariate analysis, statistically significant factors correlated with major bleeding were advanced cancer stage, high performance status, stomach cancer, and gallbladder cancer; those correlated with all-cause death were advanced cancer stage, high performance status, liver dysfunction, pancreatic cancer, and major bleeding. Cumulative events of major bleeding and recurrence between patients with prolonged DOAC therapy (≥90 days) and those with nonprolonged therapy were not significantly different. Conclusions: Preventing major bleeding is important because it is a significant risk factor for all-cause death. Major bleeding and recurrent events were comparable between prolonged and nonprolonged therapy.

Keywords: direct oral anticoagulant; isolated distal deep vein thrombosis; cancer

Citation: Ogino, Y.; Ishigami, T.; Sato, R.; Nakahashi, H.; Minamimoto, Y.; Kimura, Y.; Okada, K.; Matsuzawa, Y.; Iwahashi, N.; Hibi, K.; et al. Direct Oral Anticoagulant Therapy for Isolated Distal Deep Vein Thrombosis Associated with Cancer in Routine Clinical Practice. *J. Clin. Med.* **2021**, *10*, 4648. https://doi.org/10.3390/jcm10204648

Academic Editor: Mahboob Alam

Received: 26 August 2021
Accepted: 8 October 2021
Published: 11 October 2021

1. Introduction

The application of anticoagulant therapy for isolated distal deep vein thrombosis (IDDVT) associated with cancer remains controversial. Some previous studies reported that the high recurrence risk of cancer-associated venous thromboembolism (VTE) and effectiveness of anticoagulant therapy for IDDVT is correlated with active cancer [1,2]. According to these studies, in routine clinical practice, patients with IDDVT associated with active cancer are sometimes prescribed a direct oral anticoagulant (DOAC), especially in the preoperative period. However, in these studies, the examination for the presence of pulmonary embolism (PE) using contrast-enhanced computed tomography (CT) or ventilation–perfusion lung scintigraphy was not routinely performed. There is a paucity of data on the efficacy and bleeding complications of DOAC therapy for "real" IDDVT associated with active cancer in routine clinical practice; moreover, the safety and efficacy of prolonged DOAC therapy (≥90 days) for cancer-associated IDDVT has not been fully elucidated.

This study evaluates bleeding and recurrent complication of patients with cancer-associated IDDVT who received DOAC therapy, and validates the safety and efficacy of prolonged DOAC therapy in routine clinical practice.

2. Materials and Methods

This physician-initiated retrospective study enrolled 1641 consecutive patients with acute VTE who had received oral anticoagulant therapy, including warfarin or DOAC, between April 2014 and September 2018 at Yokohama City University Hospital and Yokohama City University Medical Center. Patient data, including age, sex, VTE etiology, VTE symptomatology, and other VTE-related factors, were collected from hospital charts. VTE diagnosis was based of symptoms and lower-limb findings on ultrasound, contrast-enhanced computed tomography, and ventilation–perfusion lung scintigraphy. For asymptomatic patients, physicians normally diagnose VTE based on the clinical course and objective results on imaging, especially lower-limb ultrasound, which is routinely used in clinical practice [3].

In the current study, IDDVT was defined as venous thrombosis of the calf veins, including peroneal, posterior tibial, anterior tibial, and soleus muscle veins below the knee. Major bleeding was defined using the International Society of Thrombosis and Hemostasis criteria: reduction in hemoglobin level by at least 2 g/dL, transfusion of at least 2 units of blood, or symptomatic bleeding in a critical area or organ [4]. In the present study, DOAC withdrawal depended on the treating physician's judgement. The timing of evaluation for recurrent VTE also depended on the judgment of each physician in the presence of the following symptoms: leg pain, leg swelling, and dyspnea. Regarding asymptomatic cases, increased D-dimer levels were an indication for objective imaging examinations to search for a new thrombus.

Patients with cancer-associated VTE included those receiving treatment for cancer, such as chemotherapy or radiotherapy; those scheduled to undergo cancer surgery; those with metastasis to other organs; and those with terminal cancer (expected life expectancy of ≤6 months) at the time of diagnosis [5]. We confirmed the specific tumor types, performance status (PS), cancer stage, and performance of chemotherapy at the time of VTE diagnosis. Cancer stage was determined using the TNM classification. Cancers with distal metastasis or the highest malignant grade were classified under stage 4. Liver dysfunction was defined as the presence of a chronic hepatic disease (e.g., cirrhosis) or biochemical evidence of significant hepatic derangement (e.g., bilirubin level of more than twice the upper limit or aspartate aminotransferase/alanine aminotransferase/alkaline phosphatase level of more than thrice the upper limit). This definition was derived from the HAS-BLED score [6]. We evaluated the incidence and characteristics of VTE recurrence, major bleeding, and all-cause death among patients with IDDVT associated with cancer who had undergone DOAC therapy. In the present study, prolonged therapy was defined as anticoagulant therapy with DOAC and/or initial intravenous anticoagulant over 3 months (90 days) according to the guideline of Japanese Circulation Society [7]. We evaluated the relationship between prolonged DOAC therapy, and events of major bleeding and recurrent VTE respectively by conducting a quasi-RCT using the inverse probability of treatment weighting (IPTW) technique [8].

This study was approved by the ethics committee of Yokohama City University Hospital and was conducted in accordance with the Declaration of Helsinki. Written informed consent was obtained from all patients.

Statistical Analysis

Continuous variables were reported as means ± SDs and categorical variables as frequencies (percentages). Unpaired t-test was used to compare the continuous variables, and the chi-squared test was used to test the difference in the qualitative variables between the groups. For all comparisons, p values of <0.05 were considered statistically significant.

In the factors that were significantly associated with major bleeding, recurrent VTE, and all-cause death by using the unpaired t-test or chi-squared test, univariate Cox regression analysis was performed. Thereafter, factors with p values of <0.05 were validated in multivariate Cox regression analysis.

For propensity score calculation, a logistic regression model was used. Multivariable models were adjusted using the IPTW method combined with logistic regression modeling to control for potential confounders: age, sex, body mass index (BMI), the primary site of cancer, cancer stage, performance status, chemotherapy, D-dimer, hemoglobin (Hb), estimated glomerular filtration ration (eGFR), blood platelet count, symptomatic state, use of single drug therapy, use of intravenous anticoagulant, history of stroke, liver dysfunction, diabetes mellitus, and hypertension. We conducted Cox hazards-models analysis to consider survival time of major bleeding and recurrent VTE. Moreover, the Kaplan–Meier method was used to evaluate the cumulative event rate of major bleeding and recurrent VTE.

SPSS ver. 26 (IBM, Armonk, NY, USA) and R 3.3.2 (R Foundation for Statistical Computing, Vienna, Austria) were used for the statistical analysis.

3. Results

Between April 2014 and September 2018, 1641 patients with acute VTE were treated with oral anticoagulant therapy at our institutions. Among them, 1244 and 397 patients were treated with DOAC and warfarin, respectively. In the DOAC group, there were 552 patients with cancer-associated VTE; 279 patients had PE and/or proximal DVT and 30 patients were not examined for the presence of PE. Nineteen patients could not be followed-up, and 24 patients received underdose off-label prescription of DOAC. After the exclusion of these patients, 200 patients with cancer-associated IDDVT remained and were evaluated (Figure 1). The mean follow-up period was 780 ± 593 days.

Table 1 shows the characteristics of the 200 patients with cancer-associated IDDVT. Regarding the primary site of cancer, digestive-organ cancers had the greatest number of cases. The number of blood-cancer cases was as follows: malignant lymphoma (n = 8) and multiple myeloma (n = 2). The number of head and neck cancer cases was as follows: pharyngeal cancer (n = 2), oral-cavity cancer (n = 2), tongue (n = 1), and nasal-cavity cancer (n = 1). Regarding treatment in the acute phase, single-drug therapy with 15 mg rivaroxaban BID or 10 mg apixaban BID was used in 6 patients. Intravenous unfractionated heparin was used in 10 patients.

Table 1. Baseline characteristics.

Baseline	n = 200
Age (years)	73.2 ± 8.9
Female sex	104 (52.0%)
Body weight (kg)	53.6 ± 11.5
Body mass index	21.6 ± 4.0
Body mass index of ≥30 kg/m^2	5 (2.5%)
Symptomatic DVT	49 (24.5%)
Primary site of cancer	
Stomach	30 (15.0%)
Colorectum	50 (25.0%)
Pancreas	33 (16.5%)
Esophagus	5 (2.5%)
Bile duct	9 (4.5%)
Gallbladder	4 (2.0%)
Liver	2 (1.0%)
Lung	14 (7.0%)
Breast	5 (2.5%)

Table 1. *Cont.*

Baseline	n = 200
Uterus	6 (3.0%)
Ovary	10 (5.0%)
Prostate	3 (1.5%)
Urinary bladder	6 (3.0%)
Kidney	3 (1.5%)
Blood	10 (5.0%)
Head and neck	6 (3.0%)
Nerve	2 (1.0%)
Skin	2 (1.0%)
Stage	
1 to 3	122 (61.0%)
4	78 (39.0%)
Performance status	
0	112 (56.0%)
1	73 (36.5%)
2	14 (7.0%)
3 to 4	1 (0.5%)
Chemotherapy	115 (57.5%)
Hypertension	78 (39.0%)
Diabetes mellitus	30 (15.0%)
Previous stroke	6 (3.0%)
Liver dysfunction	16 (8.0%)
Laboratory results at diagnosis	
D-dimer (μg/mL)	8.6 ± 14.6
eGFR (mL/min/1.73 m^2)	70.2 ± 20.3
Hemoglobin (g/dL)	11.6 ± 1.80
Platelet (×10^4/dL)	23.6 ± 9.8
Treatment in the acute phase	
Single-drug therapy	6 (3.0%)
Intravenous anticoagulant	10 (5.0%)
Drug at diagnosis	
Antiplatelet agents	8 (4.0%)
Nonsteroidal anti-inflammatory drugs	29 (14.5%)
Corticosteroids	13 (6.5%)

DVT, deep vein thrombosis; eGFR, estimated glomerular filtration ration.

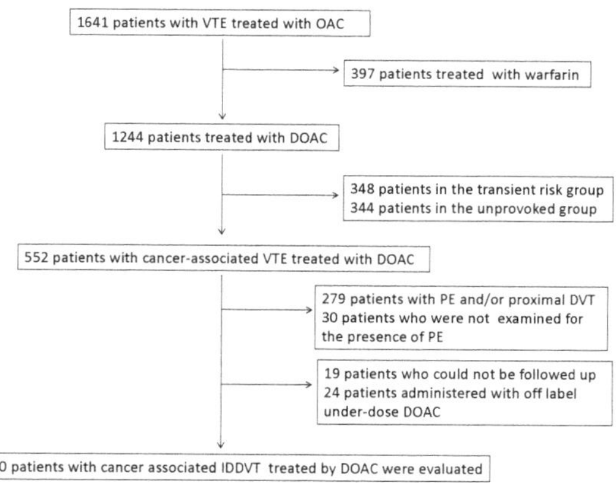

Figure 1. Flowchart of participant inclusion criteria. VTE, venous thromboembolism; OAC, oral anticoagulant; DOAC, direct oral anticoagulant; DVT, deep vein thrombosis; PE, pulmonary embolism; IDDVT, isolated distal deep vein thrombosis.

Figure 2 shows the Kaplan–Meier curve estimate of the rate of discontinuation of anticoagulation. In the follow-up period, 187 patients discontinued DOAC; 68, 66, 26, 26, and 1 patient discontinued DOAC because of difficulty of oral intake due to the progression of cancer, physician's judgement, confirmation of disappearance of thrombus, major and minor bleeding complications, and emergent surgical operation, respectively. The physician's judgement was that the duration of DOAC was sufficient for their patients without confirmation of disappearance of thrombus. Almost all these patients underwent follow-up lower-limb ultrasound to confirm the reduction of thrombus after discontinuation of DOAC.

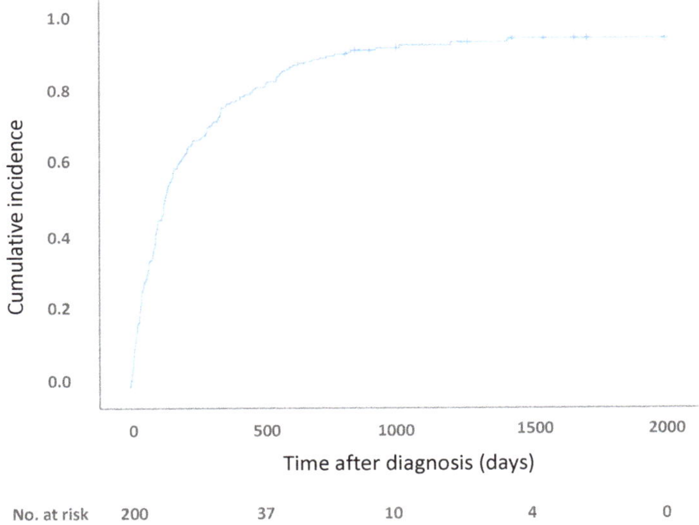

Figure 2. Kaplan–Meier curve-estimated discontinuation of DOAC therapy.

In the follow-up period, 22 (11%) patients developed major bleeding, and 11 (5.5%) patients developed recurrent VTE. A total of 11, 7, 1, 1, 1, and 1 patients had major bleeding in the upper digestive tract, lower digestive tract, brain, biliary tract, intra-abdominal, and aneurysm (rupture), respectively. Fatal bleeding complication under DOAC therapy occurred in one patient (rupture of aneurysm). Among the patients with recurrent VTE, 5, 2, and 4 had nonmassive PE, proximal DVT, and distal DVT, respectively. No patients with recurrent VTE died due to VTE. Table 2 shows the comparison between patients with and without major bleeding. Table 3 shows the comparison between the patients with and without recurrent VTE. Median duration of anticoagulant therapy between the recurrent and nonrecurrent groups was not significant. Table 4 shows the comparison between the patients who survived and those who died. In the present study, 110 patients died; 102, 3, 2, 1, 1, and 1 died from progression of cancer, natural death, aspiration pneumonitis, cerebral infarction, rupture of aorta aneurysm, and unidentified death, respectively.

Table 2. Comparison between patients with bleeding and without bleeding.

	Bleeding (*n* = 22)	No Bleeding (*n* = 178)	*p* Value
Age (years)	74.5 ± 8.8	73.0 ± 8.9	0.47
Female sex	10 (45.5%)	94 (52.8%)	0.51
Body weight (kg)	49.5 ± 8.5	54.1 ± 11.7	0.079
Body mass index	20.6 ± 3.4	21.8 ± 4.0	0.18
Body mass index of ≥30 kg/m^2	0 (0.0%)	5 (2.8%)	0.43
Symptomatic DVT	10 (45.5%)	39 (21.9%)	0.015
Primary site of cancer			
Stomach	8 (36.4%)	22 (12.4%)	0.0029
Colorectum	4 (18.2%)	46 (25.8%)	0.43
Pancreas	4 (18.2%)	29 (16.3%)	0.82
Esophagus	0 (0.0%)	5 (2.8%)	0.43
Bile duct	0 (0.0%)	9 (5.1%)	0.28
Gallbladder	2 (9.1%)	2 (1.1%)	0.012
Liver	0 (0.0%)	2 (1.1%)	0.62
Lung	1 (4.5%)	13 (7.3%)	0.63
Breast	1 (4.5%)	4 (2.2%)	0.51
Uterus	0 (0.0%)	6 (3.4%)	0.38
Ovary	2 (9.1%)	8 (4.5%)	0.35
Prostate	0 (0.0%)	3 (1.7%)	0.54
Urinary bladder	0 (0.0%)	6 (3.4%)	0.38
Kidney	0 (0.0%)	3 (1.7%)	0.54
Blood	0 (0.0%)	10 (5.6%)	0.25
Head and neck	0 (0.0%)	6 (3.4%)	0.38
Nerve	0 (0.0%)	2 (1.1%)	0.62
Skin	0 (0.0%)	2 (1.1%)	0.62
Stage			
1 to 3	8 (36.4%)	114 (64.0%)	
4	14 (63.6%)	64 (36.0%)	0.012
Performance status			
0	4 (18.2%)	108 (60.7%)	<0.001
1	14 (63.6%)	59 (33.1%)	0.005
2 to 4	4 (18.2%)	11 (6.2%)	0.044
Chemotherapy	16 (72.3%)	99 (55.6%)	0.13
Hypertension	12 (54.5%)	66 (37.1%)	0.11
Diabetes mellitus	5 (22.7%)	25 (14.0%)	0.28
Previous stroke	1 (4.5%)	5 (2.8%)	0.65
Liver dysfunction	1 (4.5%)	15 (8.4%)	0.53
Laboratory results at diagnosis			
D-dimer (μg/mL)	5.75 ± 5.2	8.96 ± 15.3	0.38
eGFR (mL/min/1.73 m^2)	67.8 ± 26.3	70.5 ± 19.5	0.57
Hemoglobin (g/dL)	11.2 ± 2.1	11.6 ± 1.8	0.30
Platelet (×10^4/dL)	26.8 ± 9.3	23.2 ± 9.8	0.11
Treatment in the acute phase			
Single-drug therapy	1 (4.5%)	5 (2.8%)	0.65
Intravenous anticoagulant	1 (4.5%)	9 (5.1%)	0.92
Drug at diagnosis			
Antiplatelet agents	1 (4.5%)	7 (3.9%)	0.89
Nonsteroidal anti-inflammatory drugs	3 (13.6%)	26 (14.6%)	0.90
Corticosteroids	0 (0.0%)	13 (7.3%)	0.19

DVT, deep vein thrombosis.

Table 3. Comparison between patients with and without bleeding.

	Recurrence (n = 11)	No Recurrence (n = 189)	p Value
Age (years)	69.5 ± 9.3	73.4 ± 8.9	0.16
Female sex	5 (45.5%)	99 (52.4%)	0.65
Body weight (kg)	56.3 ± 10.3	53.4 ± 11.6	0.42
Body mass index	22.3 ± 2.57	21.6 ± 4.0	0.56
Body mass index ≥ 30 kg/m^2	0 (0.0%)	5 (2.6%)	0.58
Symptomatic DVT	4 (36.3%)	45 (23.8%)	0.35
Primary site of cancer			
Stomach	2 (18.2%)	28 (14.8%)	0.76
Colorectum	4 (36.4%)	46 (24.3%)	0.37
Pancreas	1 (9.1%)	32 (16.9%)	0.50
Esophagus	0 (0.0%)	5 (2.6%)	0.58
Bile duct	0 (0.0%)	9 (4.8%)	0.46
Gallbladder	0 (0.0%)	4 (2.1%)	0.63
Liver	0 (0.0%)	2 (1.1%)	0.73
Lung	1 (9.1%)	13 (6.9%)	0.78
Breast	0 (0.0%)	5 (2.6%)	0.58
Uterus	0 (0.0%)	6 (3.2%)	0.55
Ovary	1 (9.1%)	9 (4.8%)	0.52
Prostate	0 (0.0%)	3 (1.6%)	0.67
Urinary bladder	1 (9.1%)	5 (2.6%)	0.22
Kidney	0 (0.0%)	3 (1.6%)	0.67
Blood	0 (0.0%)	10 (5.3%)	0.43
Head and neck	0 (0.0%)	6 (3.4%)	0.55
Nerve	1 (9.1%)	1 (0.53%)	0.006
Skin	0 (0.0%)	2 (1.1%)	0.73
Stage			
1 to 3	8 (72.7%)	114 (60.3%)	
4	3 (27.3%)	75 (39.7%)	0.41
Performance status			
0	9 (81.8%)	103 (54.5%)	0.076
1	2 (18.2%)	71 (37.6%)	0.19
2 to 4	0 (0.0%)	15 (7.9%)	0.33
Chemotherapy	6 (54.5%)	109 (57.7%)	0.84
Hypertension	6 (54.5%)	72 (38.1%)	0.28
Diabetes mellitus	2 (18.2%)	28 (14.8%)	0.76
Previous stroke	1 (9.1%)	5 (2.6%)	0.22
Liver dysfunction	1 (9.1%)	15 (7.9%)	0.89
Laboratory results at diagnosis			
D-dimer (μg/mL)	4.7 ± 4.2	8.9 ± 15.1	0.36
eGFR (mL/min/1.73 m^2)	70.5 ± 23.0	70.1 ± 20.1	0.96
Hemoglobin (g/dL)	12.5 ± 1.6	11.5 ± 1.8	0.071
Platelet (×10^4/dL)	24.9 ± 10.3	23.5 ± 9.8	0.64
Treatment in the acute phase			
Single-drug therapy	0 (0.0%)	6 (3.4%)	0.55
Intravenous anticoagulant	0 (0.0%)	10 (5.3%)	0.43
Drug at diagnosis			
Antiplatelet agents	1 (9.0%)	7 (3.7%)	0.38
Nonsteroidal anti-inflammatory drugs	2 (18.2%)	27 (14.3%)	0.72
Corticosteroids	0 (0.0%)	13 (6.9%)	0.37
Median duration of anticoagulant (days)	163	126	0.40

DVT, deep vein thrombosis.

Table 4. Comparison between patients with and without death.

	Death (n = 110)	No Death (n = 90)	p Value
Age (years)	73.0 ± 9.4	73.4 ± 8.3	0.73
Female sex	58 (52.7%)	46 (51.1%)	0.82
Body weight (kg)	52.8 ± 11.9	54.5 ± 10.9	0.31
Body mass index	21.2 ± 4.2	22.1 ± 3.4	0.13
Body mass index ≥ 30 kg/m^2	1 (0.91%)	4 (4.4%)	0.11
Symptomatic DVT	26 (23.6%)	23 (25.6%)	0.75
Primary site of cancer			
Stomach	18 (16.4%)	12 (13.3%)	0.55
Colorectum	24 (21.8%)	26 (28.9%)	0.25
Pancreas	27 (24.5%)	6 (6.7%)	<0.001
Esophagus	4 (3.6%)	1 (1.1%)	0.26
Bile duct	4 (3.6%)	5 (5.6%)	0.51
Gallbladder	4 (3.6%)	0 (0.0%)	0.068
Liver	0 (0.0%)	2 (2.2%)	0.12
Lung	7 (6.4%)	7 (7.8%)	0.70
Breast	2 (1.8%)	3 (3.3%)	0.49
Uterus	2 (1.8%)	4 (4.4%)	0.28
Ovary	4 (3.6%)	6 (6.7%)	0.33
Prostate	2 (1.8%)	1 (1.1%)	0.68
Urinary bladder	2 (1.8%)	4 (4.4%)	0.28
Kidney	0 (0.0%)	3 (3.3%)	0.054
Blood	3 (2.7%)	7 (7.8%)	0.10
Head and neck	5 (4.5%)	1 (1.1%)	0.16
Nerve	0 (0.0%)	2 (2.2%)	0.12
Skin	2 (1.8%)	0 (0.0%)	0.20
Stage			
1 to 3	39 (35.5%)	83 (92.2%)	
4	71 (64.5%)	7 (7.8%)	<0.001
Performance status			
0	35 (31.8%)	77 (85.6%)	<0.001
1	60 (54.5%)	13 (14.4%)	<0.001
2 to 4	15 (13.6%)	0 (0.0%)	<0.001
Chemotherapy	81 (73.6%)	34 (37.8%)	<0.001
Hypertension	40 (36.3%)	38 (42.2%)	0.40
Diabetes mellitus	19 (17.3%)	11 (12.2%)	0.32
Previous stroke	4 (3.6%)	2 (2.2%)	0.56
Liver dysfunction	15 (16.7%)	1 (1.1%)	0.001
Laboratory results at diagnosis			
D-dimer (μg/mL)	10.8 ± 14.9	6.16 ± 14.1	0.034
eGFR (mL/min/1.73 m^2)	72.6 ± 21.1	67.2 ± 18.9	0.063
Hemoglobin (g/dL)	11.1 ± 1.7	12.1 ± 1.8	<0.001
Platelet (×10^4/dL)	24.3 ± 9.6	22.7 ± 10.1	0.26
Treatment in the acute phase			
Single-drug therapy	3 (2.7%)	3 (3.3%)	0.80
Intravenous anticoagulant	6 (5.5%)	4 (4.4%)	0.74
Drug at diagnosis			
Antiplatelet agents	5 (4.5%)	3 (3.3%)	0.66
Nonsteroidal anti-inflammatory drugs	15 (13.6%)	14 (15.6%)	0.70
Corticosteroids	6 (5.5%)	7 (7.8%)	0.51
Major bleeding	20 (18.2%)	2 (2.2%)	<0.001
Recurrent VTE	4 (3.6%)	7 (7.8%)	0.20

DVT, deep vein thrombosis; VTE, venous thromboembolism.

Table 5 indicates the independent factors correlated with major bleeding, recurrent VTE, and all-cause death after adjustments in Cox regression analysis. In multivariate analysis, advanced cancer stage, high PS, stomach cancer, and gallbladder cancer were correlated with major bleeding. There was no factor correlated with recurrent VTE in this study. Conversely, advanced cancer stage, high PS, pancreatic cancer, liver dysfunction, and major bleeding were independently correlated with all-cause death.

Table 5. Factors correlated with major bleeding, recurrent VTE, and all-cause death.

	Univariate HR (95% CI)	p Value	Multivariate HR (95% CI)	p-Value
Major bleeding				
Symptomatic DVT	2.559 (1.105–5.924)	0.028	2.351 (0.988–5.597)	0.053
Stomach cancer	3.386 (1.417–8.091)	0.006	2.749 (1.050–7.202)	0.040
Gallbladder	15.33 (3.404–69.06)	<0.001	11.86 (2.196–64.00)	0.004
Stage 4	4.854 (1.996–11.80)	<0.001	2.686 (1.036–6.964)	0.042
Performance status	2.850 (1.797–4.518)	<0.001	2.667 (1.528–4.656)	0.001
Recurrent VTE				
Nerve	6.024 (0.765–47.46)	0.088		
All-cause death				
Pancreatic cancer	2.460 (1.587–3.811)	<0.001	1.912 (1.182–3.093)	0.008
Stage 4	7.415 (4.901–11.22)	<0.001	3.712 (2.289–6.021)	<0.001
Performance status	2.359 (1.903–2.924)	<0.001	1.860 (1.345–2.573)	<0.001
Chemotherapy	2.771 (1.809–4.246)	<0.001	1.222 (0.749–1.996)	0.422
Liver dysfunction	4.568 (2.623–7.956)	<0.001	2.513 (1.207–5.236)	0.014
D-dimer	1.013 (1.004–1.022)	0.004	1.007 (0.993–1.022)	0.321
Hemoglobin level	0.823 (0.740–0.916)	<0.001	0.893 (0.791–1.008)	0.066
Major bleeding	3.067 (1.867–5.040)	<0.001	2.149 (1.200–3.851)	0.010

VTE, venous thromboembolism; DVT, deep vein thrombosis, HR, hazard ratio; CI, confidential interval.

In the current study, we compared the prolonged-therapy group (n = 125) with nonprolonged-therapy group (n = 75). Table 6 shows the comparison between the patients with prolonged and nonprolonged therapy. A higher number of patients in the prolonged-therapy group received chemotherapy, which is a significant risk factor for VTE [9]. In the prolonged-therapy group, 44, 34, 23, 11 patients discontinued DOAC because of the difficulty of oral intake due to progression of cancer, physician's judgement, confirmation of thrombus disappearance, and major and minor bleeding complication. The 13 remaining patients in the prolonged-therapy group continued DOAC therapy in the follow-up period. In the nonprolonged-therapy group, 32, 24, 15, 3, and 1 patients discontinued DOAC because of physician's judgement, difficulty of oral intake due to the progression of cancer, major and minor bleeding complications, confirmation of thrombus disappearance, and emergent surgical operation. Figure 3 indicates the Kaplan–Meier curve-estimated outcome of major bleeding and recurrent VTE for patients who received prolonged and nonprolonged therapy. The incidences of major bleeding and recurrent VTE after diagnosis were not significantly different between the two groups. Table 7 indicates that the hazard ratio and 95% confidence interval estimated for prolonged therapy correlated with major bleeding, recurrent VTE, and all-cause death. In Cox regression analysis, after propensity matching with IPTW methods, prolonged therapy was not a significant risk factor for major bleeding, recurrent VTE, and all-cause death.

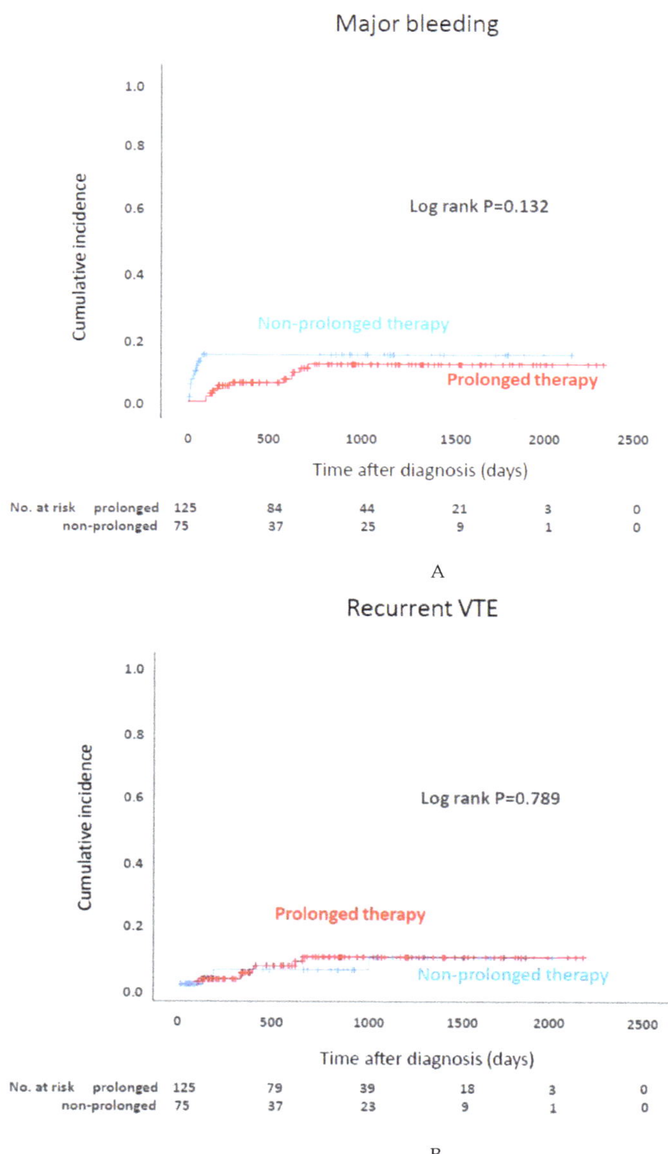

Figure 3. Kaplan–Meier curves estimating incidence of major bleeding (**A**) and recurrent venous thromboembolism (**B**) between patients who received prolonged and nonprolonged therapy.

Table 6. Comparison between patients with prolonged and nonprolonged therapy.

	Prolonged Therapy (n = 125)	Nonprolonged Therapy (n = 75)	p Value
Age (years)	73.4 ± 9.2	72.8 ± 8.4	0.62
Female sex	59 (47.2%)	45 (60%)	0.079
Body weight (kg)	55.0 ± 11.6	51.2 ± 11.0	0.028
Body mass index	22.1 ± 4.10.	20.9 ± 3.68	0.045
Body mass index ≥ 30 kg/m^2	3 (2.4%)	2 (2.7%)	0.91
Symptomatic DVT	36 (28.8%)	13 (17.3%)	0.068
Primary site of cancer			
Stomach	21 (16.8%)	9 (12.0%)	0.36
Colorectum	28 (22.4%)	22 (29.3%)	0.27
Pancreas	20 (16.0%)	13 (17.3%)	0.81
Esophagus	2 (1.6%)	3 (4.0%)	0.29
Bile duct	3 (2.4%)	6 (8.0%)	0.064
Gallbladder	1 (0.8%)	3 (4.0%)	0.12
Liver	1 (0.8%)	1 (1.3%)	0.71
Lung	10 (8.0%)	4 (5.3%)	0.47
Breast	4 (3.2%)	1 (1.3%)	0.41
Uterus	5 (4.0%)	1 (1.3%)	0.28
Ovary	8 (6.4%)	2 (2.7%)	0.24
Prostate	1 (0.8%)	2 (2.7%)	0.29
Urinary bladder	6 (4.8%)	0 (0.0%)	0.054
Kidney	3 (2.4%)	0 (0.0%)	0.18
Blood	6 (4.8%)	4 (5.3%)	0.87
Head and neck	5 (4.0%)	1 (1.3%)	0.28
Nerve	0 (0.0%)	2 (2.7%)	0.067
Skin	1 (0.8%)	1 (1.3%)	0.71
Stage			
1 to 3	78 (62.4%)	44 (58.7%)	
4	47 (37.6%)	31 (41.3%)	0.60
Performance status			
0	73 (58.4%)	39 (52.0%)	0.38
1	46 (36.8%)	27 (36.0%)	0.91
2 to 4	6 (4.8%)	9 (12.0%)	0.061
Chemotherapy	80 (64.0%)	35 (46.7%)	0.016
Hypertension	50 (40.0%)	28 (37.3%)	0.71
Diabetes mellitus	21 (16.8%)	9 (12.0%)	0.36
Previous stroke	3 (2.4%)	3 (4.0%)	0.52
Liver dysfunction	6 (4.8%)	10 (13.3%)	0.031
Laboratory results at diagnosis			
D-dimer (μg/mL)	7.55 ± 13.5	10.5 ± 16.3	0.20
eGFR (mL/min/1.73 m^2)	70.6 ± 18.4	69.5 ± 23.2	0.70
Hemoglobin (g/dL)	11.6 ± 1.70	11.4 ± 1.92	0.42
Platelet (×10^4/dL)	23.9 ± 10.0	23.2 ± 9.5	0.62
Treatment in the acute phase			
Single-drug therapy	6 (4.8%)	0 (0.0%)	0.054
Intravenous anticoagulant	9 (7.2%)	1 (1.3%)	0.065
Drug at diagnosis			
Antiplatelet agents	6 (4.8%)	2 (2.7%)	0.46
Nonsteroidal anti-inflammatory drugs	18 (14.4%)	11 (14.7%)	0.96
Corticosteroids	9 (7.2%)	4 (5.3%)	0.60
Median duration of anticoagulant (days)	281	35	<0.01

DVT, deep vein thrombosis.

Table 7. Validation of prolonged therapy for major bleeding, recurrent VTE, and all-cause death after propensity matching with IPTW method.

	Hazard Ratio	95% CI	*p*-Value
Major bleeding	0.62	0.207–1.884	0.40
Recurrent VTE	2.01	0.423–9.50	0.40
All-cause death	0.99	0.512–1.930	0.98

VTE, venous thromboembolism; IPTW, inverse probability of treatment weighting; CI, confidential interval.

4. Discussion

Prior studies revealed that IDDVT associated with active cancer had a high risk to develop proximal DVT and PE [1,10]. In fact, the American College of Chest Physicians (ACCP) guideline recommends that the management of patients with active cancer should be the same as that for patients with acute proximal DVT [11]. However, due to the lack of routine objective imaging to confirm the presence of PE in some cases, patients included in these studies were not stratified on the basis of whether they had only IDDVT or had both IDDVT and PE, especially asymptomatic PE. Nevertheless, one epidemiological study reported that 29% of distal DVT had concomitant PE [12]. Moreover, in the Italian Master registry, the presence of PE was frequently associated with IDDVT rather than proximal DVT [13]. Our study evaluated the patients who had only IDDVT and were not screened for presence of PE using contrast-enhanced CT or ventilation–perfusion lung scintigraphy. To the best of our knowledge, studies similar to ours are rare.

SELECT-D, Hokusai-VTE cancer, and CARABAGGIO trials, which compared DOAC with dalteparin for cancer-associated VTE, reported the rate of major bleeding of the DOAC group, which ranged approximately from 4.0% to 7.0% [14–16]. These randomized control trials (RCTs) included proximal DVT and/or PE and excluded IDDVT. In the current study, even though only IDDVT was included, the rate of major bleeding was higher compared with in these RCTs. In routine clinical practice in Japan, major bleeding events may be higher compared with in Western countries. This may mainly be attributed to the higher incidence of stomach cancer in the current study, as our previous study reported [17]. Regarding stomach cancer, the International Society of Thrombosis suggests LMWH therapy instead of DOACs in patients with gastrointestinal cancer because of their high risk of bleeding [18]. However, LMWH is not permitted to use for the treatment of VTE and is just approved for the prevention of VTE after surgery in Japan. For this reason, in the current study, DOAC therapy was selected even though it was for patients with gastrointestinal cancer. In addition, the low body weight of Japanese people who are affected with cancer might be one reason for the higher rate of major bleeding. For example, the average body weight in the current study was 53.6 kg, compared with 75.7–78.8 kg reported in the Hokusai VTE cancer and CARAVAGGIO trials. Individuals with a higher prevalence of stomach cancer and low body weight, such as Japanese people, should use DOACs cautiously. In this study, gallbladder cancer was also a risk factor for major bleeding. However, the number of gallbladder-cancer cases was too small to ascertain their significance.

Regarding recurrent VTE, there was no fatal PE in the current study. IDDVT has a low risk to develop proximal DVT and PE [19,20]. Even for cancer-associated IDDVT, there is low risk of fatal recurrent VTE under DOAC therapy. Unfortunately, factors correlated with recurrent VTE could not be determined in this study. Further validation on larger numbers of patients is needed to estimate the factors correlated with recurrent VTE.

In Cox regression analysis, major bleeding was an independent risk factor for all-cause death. Among patients with major bleeding, only one had fatal bleeding (rupture of aneurysm). However, major bleeding was associated with prognosis. This might mainly be because therapy for cancer such as chemotherapy or surgery was transiently stopped once major bleeding had developed. The discontinuation of therapy for active cancer might be correlated with shortening of life expectancy. We should pay more attention to avoiding bleeding complications during DOAC therapy for cancer-associated VTE by accordingly adjusting the DOAC dose and the duration of DOAC therapy.

JCS guidelines recommend anticoagulant therapy for over 3 months (prolonged therapy) for cancer-associated VTE, but prolonged therapy is not recommended for IDDVT [7]. Evidence on the efficacy and safety of prolonged DOAC therapy for IDDVT associated with cancer is scarce, and as such, in routine clinical practice, the duration of DOAC therapy for IDDVT associated with cancer is totally dependent on the judgement of the treating physician. In the current study, physicians tended to select prolonged therapy for patients who receive chemotherapy, which is significant risk factor for VTE. The Kaplan–Meier curve demonstrated the same incidence for recurrent VTE between the prolonged- and nonprolonged-therapy groups in the follow-up period. Patients who develop major bleeding within 90 days stop the anticoagulant within 90 days, and all these patients were included in the nonprolonged-therapy group. For this reason, in the Kaplan–Meier curve estimating major bleeding, the number of major bleeding event within 90 days was larger in the nonprolonged-therapy group compared with the prolonged-therapy group. However, cumulative major bleeding events in the follow-up period were comparable between them. Moreover, prolonged therapy in quasi-RCT was not a significant risk factor for either major bleeding or recurrent VTE in this study. Because the duration of anticoagulant therapy individually varied in this study, the fact that the incidence of major bleeding and recurrence were comparable may have changed in another study design. However, at least in the routine clinical situation where each treating physician decided the duration of DOAC therapy for IDDVT associated with cancer, the incidence of major bleeding and recurrence were comparable by the Kaplan–Meier method in our analysis.

The application of anticoagulant therapy for IDDVT associated with cancer, especially asymptomatic IDDVT, is still controversial. In fact, 151 out of 200 patients (75.5%) had asymptomatic IDDVT in this study. As described in Section 1, previous studies reported that the high recurrence risk of VTE and effectiveness of anticoagulant therapy for IDDVT associated with active cancer, even though IDDVT was not symptomatic. Moreover, Ro et al. estimated that thrombi propagate to the proximal vein from the soleus muscle vein in autopsy cases with massive PE, and reported the importance of preventing soleus vein thrombus [21]. In addition, the ACCP guideline recommends that the management of patients with active cancer should be the same as that for patients with acute proximal DVT. According to these studies and guideline, 200 patients with IDDVT associated with active cancer in the current study were prescribed DOAC. Further prospective studies that research the validity of DOAC therapy for IDDVT associated with cancer are needed.

This study had several limitations. First, both cancer itself, and daily lifestyle factors such as the length of sitting time and drinking behavior affect the formation of IDDVT [22]. The data of lifestyle factors in the current study are limited because it is retrospective. PS, cancer stage, and chemotherapy, which were included in our analysis, might help to to partially predict the daily lifestyle of cancer patients. A prospective study that includes the data of lifestyle factors is needed. Second, this was a retrospective observational study; decisions regarding the validation of recurrent VTE and continuation of anticoagulant therapy depended on the attending physician. This could mainly affect the incidence of recurrent VTE. Third, given that this study only involved two Japanese centers, the number of analyzed patients was relatively small, and most intended patients were Japanese. Fourth, in this study, 158 patients were prescribed edoxaban, 26 rivaroxaban, and 16 were apixaban. Because the numbers of those prescribed rivaroxaban and apixaban were small, we could not evaluate the statistical deference between DOACs. Lastly, compliance to medications was unclear.

5. Conclusions

Preventing major bleeding is important because it is a significant risk factor for all-cause death. Major bleeding and recurrent events were comparable between prolonged and nonprolonged therapy.

Author Contributions: Y.O., study idea, data collection and evaluation, manuscript drafting. R.S., H.N., Y.M. (Yugo Minamimoto), Y.K., K.O., Y.M. (Yasushi Matsuzawa), N.I., K.H., M.K., T.E., T.I. (Toshiyuki Ishikawa), K.T., and K.K., data acquisition. T.I. (Tomoaki Ishigami), data analysis and interpretation. All authors have read and agreed to the published version of the manuscript.

Funding: This research received no external funding.

Institutional Review Board Statement: The study was conducted according to the guidelines of the Declaration of Helsinki, and approved by Yokohama City University, Center for Novel and Exploratory Clinical Trials (reference number, B160401015).

Informed Consent Statement: Informed consent was obtained from all subjects involved in the study.

Data Availability Statement: Deidentified participant data will not be shared.

Acknowledgments: Kino Tabito, research scholar of Cardiovascular Research Center Lewis Katz School of Medicine at Temple University, helped us to analyze the data.

Conflicts of Interest: The authors declare no conflict of interest.

References

1. Dentali, F.; Pegoraro, S.; Barco, S.; Minno, M.; Mastroiacovo, D.; Pomero, F.; Lodigiani, C.; Bagna, F.; Sartori, M.; Barillari, G.; et al. Clinical course of isolated distal deep vein thrombosis in patients with active cancer: A multicenter cohort study. *J. Thromb. Haemost.* **2017**, *15*, 1757–1763. [CrossRef]
2. Yamashita, Y.; Shiomi, H.; Morimoto, T.; Yoneda, T.; Yamada, C.; Makiyama, T.; Kato, T.; Saito, N.; Shizuta, S.; Ono, K.; et al. Asymptomatic lower extremity deep vein thrombosis- clinical characteristics, management strategies, and long-term outcomes. *Circ. J.* **2017**, *81*, 1936–1944. [CrossRef]
3. Ohgi, S.; Kanaoka, Y. Ultrasound diagnosis of deep vein thrombosis as embolic sources. *Jpn. J. Med. Ultrasonics.* **2004**, *31*, 337–346.
4. Schulman, S.; Kearon, C. Subcommittee on Control of Anticoagulation of the Scientific and Standardization Committee of the International Society on Thrombosis and Haemostasis. Definition of major bleeding in clinical investigations of antihemostatic medicinal products in non-surgical patients. *J. Thromb. Haemost.* **2005**, *3*, 692–694.
5. Yamashita, Y.; Morimoto, T.; Amano, H.; Takase, T.; Hiramori, S.; Kim, K.; Konishi, T.; Akao, M.; Kobayashi, Y.; Inoueet, T.; et al. Anticoagulation therapy for venous thromboembolism in the real world: From the COMMAND VTE Registry. *Circ. J.* **2018**, *82*, 1262–1270. [CrossRef]
6. Pisters, R.; Lane, D.A.; Nieuwlaat, R.; de Vos, C.B.; Crijns, H.J.; Lip, G.Y. A novel user-friendly score (HAS-BLED) to assess 1-year risk of major bleeding in patients with atrial fibrillation: The Euro Heart Survey. *Chest* **2010**, *138*, 1093–1100. [CrossRef] [PubMed]
7. JCS Joint Working Group. Guidelines for Diagnosis, Treatment and Prevention of Pulmonary Thromboembolism and Deep Vein Thrombosis (JCS 2017). Available online: http://www.j-circ.or.jp/guideline/pdf/JCS2017_ito_h.pdf.2018.12.10 (accessed on 8 October 2020).
8. McCaffrey, D.F.; Griffin, B.A.; Almirall, D.; Slaughter, M.E.; Ramchand, R.; Burgette, L.F. A tutorial on propensity score estimation for multiple treatments using generalized boosted models. *Stat. Med.* **2013**, *32*, 3388–3414. [CrossRef]
9. Zamorano, J.L.; Lancellotti, P.; Rodriguez, M.D.; Aboyans, V.; Asteggiano, R.; Galderisi, M.; Habib, G.; Lenihan, D.J.; Lip, G.Y.H.; Lyon, A.R.; et al. 2016 ESC Position Paper on cancer treatments and cardiovascular toxicity developed under the auspices of the ESC Committee for Practice Guidelines: The Task Force for cancer treatments and cardiovascular toxicity of the European Society of Cardiology (ESC). *Eur. Heart J.* **2016**, *37*, 2768–2801. [CrossRef] [PubMed]
10. Singh, K.; Yakoub, D.; Giangola, P.; DeCicca, M.; Patel, C.A.; Marzouk, F.; Giangola, G. Early follow-up and treatment recommendations for isolated calf deep venous thrombosis. *J. Vasc. Surg.* **2012**, *55*, 136–140. [CrossRef] [PubMed]
11. Kearon, C.; Akl, E.A.; Comerota, A.J.; Prandoni, P.; Bounameaux, H.; Goldhaber, S.Z.; Nelson, M.E.; Wells, P.S.; Gould, M.K.; Dentali, F.; et al. Antithrombotic therapy for VTE disease: Antithrombotic Therapy and Prevention of Thrombosis, 9th ed: American College of Chest Physicians Evidence-Based Clinical Practice Guidelines. *Chest* **2012**, *141*, e419S–e496S. [CrossRef]
12. Seinturier, C.; Bosson, J.L.; Colonna, M.; Imbert, B.; Carpentier, P.H. Site and clinical outcome of deep vein thrombosis of the lower limbs: An epidemiological study. *J. Thromb. Haemost.* **2005**, *3*, 1362–1367. [CrossRef] [PubMed]
13. Palareti, G.; Agnelli, G.; Imberti, D.; Moia, M.; Ageno, W.; Pistelli, R.; Rossi, R.; Verso, M. Do Italian vascular centers look for isolated calf deep vein thrombosis? Analysis of isolated calf deep vein thromboses included in the "Master" Registry. *Int. Angiol.* **2008**, *27*, 482–488. [PubMed]
14. Young, A.M.; Marshall, A.; Thirlwall, J.; Chapman, O.; Lokare, A.; Hill, C.; Hale, D.; Dunn, J.A.; Lyman, G.H.; Hutchinson, C. Comparison of an oral factor Xa inhibitor with low molecular weight heparin in patients with cancer with venous thromboembolism: Results of a randomized trial (SELECT-D). *J. Clin. Oncol.* **2018**, *36*, 2017–2023. [CrossRef] [PubMed]
15. Raskob, G.E.; van Es, N.; Verhamme, P.; Carrier, M.; Di Nisio, M.; Garcia, D.; Michael, A.; Grosso, M.A.; Kakkar, A.K.; Kovacs, M.J.; et al. Edoxaban for the Treatment of Cancer-Associated Venous Thromboembolism. *N. Engl. J. Med.* **2018**, *378*, 615–624. [CrossRef]

16. Agnelli, G.; Becattini, C.; Meyer, G.; Muñoz, A.; Huisman, M.V.; Connors, J.M.; Cohen, A.; Bauersachs, R.; Brenner, B.; Torbicki, A.; et al. Apixaban for the Treatment of Venous Thromboembolism Associated with Cancer. *N. Engl. J. Med.* **2020**, *382*, 1599–1607. [CrossRef] [PubMed]
17. Ogino, Y.; Ishigami, T.; Minamimoto, Y.; Kimura, Y.; Akiyama, E.; Okada, K.; Matsuzawa, K.; Maejima, N.; Iwahashi, N.; Hibi, K.; et al. Direct Oral Anticoagulant Therapy for Cancer-Associated Venous Thromboembolism in Routine Clinical Practice. *Circ. J.* **2020**, *84*, 1330–1338. [CrossRef]
18. Khorana, A.A.; Noble, S.; Lee, A.Y.Y.; Soff, G.; Meyer, G.; O'Connell, C.; Carrier, M. Role of direct oral anticoagulants in the treatment of cancer-associated venous thromboembolism: Guidance from the SSC of the ISTH. *J. Thromb. Haemost.* **2018**, *16*, 1891–1894. [CrossRef]
19. Macdonald, P.S.; Kahn, S.R.; Miller, N.; Obrand, D. Short-term natural history of isolated gastrocnemius and soleal vein thrombosis. *J. Vasc. Surg.* **2003**, *37*, 523–527. [CrossRef]
20. Schwarz, T.; Buschmann, L.; Beyer, J.; Halbritter, K.; Rastan, A.; Schellong, S. Therapy of isolated calf muscle vein thrombosis: A randomized, controlled study. *J. Vasc. Surg.* **2010**, *52*, 1246–1250. [CrossRef] [PubMed]
21. Ro, A.; Kageyama, N. Clinical significance of the soleal vein and related drainage veins, in calf vein thrombosis in autopsy cases with massive pulmonary thromboembolism. *Ann. Vasc. Dis.* **2016**, *9*, 15–21. [CrossRef] [PubMed]
22. Mukai, M.; Oka, T. Mechanism and management of cancer-associated thrombosis. *J. Cardiol.* **2018**, *72*, 89–93. [CrossRef]

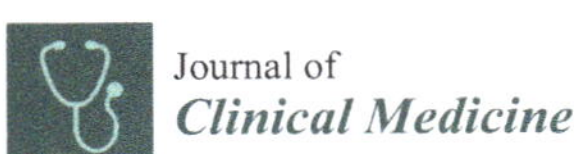
Journal of
Clinical Medicine
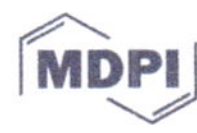

Review

Effects of SGLT2 Inhibitors on Atherosclerosis: Lessons from Cardiovascular Clinical Outcomes in Type 2 Diabetic Patients and Basic Researches

Jing Xu [1,†], Taro Hirai [1,†], Daisuke Koya [1,2,3] and Munehiro Kitada [1,2,*]

1 Department of Diabetology and Endocrinology, Kanazawa Medical University, Uchinada, Ishikawa 920-0293, Japan; xujing@kanazawa-med.ac.jp (J.X.); taro-h@kanazawa-med.ac.jp (T.H.); koya0516@kanazawa-med.ac.jp (D.K.)
2 Division of Anticipatory Molecular Food Science and Technology, Medical Research Institute, Kanazawa Medical University, Uchinada, Ishikawa 920-0293, Japan
3 Omi Medical Center, Omi General Hospital, Kusatsu, Shiga 525-8585, Japan
* Correspondence: kitta@kanazawa-med.ac.jp; Tel.: +81-76-2211
† These authors contributed equally to this work.

Abstract: Atherosclerosis-caused cardiovascular diseases (CVD) are the leading cause of mortality in type 2 diabetes mellitus (T2DM). Sodium-glucose cotransporter 2 (SGLT2) inhibitors are effective oral drugs for the treatment of T2DM patients. Multiple pre-clinical and clinical studies have indicated that SGLT2 inhibitors not only reduce blood glucose but also confer benefits with regard to body weight, insulin resistance, lipid profiles and blood pressure. Recently, some cardiovascular outcome trials have demonstrated the safety and cardiovascular benefits of SGLT2 inhibitors beyond glycemic control. The SGLT2 inhibitors empagliflozin, canagliflozin, dapagliflozin and ertugliflozin reduce the rates of major adverse cardiovascular events and of hospitalization for heart failure in T2DM patients regardless of CVD. The potential mechanisms of SGLT2 inhibitors on cardioprotection may be involved in improving the function of vascular endothelial cells, suppressing oxidative stress, inhibiting inflammation and regulating autophagy, which further protect from the progression of atherosclerosis. Here, we summarized the pre-clinical and clinical evidence of SGLT2 inhibitors on cardioprotection and discussed the potential molecular mechanisms of SGLT2 inhibitors in preventing the pathogenesis of atherosclerosis and CVD.

Keywords: SGLT2 inhibitors; atherosclerosis; cardiovascular disease; diabetes

Citation: Xu, J.; Hirai, T.; Koya, D.; Kitada, M. Effects of SGLT2 Inhibitors on Atherosclerosis: Lessons from Cardiovascular Clinical Outcomes in Type 2 Diabetic Patients and Basic Researches. *J. Clin. Med.* **2022**, *11*, 137. https://doi.org/10.3390/jcm11010137

Academic Editor: Tomoaki Ishigami

Received: 1 December 2021
Accepted: 24 December 2021
Published: 27 December 2021

Publisher's Note: MDPI stays neutral with regard to jurisdictional claims in published maps and institutional affiliations.

1. Introduction

Atherosclerosis is a chronic progressive disease characterized by the accumulation and deposition of lipids and fibrous elements in large arteries [1]. Generally, the formation of atherosclerotic plaques is divided into four stages: fatty streaks, atheromatous plaques, complicated atheromatous plaques and clinical complications [2]. Plaque rupture and thromboembolism may lead to severe cardiovascular diseases (CVD), including acute coronary syndrome (ACS), myocardial infarction (MI) or stroke [1,3]. CVD caused by atherosclerosis is the main cause of mortality in metabolic-related diseases, especially in type 2 diabetes mellitus (T2DM) [4–6]. Correspondingly, compared with non-diabetic individuals, T2DM patients have a higher risk of atherosclerosis and CVD [7,8]. Over the last decade, CVD globally affected approximately 32.2% of T2DM patients, accounting for 9.9% of deaths among them [9]. Therefore, in recent years, clinical trials of anti-diabetic agents have not only focused on hypoglycemic benefits but on cardiovascular safety and cardioprotective effects as well.

Sodium-glucose cotransporter 2 (SGLT2) is mainly localized in the proximal tubule, which is responsible for reabsorbing 80–90% of filtered glucose under physiological conditions [10,11]. The direct effect of SGLT2 inhibitors is to block glucose transportation in the kidney, which may depend on two distinct mechanisms: (1) by augmenting renal glucose excretion and (2) by ameliorating glucotoxicity [10]. Multiple clinical trials have demonstrated that SGLT2 inhibitors reduce blood glucose by inhibiting the reabsorption of filtered glucose in the proximal tubules independent of insulin. SGLT2 inhibitors slow the progression of macroalbuminuria, reduce the doubling of the serum creatinine level, sustain 40% reduction in the estimated glomerular filtration rate (eGFR) and further protect from inevitable renal replacement therapy or death from renal disease [12–16]. These renoprotective benefits of SGLT2 inhibitors may be attributed to glycemic control, reducing body weight, lipid profiles, blood pressure and uric acid and improving insulin resistance. Moreover, due to the improvement of these cardiovascular risk factors, SGLT2 inhibitors also present cardioprotective effects [10–19].

In this review, we summarized the clinical evidence of SGLT2 inhibitors on cardioprotection and discussed the potential molecular mechanisms of SGLT2 inhibitors in preventing the pathogenesis of atherosclerosis and CVD.

2. Pathophysiological and Pharmacologic Roles of SGLT2 Inhibition

The kidney is a crucial organ for maintaining glucose metabolism. In healthy individuals, the human kidney filters more than 180 g of glucose per day. SGLT2 is a 75 kilodalton (kDa) protein coded by the solute carrier family 5 (SLC5A2) gene in humans and is mainly localized in the kidney proximal tubule [20]. A total of 80–90% of filtered glucose is reabsorbed by SGLT2 in the early proximal tubule, while the remaining 10–20% is absorbed by SGLT1. The energy for the transport capacity of SGLT2 and SGLT1 is derived from the Na^+/K^+ ATPase pump located in the basolateral membrane of the proximal tubule. Therefore, the reabsorption of filtered glucose is also accompanied by Na^+ reabsorption [10,18,21]. SGLT2 knockout mice had glucosuria and polyuria compared with wildtype mice [22]. In patients with T2DM, the reabsorption of filtered glucose in the proximal tubules is significantly increased, contributing to elevated SGLT2 expression [23,24]. Meanwhile, the elevated reabsorption of Na^+ activates the local renin-angiotensin system, stimulating the constriction of the adjacent efferent arteriole and dilation of the afferent arteriole, which leads to increases in intraglomerular pressure and glomerular filtration rate (GFR), which ultimately results in glomerular damage [10]. This evidence indicates that the inhibition of SGLT2 is a potential target for glycemic control and conferring renoprotection in treating T2DM.

The first natural SGLT inhibitor, called phlorizin, is derived from fruit trees. Phlorizin functions as a competitive inhibitor of SGLT1/2 to block glucose absorption in the proximal renal tubule and mucosa of the small intestine [25,26]. However, due to poor solubility in water, poor oral bioavailability, the non-selective inhibition of both SGLT1 and SGLT2 and a short half-life, effective studies on the mechanisms of specific SGLT2 inhibition by phlorizin are limited [25,27]. Subsequently, more novel selective SGLT2 inhibitors have been identified. Compared with phlorizin, these SGLT2 inhibitors are structurally improved. Dapagliflozin contains C-glucoside, while canagliflozin and empagliflozin contain C-glycosylated diarylmethane pharmacophore. These structures are resistant to hydrolysis by β-glucosidases to increase their half-life and specificity to SGLT2 [27,28]. To date, empagliflozin, canagliflozin, dapagliflozin and ertugliflozin have been approved by the United States Food and Drug Administration (FDA) and the European Medicines Agency (EMA) for the treatment of T2DM [26]. Some other novel SGLT2 inhibitors, such as ipragliflozin and luseogliflozin, have been approved in Japan and other countries [29,30].

3. Mechanisms of SGLT2 Inhibitors against Atherosclerosis

During the formation of atherosclerotic plaques, three types of cells, endothelial cells (ECs), vascular smooth muscle cells (VSMCs) and monocytes/macrophages, play crucial roles. At the first stage, due to endothelial dysfunction, excessive lipids and lipoproteins accumulate in the subendothelial matrix. This process is triggered by the accumulation of oxidized low-density lipoprotein (Ox-LDL), which stimulates the release of pro-inflammatory cytokines, including interleukin 8 (IL-8) and adhesion molecules such as intercellular cell adhesion molecule-1 (ICAM-1), Vascular cell adhesion protein 1 (VCAM-1), monocyte chemoattractant protein 1 (MCP-1) and macrophage colony-stimulating factor (M-CSF). Then, circulating monocytes migrate to the intima, where they proliferate, differentiate into macrophages and combine with lipoproteins to form foam cells. Monocytes/macrophages express pro-inflammatory cytokines, including IL-1 and tumor necrosis factor α (TNFα). VSMCs migrating from the medial layer can also secret pro-fibrosis molecules. With the continuous migration of monocytes into the intima and the accumulation of lipids and lipoproteins, foam cells and SMCs die to form necrotic cores. Platelets will recruit to form thrombi and eventually develop atherosclerotic plaques. Vascular occlusion or plaque rupture may result in acute cardiovascular and cerebrovascular events [1,3,31].

Some metabolic characteristics, including obesity, dyslipidemia, hyperglycemia and hypertension, are independent risk factors for atherosclerosis [32]. These metabolic disorders, which may lead to endothelial dysfunction, oxidative stress, inflammation and the impairment of autophagy, participate in the formation of plaques and the pathogenesis of atherosclerosis [33]. A series of basic studies have confirmed that SGLT2 inhibitors have cardioprotective effects beyond glucose control in animal models of atherosclerosis [34–38]. The underlying mechanisms of SGLT2 inhibitors may be related to protecting endothelial function, anti-oxidative stress, anti-inflammation and maintaining basal and adaptive autophagy (Figure 1).

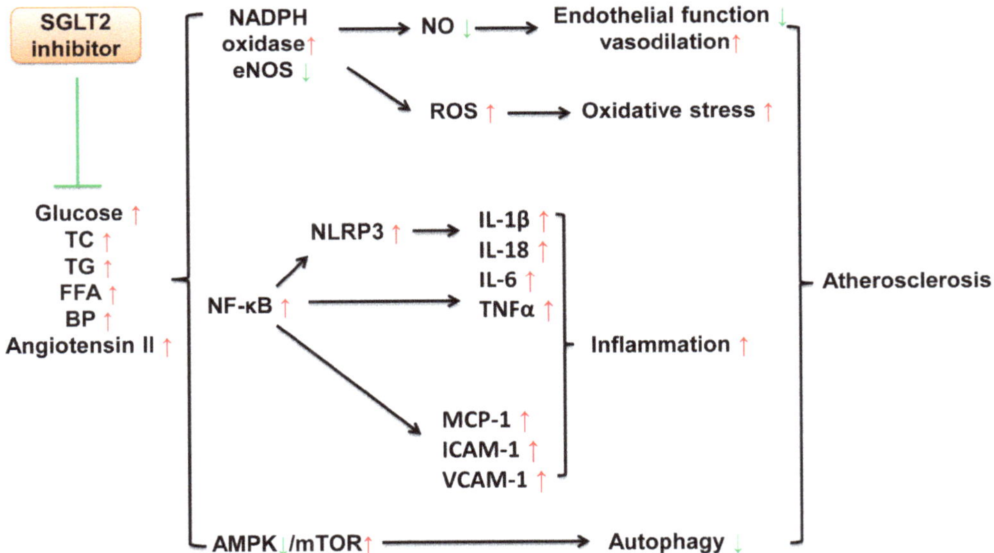

Figure 1. Mechanisms of SGLT2 inhibitors against atherosclerosis. Elevated metabolic characteristics including glucose, TC, TG, FFA, BP and angiotensin II accelerate the progression of atherosclerosis via the dysregulation of endothelial function, vasodilation and autophagy and activating oxidative stress and inflammation. SGLT2 inhibitors attenuate the alterations caused by these metabolic changes. TC, total cholesterol; TG, triglyceride; FFA, free fatty acid; BP, blood pressure; NADPH, nicotinamide adenine dinucleotide phosphate; NO, nitric oxide; eNOS, endothelial nitric oxide synthase; ROS, reactive oxygen species; NF-κB, nuclear factor kappa-B; NLRP3, nucleotide-binding oligomerization domain-like receptor family pyrin domain containing 3; IL, interleukin; TNFα, tumor necrosis factor α; MCP-1, monocyte chemoattractant protein 1; ICAM-1, intercellular cell adhesion molecule-1; VCAM-1, vascular cell adhesion protein 1; AMPK, AMP-activated protein kinase; mTOR, mechanistic target of rapamycin; ↑, increase; ↓, decrease.

3.1. Maintaining Endothelial Function

Endogenous nitric oxide (NO) is a vasodilatory molecule produced by NO synthase (NOS), which presents antiatherosclerotic effects [39]. SGLT2 inhibitors inhibit cardiac Na^+/K^+ exchange to induce vasodilation [40]. Previous studies have shown that SGLT2 inhibitors can participate in the regulation of vasodilation by increasing the anabolism and bioavailability of NO. Both empagliflozin and canagliflozin ameliorated aortic stiffness and improved vasodilation via endothelial NOS (eNOS) phosphorylation in db/db mice and non-diabetic rats [41,42]. Empagliflozin and dapagliflozin restored NO bioavailability by suppressing reactive oxygen species (ROS) generation in TNFα-induced ECs [43].

3.2. Anti-Oxidative Stress

An imbalance between the production and scavenging of ROS results in oxidative stress, which plays crucial roles in the progression of atherosclerosis [44]. Multiple risk factors of atherosclerosis, such as high glucose, elevated free fatty acids (FFA) and triglyceride (TG), can increase ROS production via activating nicotinamide adenine dinucleotide phosphate (NADPH) oxidases (NOX1-5, p22phox, p47phox), inhibiting NOS and suppressing glyceraldehyde 3-phosphate dehydrogenase (GAPDH) activity, and then by further amplifying oxidative stress in macrophages, ECs and adipocytes and accelerating the formation of atherosclerotic plaques [45–48].

Both in vitro and in vivo experiments have confirmed the anti-oxidative stress effects of SGLT2 inhibitors. Angiotensin II can induce SGLT2 expression in ECs, which leads to the activation of oxidative stress due to NADPH oxidase. Empagliflozin presented anti-oxidant effects to protect against endothelial senescence and dysfunction via suppressing the NADPH oxidase/SGLT2 pathway [49]. Canagliflozin reduced the expression of NADPH oxidase, including NOX2, NOX4, p22phox and p47phox, and reduced the urinary excretion of 8-hydroxy-2′ -deoxyguanosine (8-OHdG) in diabetic Apolipoprotein E-deficient ($ApoE^{-/-}$) mice [50]. Both empagliflozin and dapagliflozin inhibited the production of ROS, ameliorated TNFα-induced oxidative stress and restored impaired NO bioavailability in human umbilical vein endothelial cells (HUVECs) and human coronary arterial endothelial cells (HCAECs) [43]. SGLT2 inhibitors, including canagliflozin, dapagliflozin and empagliflozin, protected from high-glucose-induced vasodilation disorders via suppressing NAPDH oxidase/ROS signaling in cultured ECs [51].

3.3. Anti-Inflammation

Inflammatory cytokines and inflammatory cascade reactions throughout participate in the formation, progression and rupture of atherosclerotic plaque [1,31]. Previous studies have revealed that SGLT2 inhibitors, including dapagliflozin, empagliflozin, canagliflozin and luseogliflozin, reduced a series of pro-inflammatory cytokines, including IL-1β, IL-18 [34], IL-6 and TNFα [35], and adhesion molecules such as MCP-1 [35,38,52,53], ICAM-1 [36,50] and VCAM-1 [50,52,53] in atherosclerosis animal models with or without diabetes. In vitro studies have explored the potential mechanisms of the anti-inflammatory effects of SGLT2 inhibitors. Dapagliflozin may inhibit high glucose-induced TNFα, MCP-1 and VCAM-1 via suppressing the nuclear factor kappa-B (NF-κB) pathway in human vascular endothelial cells [54]. Canagliflozin suppressed IL-1β-activated cytokine and chemokine, such as IL-6 and MCP-1, partly via AMP-activated protein kinase (AMPK) activation [55].

In addition to inflammatory pathways, inflammasome-mediated inflammatory pathways are also involved in the pathogenesis of atherosclerosis [56–58]. Ox-LDL and high glucose are responsible for the activation of the nucleotide-binding oligomerization domain-like receptor family pyrin domain containing 3 (NLRP3) inflammasome [56,59]. NLRP3 is essential for activating the precursors of IL-1β and IL-18 into their mature forms, which recruit in vascular endothelial cells, leading to atherothrombosis [58]. NF-κB promotes the transcription of NLRP3 and participates in cardiac inflammation [60], which links inflammasome and the inflammatory pathway. Moreover, TG and very low-density lipoprotein (VLDL)-related arterial inflammation are closely related to the nucleotide-binding oligomerization domain-like receptor family pyrin domain containing 1 (NLRP1) inflammasome activation in ECs [61]. Dapagliflozin inhibited IL-1β expression via NLRP3/caspase 1 signaling in streptozotocin (STZ)-induced diabetic ApoE$^{-/-}$ mice and T2DM rodent models [34,62,63]. Empagliflozin suppressed IL-17A-induced IL-1β and IL-18 secretions via NLRP3/caspase1 signaling and further inhibited the cell proliferation and migration of human aortic SMCs [64] and decreased the expression of IL-1β via suppressing NF-κB phosphorylation/NLRP3 signaling in human macrophages [62].

3.4. Regulation of Autophagy

Autophagy plays a complex role in the pathogenesis of atherosclerosis. Basal and mild adaptive autophagy to stress can maintain the endothelial functions of ECs, VSMCs and macrophages and protect against the formation of atherosclerotic plaques, while both deficient and excessive autophagy are related to inflammation, oxidative stress and apoptosis, which may contribute to autophagy-dependent cell death, aggravate vascular injury and lead to plaque instability or rupture [33,65,66]. Therefore, the precise regulation of autophagy is essential to prevent the development of atherosclerosis.

The SGLT2 inhibitors empagliflozin and dapagliflozin have been identified to restore autophagy deficiency in diabetic or obese rodent models, which mainly depends on the activation of nutrient-sensing pathways, such as the AMPK/mTOR (mechanistic target of rapamycin) signaling pathway [67,68]. In vitro studies have also identified several potential mechanisms. Empagliflozin restored autophagic flux impairment via activating AMPK and suppressing mTOR in H9c2 cells (rat cardiac myoblast) [69], RAW264.7 and THP-1 cells (macrophage cell lines) [70]. Our previous study also indicated that dapagliflozin had similar effects on autophagy restoration via AMPK/mTOR signaling in high-glucose-treated proximal tubular cells [71].

4. Improvements of Indicators Related to CVD by SGLT2 Inhibitor

Disorders of metabolic-related characteristics, including glucose, lipid profiles, blood pressure, uric acid, etc., contribute to increased risks of developing atherosclerosis and CVD [33]. Beyond the benefits from glycemic control, multiple clinical and rodent research studies have demonstrated that the cardiovascular benefits of SGLT2 inhibitors are closely related to the improvement of these metabolic-related characteristics.

4.1. Pre-Clinical Evidence

ApoE$^{-/-}$ mice and low density lipoprotein receptor knockout (Ldlr$^{-/-}$) mice are well-established and extensively used rodent models of atherosclerosis [72]. Multiple studies have demonstrated that SGLT2 inhibitors, including dapagliflozin, empagliflozin, canagliflozin, luseogliflzin and ipragliflozin, reduce metabolic indicators to protect from the progression of atherosclerosis (Table 1). Dapagliflozin reduced fasting blood glucose (FBG), total cholesterol (TC) and TG [34], body weight, and glycosylated hemoglobin (HbA1c) [73] in STZ-induced diabetic ApoE$^{-/-}$ mice and STZ-induced diabetic Ldlr$^{-/-}$ mice [37]. Empagliflozin ameliorated FBG, TC, heart rate, blood pressure (BP) [53], TG, LDL [74], urinary microalbumin, body weight and fat mass [35,74] in high fat diet (HFD)-fed ApoE$^{-/-}$ mice and reduced body weight and TG in STZ-induced diabetic ApoE$^{-/-}$ mice [38]. Canagliflozin decreased glucose, TC, TG, LDL and heart rate in HFD-fed diabetic ApoE$^{-/-}$ mice [52] and reduced TC and glucose in STZ-induced diabetic ApoE$^{-/-}$ mice [50]. Luseogliflozin reduced body weight, TC, TG, BP and glucose in HFD-fed mice [75] and nicotinamide in STZ-induced diabetic ApoE$^{-/-}$ mice [36]. Ipragliflozin decreased body weight and glucose to inhibit vascular remodeling in HFD-fed mice [76]. All these metabolic changes ameliorate vascular remodeling, reduce plaque size and increase plaque stability to protect from the progression of atherosclerosis.

Table 1. Benefits of SGLT2 inhibitors in atherosclerotic rodents.

SGLT2 Inhibitors	Atherosclerotic Rodents	Changes of Metabolic Characteristics	References
Dapagliflozin	STZ-induced diabetic ApoE$^{-/-}$ mice	FBG↓, TC↓, TG↓ body weight↓, HbA1c↓	[34,73]
Dapagliflozin	STZ-induced diabetic Ldlr$^{-/-}$ mice	FBG↓, TC↓, TG↓ body weight↓	[37]
Empagliflozin	HFD-fed ApoE$^{-/-}$ mice	FBG↓, TC↓, heart rate↓, BP↓ TG↓, LDL↓, urinary microalbumin↓, body weight↓	[35,53,74]
Empagliflozin	STZ-induced diabetic ApoE$^{-/-}$ mice	body weight↓, TG↓	[38]
Canagliflozin	HFD-fed diabetic ApoE$^{-/-}$ mice	glucose↓, TC↓, TG↓, LDL↓, heart rate↓	[52]
Canagliflozin	STZ-induced diabetic ApoE$^{-/-}$ mice	TC↓, glucose↓	[50]
Luseogliflozin	HFD-fed mice	body weight↓, TC↓, TG↓, BP↓, glucose↓	[75]
Luseogliflozin	STZ-induced diabetic ApoE$^{-/-}$ mice	body weight↓, TC↓, TG↓, BP↓, glucose↓	[36]
Ipragliflozin	HFD-fed mice	body weight↓, glucose↓	[76]

↓, decrease; STZ, streptozotocin; Apo E, Apolipoprotein E; Ldlr, low density lipoprotein receptor; HFD, high fat diet; FBG, fasting blood glucose; TC, total cholesterol; TG, triglycerides; HbA1c, glycosylated hemoglobin; LDL, low-density lipoprotein; BP, blood pressure.

In addition to these risk factors of CVD, T2DM patients treated with SGLT2 inhibitors showed elevated plasma ketone levels [77]. SGLT2 inhibitors reduce plasma glucose concentration by increasing renal glucose excretion. To meet the energy requirements of cellules, lipid oxidation is activated, leading to the increasing of acetyl coenzyme A (CoA). Acetyl CoA can enter the Krebs cycle to be converted to ketones (acetoacetate and β-hydroxybutyrate). Moreover, enhanced lipolysis in the adipocyte leads to the increase of plasma FFA, which can also be converted to acetyl CoA via β oxidation and subsequently to ketones in the liver [10]. The elevated ketones may improve the energy metabolism of the heart. Previous studies indicated that β-hydroxybutyrateas is a strong anti-inflammatory factor. Empagliflozin can significantly increase serum β-hydroxybutyrateas to inhibit NLRP3 inflammasome and reduce the expression of IL-1β levels, which benefit from CVD [62] (Figure 2).

4.2. Clinical Evidence

SGLT2 inhibitors not only reduce high glucose independent of insulin but also improve systolic blood pressure (SBP), body weight, lipid profile and uric acid, which are considered high risk factors for CVD [10] (Figure 2). The improvement of these metabolic indicators may play a crucial role in protecting against the pathogenesis of atherosclerosis and CVD. Numerous clinical trials have confirmed that SGLT2 inhibitors can effectively reduce body weight, which may be related to increases in fat utilization, reductions in adipose tissue mass and browning in white adipose tissue, further attenuating obesity-induced insulin resistance [78–82]. Treatment with empagliflozin [83–85], canagliflozin [82,86–88] and ertugliflozin [89] reduced SBP in patients with T2DM and hypertension or patients with T2DM and chronic kidney disease (CKD). This benefit may be related to minimal natriuresis and urinary glucose excretion, which lead to weight loss, osmotic diuresis, reduced plasma volume and arterial stiffness [90]. SGLT2 inhibitors also lead to a small decrease in plasma TG, increases in high-density lipoprotein cholesterol (HDL-C) and a small increase in LDL [82,91–93]. A potential mechanism of increased LDL and decreased

TG with SGLT2 inhibition may be related to the reduction of LDL clearance, the greater lipolysis of triglyceride-rich lipoproteins [94] and the effect of switching energy metabolism from carbohydrate to lipid utilization [95]. Elevated circulating uric acid is associated with the risk of hypertension and CVD. Multiple studies have demonstrated that SGLT2 inhibitors can reduce circulating uric acid via enhancing urinary uric acid excretion in association with increased urinary glucose [96–98], which may benefit patients with CVD.

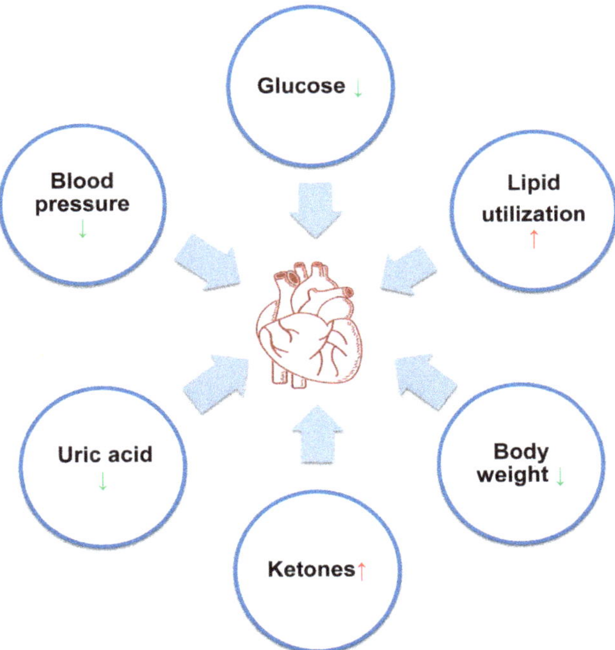

Figure 2. Improvements of some CVD-related clinical indicators by SGLT2 inhibitors. SGLT2 inhibitors not only reduce high glucose independent of insulin but also improve blood pressure, body weight, lipid profile and ketones and uric acid to present cardioprotective effects; ↑, increase; ↓, decrease.

5. Clinical Evidence of SGLT2 Inhibitors against CVD

Since 2008, the FDA has required that cardiovascular outcome trials (CVOTs) be carried out for new anti-diabetic drugs due to the significance of cardioprotection on T2DM patients. All potential drugs should exclude the major adverse cardiovascular events (MACE) defined in the FDA guidance, including non-fatal myocardial infarction, non-fatal stroke and cardiovascular death [99,100]. Furthermore, the effect of SGLT2 inhibitors on cardiovascular outcomes, including hospitalization for heart failure, death and CVD, compared to other glucose-lowering drugs, was also verified in a real clinical practice [101,102].

5.1. Randomized Controlled Trials (RCTs)

A meta-analysis that summarized 6 regulatory submissions and 57 published trials revealed that seven different SGLT2 inhibitors reduced the risk of Major Adverse Cardiovascular Events (MACEs) and death from any cause [103]. In this section, we summarized some landmark CVOTs of SGLT2 inhibitors (Table 2).

Table 2. Reported cardiovascular outcome trials of SGLT2 inhibitors.

	EMPA-REG OUTCOME [104]	EMPEROR-Reduced [105,106]	EMPEROR-Preserved [107]	CANVAS [19]	CREDENCE [14]	DECLARE- TIMI 58 [108]	DAPA-HF [109]	VERTIS CV [110]	SOLOIST-WHF [111]	SCORED [112]
Drug	empagliflozin	empagliflozin	empagliflozin	canagliflozin	canagliflozin	dapagliflozin	dapagliflozin	ertugliflozin	sotaglflozin	sotaglflozin
Patients	7020 (T2DM and CVD)	3730 (NYHA class II, III, or IV heart failure, EF ≤ 40%, 50% were DM)	5988 (NYHA class II-IV and EF ≥ 40%)	10,142 (T2DM)	4401 (T2DM and CKD)	17,160 (T2DM)	4744 (NYHA class II, III, or IV heart failure, EF ≤ 40%, 45% were T2DM)	8238 (T2DM and CVD)	1222 (T2DM and heart failure	10,584 (T2DM and CKD)
Duration of diabetes	≥10 years	-	-	13.5 ± 7.8	15.8 ± 8.6	11 (6–16)	-	12.9 ± 8.3	-	-
Median follow-up	3.1 years	16 months	26.2 months	126.1 weeks	2.62 years	4.2 years	3.5 years	3.5 years	9.0 months	16 months
Primary outcome *	0.86 (0.74–0.99)	0.76 (0.67–0.87)	0.79 (0.69–0.90)	0.86 (0.75–0.97)	0.70 (0.59–0.82)	0.93 (0.84–1.03)	0.74 (0.65–0.85)	0.97 (0.85–1.11)	0.67 (0.52–0.85)	0.74 (0.63–0.88)
Cardiovascular death	0.62 (0.49–0.77)	-	0.91 (0.76–1.09)	0.87 (0.72–1.06)	0.78 (0.61–1.00)	0.98 (0.82–1.17)	0.82 (0.69–0.98)	0.92 (0.77–1.11)	0.84 (0.58–1.22)	0.90 (0.73–1.12)
Nonfatal MI	0.87 (0.70–1.09)	-	-	0.85 (0.69–1.05)	-	0.89 (0.77–1.01)	-	1.04 (0.86–1. 27)	-	-
Nonfatal stroke	1.24 (0.92–1.67)	-	-	0.90 (0.71–1.15)	-	1.01 (0.84–1.21)	-	1.00 (0.76–1.32)	-	-
Death from any cause	0.68 (0.57–0.82)	-	1.00 (0.87–1.15)	0.87 (0.74–1.01)	0.83 (0.68–1.02)	0.93 (0.82–1.04)	0.83 (0.71–0.97)	0.93 (0.80–1.08)	0.82 (0.59–1.14)	0.99 (0.83–1.18)
Hospitalization for heart failure	0.65 (0.50–0.85)	0.70 (0.58–0.85)	0.71 (0.60–0.83)	0.67 (0.52–0.87)	0.61 (0.47–0.80)	0.73 (0.61–0.88)	0.70 (0.59–0.83)	0.70 (0.54–0.90)	0.64 (0.49–0.83)	0.67 (0.55–0.82)

EMPA-REG OUTCOME, Empagliflozin Cardiovascular Outcome Event Trial in Type 2 Diabetes Mellitus Patients–Removing Excess Glucose; EMPEROR-Reduced, Empagliflozin Outcome Trial in Patients with Chronic Heart Failure with Reduced Ejection Fraction; EMPEROR-Preserved, Empagliflozin Outcome Trial in Patients with Chronic Heart Failure with Preserved Ejection Fraction; CANVAS, Canagliflozin Cardiovascular Assessment Study; CREDENCE, Canagliflozin and Renal Events in Diabetes with Established Nephropathy Clinical Evaluation; DECLARE–TIMI 58, Dapagliflozin Effect on Cardiovascular Events–Thrombolysis in Myocardial Infarction 58; DAPA-HF, Dapagliflozin and Prevention of Adverse Outcomes in Heart Failure; VERTIS CV, Ertugliflozin Efficacy and Safety Cardiovascular Outcomes Trial; SOLOIST-WHF, the Effect of Sotagliflozin on Cardiovascular Events in Patients with Type 2 Diabetes Post Worsening Heart Failure; SCORED, the Effect of Sotagliflozin on Cardiovascular and Renal Events in Patients with Type 2 Diabetes and Moderate Renal Impairment Who Are at Cardiovascular Risk; T2DM, type 2 diabetes mellitus; CKD, chronic kidney diseases; NYHA, New York Heart Association; CVD, cardiovascular diseases; EF, ejection fraction; MI, myocardial infarction. * Primary outcomes of RCTs: EMPA-REG OUTCOME, CANVAS, CREDENCE, DECLARE–TIMI 58, VERTIS CV: MACE (the major adverse cardiovascular events including a composite of death from cardiovascular causes, nonfatal myocardial infarction or nonfatal stroke); EMPEROR-Reduced, EMPEROR-Preserved: the composite of cardiovascular death or hospitalization for heart failure; DAPA-HF: a composite of worsening heart failure (hospitalization or an urgent visit resulting in intravenous therapy for heart failure) or cardiovascular death; SOLOIST-WHF, SCORED: the total number of deaths from cardiovascular causes and hospitalizations and urgent visits for heart failure.

The Empagliflozin Cardiovascular Outcome Event Trial in Type 2 Diabetes Mellitus Patients–Removing Excess Glucose trial (EMPA-REG OUTCOME) was the first CVOT to determine the cardiovascular benefits of SGLT2 inhibitors. This trial enrolled T2DM patients, who were treated with either empagliflozin or placebo. The primary composite outcome was MACEs. Compared with the placebo group, the empagliflozin group showed a significant reduction in death from MACEs, hospitalization for heart failure and death from any cause. However, there were no significant benefits for MI and stroke [104]. Subsequently, two trials demonstrated cardiovascular benefits in patients with heart failure and a reduced ejection fraction. The Empagliflozin Outcome Trial in Patients with Chronic Heart Failure with Reduced Ejection Fraction (EMPEROR-Reduced) enrolled 3730 patients (50% diagnosed as diabetes) with New York Heart Association (NYHA) class II to IV heart failure or with an ejection fraction (EF) $\leq$40%. Compared with the placebo group, the empagliflozin group had a lower risk of any inpatient or outpatient worsening heart failure event regardless of T2DM [105,106]. The Empagliflozin Outcome Trial in Patients with Chronic Heart Failure with Preserved Ejection Fraction (EMPEROR-Preserved) trial also identified the benefits of empagliflozin on heart failure in patients with NYHA class II to IV and an EF $\geq$40% [107].

The cardiovascular benefits of canagliflozin were demonstrated by the Canagliflozin Cardiovascular Assessment Study (CANVAS) and Canagliflozin and Renal Events in Diabetes with Established Nephropathy Clinical Evaluation (CREDENCE). CANVAS involved patients with T2DM, who were treated with canagliflozin or placebo. The primary outcome was also MACEs. Similar to empagliflozin, canagliflozin showed a significant reduction in MACEs, hospitalization for heart failure and death from any cause [19]. CREDENCE confirmed the cardio and renal benefits of canagliflozin in patients with T2DM and chronic kidney disease (CKD). The primary outcome was a composite of end-stage kidney disease or death from renal or cardiovascular disease. Patients in the canagliflozin group had a lower risk of cardiovascular death, MI, stroke and hospitalization for heart failure [14].

The Dapagliflozin Effect on Cardiovascular Events–Thrombolysis in Myocardial Infarction 58 (DECLARE–TIMI 58) evaluated the cardiovascular benefits of dapagliflozin on T2DM patients. The primary outcome was MACEs. Although dapagliflozin was not found to reduce the risk of MACEs, it reduced the risk of hospitalization for heart failure [108]. Another trial, named the Dapagliflozin and Prevention of Adverse Outcomes in Heart Failure (DAPA-HF) trial, confirmed this benefit. DAPA-HF enrolled patients with heart failure and reduced ejection fraction. The primary outcome was a composite of worsening heart failure or death from cardiovascular causes. This trial also demonstrated that dapagliflozin reduced the risk of heart failure hospitalization and cardiovascular death regardless of diabetes [109].

Ertugliflozin has also completed the assessment of cardiovascular events recently. The Evaluation of Ertugliflozin Efficacy and Safety Cardiovascular Outcomes Trial (VERTIS CV) enrolled patients with T2DM and established CVD. The primary outcome was MACEs. Similar to dapagliflozin, ertugliflozin was not found to reduce the risk of MACEs, but it did reduce the risk of hospitalization for heart failure [110].

In addition to the above SGLT2 inhibitors approved by the FDA and EMA for cardiovascular indications, another SGLT2 inhibitor, sotaliflozin, also present benefits for cardiovascular death and heart failure. The Effect of Sotagliflozin on Cardiovascular Events in Patients with Type 2 Diabetes Post Worsening Heart Failure (SOLOIST-WHF) and the Effect of Sotagliflozin on Cardiovascular and Renal Events in Patients with Type 2 Diabetes and Moderate Renal Impairment Who Are at Cardiovascular Risk (SCORED) trial demonstrated that, compared with placebo, sotaliflozin treatment significantly reduced the total number of deaths from cardiovascular causes and hospitalizations and urgent visits for heart failure in T2DM patients with recent worsening heart failure [111] and T2DM patients with chronic kidney disease regardless of albuminuria [112].

According to these hallmark CVOTs, the effects of SGLT2 inhibitors on atherosclerotic cardiovascular events, such as MI and strokes, are less impressive than the effects on heart failure (Table 2). A possible reason is the heterogeneity in the CVD risk of the study populations. Besides, SGLT2 inhibitors may primarily target on ameliorating cardiac structure and function ("the pump") and not on the "pipes" (coronary arteries) [113,114]. Patients with T2DM and cardiac hypertrophy, diastolic or systolic dysfunction or with a hypervolemic state (regardless of cardiac or renal origin) are the best candidates for treatment with SGLT2 inhibitors [114].

5.2. Multinational Observational Cohort Study

The effects of drugs may be different between the RCTs and real-world practice [115,116]. Because the characteristics of patients in the RCTs do not necessarily match the standard population with T2DM, these results are difficult to be generalized.

The Comparative Effectiveness of Cardiovascular Outcomes in New Users of SGLT2 inhibitors (CVD-REAL) Study is a multinational (USA, Sweden, Norway and Denmark) observational study. In this study, 309,056 patients newly initiated on either SGLT2 inhibitors, including empagliflozin, canagliflozin and dapagliflozin, or other glucose lowering drugs were analyzed on the risk for hospitalization for heart failure and death in patients with T2DM, using clinical data in real-world practice after propensity score matching [101]. There were 961 hospitalizations for heart failure cases during 190,164 person-years follow-up in 6 countries, and, of 215,622 patients in the United States, Norway, Denmark, Sweden and the United Kingdom, death occurred in 1334. The use of SGLT2 inhibitors was significantly associated with lower rates of hospitalization for heart failure and death, with no significant heterogeneity by country, compared to other glucose-lowering drugs (Table 3). In addition, the sub-analysis of the CVD-REAL study exhibited an association between the initiation of SGLT2 inhibitors versus other glucose-lowering drugs and the rates of MI and stroke. Overall, 205,160 patients were included, and, in the intent-to-treat analysis, over 188,551 and 188,678 person-years of follow-up (MI and stroke, respectively), there were 1077 MI and 968 stroke events. The initiation of SGLT2 inhibitors was associated with a modestly lower risk of MI and stroke [102] (Table 3).

Table 3. Reported real world evidence of SGLT2 inhibitors for CVD.

	CVD-REAL [101]	**Sub-Analysis of CVD-REAL [102]**	**CVD-REAL 2 [117]**	**Sub-Analysis of CVD-REAL 2 Study [118]**	**Retrospective Cohort Study on PAD Patients [119]**
Drug	empagliflozin, canagliflozin and dapagliflozin	empagliflozin, canagliflozin and dapagliflozin	canagliflozin, dapagliflozin, empagliflozin, in all countries; ipragliflozin in South Korea and Japan; tofogliflozin, luseogliflozin in Japan	canagliflozin, dapagliflozin and empagliflozin in all countries apart from South Korea; ipragliflozin in South Korea and Japan; Tofogliflozin and luseogliflozin in Japan only	empagliflozin and dapa gliflozin
Patients	309,056	205,160	470,128	386,248	22,862
Regions	European and North American regions	European and North American regions	the Asia-Pacific, Middle East and North American regions	the Asia-Pacific, Middle East, European and North American regions	the Asia-Pacific region
Duration of diabetes	≥1 years	≥1 years	≥1 years	≥1 years	-

Table 3. *Cont.*

	CVD-REAL [101]	Sub-Analysis of CVD-REAL [102]	CVD-REAL 2 [117]	Sub-Analysis of CVD-REAL 2 Study [118]	Retrospective Cohort Study on PAD Patients [119]
Mean follow-up *	239 days/ 211 days	254 days/ 232 days	374 days/ 392 days	Varied by country and regions	0.96 years/ 0.66 years
MI	-	0.85 (0.72–1.00)	0.81 (0.74–0.88)	0.88 (0.80–0.98)	0.84 (0.58–1.23)
Stroke	-	0.83 (0.71–0.97)	0.68 (0.55–0.84)	0.85 (0.77–0.93)	0.81 (0.62–1.06)
Death from any cause	0.49 (0.41–0.57)	-	0.51(0.37–0.70)	0.59 (0.52–0.67)	0.58 (0.49–0.67)
Hospitalizationfor heart failure	0.61 (0.51–0.73)	-	0.64 (0.50–0.82)	0.69 (0.61–0.77)	0.66 (0.49–0.89)

CVD-REAL, The Comparative Effectiveness of Cardiovascular Outcomes in New Users of SGLT2 inhibitors; PAD, peripheral artery disease; MI, myocardial infarction.* Mean follow-up: the mean follow-up time of SGLT2 inhibitors/ other glucose lowering drugs.

The CVD-REAL2 study is a similar study design to the CVD-REAL and was conducted in six countries: South Korea, Japan, Singapore, Israel, Australia and Canada [117]. After propensity score matching, the risks for death, hospitalization for heart failure, MI and stroke were analyzed in 235,064 patients of each group, newly initiated on either SGLT2 inhibitors (dapagliflozin, empagliflozin, ipragliflozin, canagliflozin, tofogliflozin and luseogliflozin) or other glucose-lowering drugs. In total, 74% of patients had no history of CVD, and patient characteristics were well-balanced in both groups. The initiation of SGLT2 inhibitors significantly reduced the risk for death, hospitalization for heart failure, MI and stroke [117] (Table 3).

In addition, a sub-analysis of the CVD-REAL-2 study showed that the initiation of SGLT2 inhibitors was associated with substantially lower risks of hospitalization for heart failure (HR 0.69, 95% CI 0.61–0.77; $p < 0.0001$), all-cause death (0.59, 0.52–0.67; $p < 0.0001$) and the composite of hospitalization for heart failure or all-cause death (0.64, 0.57–0.72; $p < 0.0001$) compared to dipeptidyl peptide-4 (DPP-4)-4 inhibitors [118]. Furthermore, in another retrospective cohort study, each of the 11,431 T2DM patients with peripheral artery disease (PAD) taking the SGLT2 inhibitor or DPP-4 inhibitor were analyzed for the risk for ischemic stroke and acute MI after propensity score matching. The use of the SGLT2 inhibitor had comparable risks of ischemic stroke and acute MI. However, the SGLT2 inhibitor group showed lower risks of congestive heart failure (HR: 0.66; 95% CI 0.49–0.89; $p = 0.0062$), lower limb ischemia requiring revascularization (HR: 0.73; 95% CI 0.54–0.98; $p = 0.0367$) or amputation (HR: 0.43; 95% CI 0.30–0.62; $p < 0.0001$) and cardiovascular death (HR: 0.67; 95% CI 0.49–0.90; $p = 0.0089$) compared to those in the DPP-4 inhibitor group. [119].

6. Perspectives and Conclusions

In recent years, as effective anti-diabetic agents, SGLT2 inhibitors have not only achieved significant results in glycemic control via increasing urinary glucose excretion independent of insulin but have also presented cardiovascular protective effects, especially in reducing the risk of MACEs and hospitalization from heart failure. Although data from the CVOTs indicated less impressive results on atherosclerotic cardiovascular events such as MI and stroke than on heart failure, some real-world practice indicated the benefits on them (Table 2). This may be related to the significant heterogeneity in the CVD risk of the study populations [113]. Clinical studies have confirmed the cardiovascular safety of SGLT2 inhibitors [19,104,108,110]. Although some common adverse events, including polyuria, genital mycotic infections, urinary tract infections and ketoacidosis, need to be carefully monitored for [19,104,108], they will not cause severe or fatal consequences. Besides, although patients need to be alerted to some other risks, such as amputation and fractures related to canagliflozin [19], there have not been significantly higher incidences than of other anti-diabetic drugs, such as glucagon-like peptide 1 receptor agonists (GLP-1RA) and

DPP-4 inhibitors [120]. Based on the safety, efficiency and cardiovascular benefits, pharmacologic recommendations from the guidelines of American Diabetes Association (ADA) recommend listing SGLT2 inhibitors for the treatment of T2DM patients with established high risk factors of atherosclerotic cardiovascular disease (ASCVD), ASCVD and heart failure [121]. The underlying mechanisms of SGLT2 inhibitors on cardioprotection may be related to improving the function of vascular endothelial cells, suppressing oxidative stress, inhibiting inflammation and regulating autophagy, which further protects from the progression of atherosclerosis. More studies are needed, however, to elucidate the underlying mechanisms.

Author Contributions: J.X., T.H., M.K. and D.K. contributed to drafting and writing the article. J.X., T.H., M.K. and D.K. contributed to the discussion of the review. M.K. and D.K. are responsible for the integrity of the content. All authors have read and agreed to the published version of the manuscript.

Funding: This research received no external funding.

Institutional Review Board Statement: Not applicable.

Informed Consent Statement: Not applicable.

Acknowledgments: Boehringer Ingelheim, Mitsubishi Tanabe Pharma, Taisho Pharmaceutical Co. and Ono Pharmaceutical Co. contributed to establishing the Division of Anticipatory Molecular Food Science and Technology. The authors declare that there are no conflicts of interest associated with this manuscript. The funders had no role in the interpretation or writing of the manuscript.

Conflicts of Interest: The authors declare that they have no conflict of interest.

References

1. Lusis, A.J. Atherosclerosis. *Nature* **2000**, *407*, 233–241. [CrossRef] [PubMed]
2. Hassanpour, M.; Rahbarghazi, R.; Nouri, M.; Aghamohammadzadeh, N.; Safaei, N.; Ahmadi, M. Role of autophagy in atherosclerosis: Foe or friend? *J. Inflam.* **2019**, *16*, 8. [CrossRef] [PubMed]
3. Weber, C.; Noels, H. Atherosclerosis: Current pathogenesis and therapeutic options. *Nat. Med.* **2011**, *17*, 1410–1422. [CrossRef]
4. Schneider, A.L.; Kalyani, R.R.; Golden, S.; Stearns, S.C.; Wruck, L.; Yeh, H.C.; Coresh, J.; Selvin, E. Diabetes and Prediabetes and Risk of Hospitalization: The Atherosclerosis Risk in Communities (ARIC) Study. *Diabetes Care* **2016**, *39*, 772–779. [CrossRef] [PubMed]
5. Lovren, F.; Teoh, H.; Verma, S. Obesity and atherosclerosis: Mechanistic insights. *Can. J. Cardiol.* **2015**, *31*, 177–183. [CrossRef]
6. Frohlich, E.D.; Susic, D. Blood pressure, large arteries and atherosclerosis. *Adv. Cardiol.* **2007**, *44*, 117–124. [CrossRef]
7. Low Wang, C.C.; Hess, C.N.; Hiatt, W.R.; Goldfine, A.B. Clinical Update: Cardiovascular Disease in Diabetes Mellitus: Atherosclerotic Cardiovascular Disease and Heart Failure in Type 2 Diabetes Mellitus—Mechanisms, Management, and Clinical Considerations. *Circulation* **2016**, *133*, 2459–2502. [CrossRef] [PubMed]
8. Beckman, J.A.; Creager, M.A. Vascular Complications of Diabetes. *Circul. Res.* **2016**, *118*, 1771–1785. [CrossRef] [PubMed]
9. Einarson, T.R.; Acs, A.; Ludwig, C.; Panton, U.H. Prevalence of cardiovascular disease in type 2 diabetes: A systematic literature review of scientific evidence from across the world in 2007–2017. *Cardiovasc. Diabetol.* **2018**, *17*, 83. [CrossRef]
10. DeFronzo, R.A.; Norton, L.; Abdul-Ghani, M. Renal, metabolic and cardiovascular considerations of SGLT2 inhibition. *Nat. Rev. Nephrol.* **2017**, *13*, 11–26. [CrossRef]
11. Fioretto, P.; Zambon, A.; Rossato, M.; Busetto, L.; Vettor, R. SGLT2 Inhibitors and the Diabetic Kidney. *Diabetes Care* **2016**, *39* (Suppl. 2), S165–S171. [CrossRef]
12. Wanner, C.; Inzucchi, S.E.; Lachin, J.M.; Fitchett, D.; von Eynatten, M.; Mattheus, M.; Johansen, O.E.; Woerle, H.J.; Broedl, U.C.; Zinman, B. Empagliflozin and Progression of Kidney Disease in Type 2 Diabetes. *N. Engl. J. Med.* **2016**, *375*, 323–334. [CrossRef] [PubMed]
13. Mosenzon, O.; Wiviott, S.D.; Cahn, A.; Rozenberg, A.; Yanuv, I.; Goodrich, E.L.; Murphy, S.A.; Heerspink, H.J.L.; Zelniker, T.A.; Dwyer, J.P.; et al. Effects of dapagliflozin on development and progression of kidney disease in patients with type 2 diabetes: An analysis from the DECLARE-TIMI 58 randomised trial. *Lancet. Diabetes Endocrinol.* **2019**, *7*, 606–617. [CrossRef]
14. Perkovic, V.; Jardine, M.J.; Neal, B.; Bompoint, S.; Heerspink, H.J.L.; Charytan, D.M.; Edwards, R.; Agarwal, R.; Bakris, G.; Bull, S.; et al. Canagliflozin and Renal Outcomes in Type 2 Diabetes and Nephropathy. *N. Engl. J. Med.* **2019**, *380*, 2295–2306. [CrossRef] [PubMed]
15. Cherney, D.Z.I.; Cosentino, F.; Dagogo-Jack, S.; McGuire, D.K.; Pratley, R.; Frederich, R.; Maldonado, M.; Liu, C.C.; Liu, J.; Pong, A.; et al. Ertugliflozin and Slope of Chronic eGFR: Prespecified Analyses from the Randomized VERTIS CV Trial. *Clin. J. Am. Soc. Nephrol. CJASN* **2021**, *16*, 1345–1354. [CrossRef]

16. Perkovic, V.; de Zeeuw, D.; Mahaffey, K.W.; Fulcher, G.; Erondu, N.; Shaw, W.; Barrett, T.D.; Weidner-Wells, M.; Deng, H.; Matthews, D.R.; et al. Canagliflozin and renal outcomes in type 2 diabetes: Results from the CANVAS Program randomised clinical trials. *Lancet Diabetes Endocrinol.* **2018**, *6*, 691–704. [CrossRef]
17. Vallon, V.; Thomson, S.C. Targeting renal glucose reabsorption to treat hyperglycaemia: The pleiotropic effects of SGLT2 inhibition. *Diabetologia* **2017**, *60*, 215–225. [CrossRef] [PubMed]
18. Sen, T.; Heerspink, H.J.L. A kidney perspective on the mechanism of action of sodium glucose co-transporter 2 inhibitors. *Cell Metab.* **2021**. [CrossRef]
19. Neal, B.; Perkovic, V.; Mahaffey, K.W.; de Zeeuw, D.; Fulcher, G.; Erondu, N.; Shaw, W.; Law, G.; Desai, M.; Matthews, D.R. Canagliflozin and Cardiovascular and Renal Events in Type 2 Diabetes. *N. Engl. J. Med.* **2017**, *377*, 644–657. [CrossRef] [PubMed]
20. Wright, E.M. Renal Na^+-glucose cotransporters. *Am. J. Physiol. Renal. Physiol.* **2001**, *280*, F10–F18. [CrossRef]
21. DeFronzo, R.A.; Reeves, W.B.; Awad, A.S. Pathophysiology of diabetic kidney disease: Impact of SGLT2 inhibitors. *Nat. Rev. Nephrol.* **2021**, *17*, 319–334. [CrossRef]
22. Vallon, V.; Platt, K.A.; Cunard, R.; Schroth, J.; Whaley, J.; Thomson, S.C.; Koepsell, H.; Rieg, T. SGLT2 mediates glucose reabsorption in the early proximal tubule. *J. Am. Soc. Nephrol.* **2011**, *22*, 104–112. [CrossRef] [PubMed]
23. Wang, X.X.; Levi, J.; Luo, Y.; Myakala, K.; Herman-Edelstein, M.; Qiu, L.; Wang, D.; Peng, Y.; Grenz, A.; Lucia, S.; et al. SGLT2 Protein Expression Is Increased in Human Diabetic Nephropathy: Sglt2 Protein Inhibition Decreases Renal Lipid Accumulation, Inflammation, And The Development Of Nephropathy In Diabetic Mice. *J. Biol. Chem.* **2017**, *292*, 5335–5348. [CrossRef]
24. Rahmoune, H.; Thompson, P.W.; Ward, J.M.; Smith, C.D.; Hong, G.; Brown, J. Glucose transporters in human renal proximal tubular cells isolated from the urine of patients with non-insulin-dependent diabetes. *Diabetes* **2005**, *54*, 3427–3434. [CrossRef]
25. Ehrenkranz, J.R.; Lewis, N.G.; Kahn, C.R.; Roth, J. Phlorizin: A review. *Diabetes Metabol. Res. Rev.* **2005**, *21*, 31–38. [CrossRef]
26. Choi, C.I. Sodium-Glucose Cotransporter 2 (SGLT2) Inhibitors from Natural Products: Discovery of Next-Generation Antihyperglycemic Agents. *Molecules* **2016**, *21*, 1136. [CrossRef] [PubMed]
27. Rieg, T.; Vallon, V. Development of SGLT1 and SGLT2 inhibitors. *Diabetologia* **2018**, *61*, 2079–2086. [CrossRef] [PubMed]
28. Grempler, R.; Thomas, L.; Eckhardt, M.; Himmelsbach, F.; Sauer, A.; Sharp, D.E.; Bakker, R.A.; Mark, M.; Klein, T.; Eickelmann, P. Empagliflozin, a novel selective sodium glucose cotransporter-2 (SGLT-2) inhibitor: Characterisation and comparison with other SGLT-2 inhibitors. *Diabetes, Obes. Metabol.* **2012**, *14*, 83–90. [CrossRef]
29. Poole, R.M.; Dungo, R.T. Ipragliflozin: First global approval. *Drugs* **2014**, *74*, 611–617. [CrossRef]
30. Markham, A.; Elkinson, S. Luseogliflozin: First global approval. *Drugs* **2014**, *74*, 945–950. [CrossRef]
31. Mizuno, Y.; Jacob, R.F.; Mason, R.P. Inflammation and the development of atherosclerosis. *J. Atherosc. Thromb.* **2011**, *18*, 351–358. [CrossRef]
32. Aboonabi, A.; Meyer, R.R.; Singh, I. The association between metabolic syndrome components and the development of atherosclerosis. *J. Hum. Hypertens.* **2019**, *33*, 844–855. [CrossRef]
33. Xu, J.; Kitada, M.; Ogura, Y.; Koya, D. Relationship Between Autophagy and Metabolic Syndrome Characteristics in the Pathogenesis of Atherosclerosis. *Front. Cell Dev. Biol.* **2021**, *9*, 641852. [CrossRef]
34. Leng, W.; Ouyang, X.; Lei, X.; Wu, M.; Chen, L.; Wu, Q.; Deng, W.; Liang, Z. The SGLT-2 Inhibitor Dapagliflozin Has a Therapeutic Effect on Atherosclerosis in Diabetic $ApoE^{-/-}$ Mice. *Med. Inflamm.* **2016**, *2016*, 6305735. [CrossRef]
35. Han, J.H.; Oh, T.J.; Lee, G.; Maeng, H.J.; Lee, D.H.; Kim, K.M.; Choi, S.H.; Jang, H.C.; Lee, H.S.; Park, K.S.; et al. The beneficial effects of empagliflozin, an SGLT2 inhibitor, on atherosclerosis in $ApoE^{-/-}$ mice fed a western diet. *Diabetologia* **2017**, *60*, 364–376. [CrossRef]
36. Nakatsu, Y.; Kokubo, H.; Bumdelger, B.; Yoshizumi, M.; Yamamotoya, T.; Matsunaga, Y.; Ueda, K.; Inoue, Y.; Inoue, M.K.; Fujishiro, M.; et al. The SGLT2 Inhibitor Luseogliflozin Rapidly Normalizes Aortic mRNA Levels of Inflammation-Related but Not Lipid-Metabolism-Related Genes and Suppresses Atherosclerosis in Diabetic ApoE KO Mice. *Int. J. Mol. Sci.* **2017**, *18*, 1704. [CrossRef] [PubMed]
37. Al-Sharea, A.; Murphy, A.J.; Huggins, L.A.; Hu, Y.; Goldberg, I.J.; Nagareddy, P.R. SGLT2 inhibition reduces atherosclerosis by enhancing lipoprotein clearance in $Ldlr^{-/-}$ type 1 diabetic mice. *Atherosclerosis* **2018**, *271*, 166–176. [CrossRef]
38. Ganbaatar, B.; Fukuda, D.; Shinohara, M.; Yagi, S.; Kusunose, K.; Yamada, H.; Soeki, T.; Hirata, K.I.; Sata, M. Empagliflozin ameliorates endothelial dysfunction and suppresses atherogenesis in diabetic apolipoprotein E-deficient mice. *Eur. J. Pharmacol.* **2020**, *875*, 173040. [CrossRef]
39. Förstermann, U.; Sessa, W.C. Nitric oxide synthases: Regulation and function. *Eur. Heart J.* **2012**, *33*, 829–837, 837a–837d. [CrossRef] [PubMed]
40. Uthman, L.; Baartscheer, A.; Bleijlevens, B.; Schumacher, C.A.; Fiolet, J.W.T.; Koeman, A.; Jancev, M.; Hollmann, M.W.; Weber, N.C.; Coronel, R.; et al. Class effects of SGLT2 inhibitors in mouse cardiomyocytes and hearts: Inhibition of Na^+/H^+ exchanger, lowering of cytosolic Na^+ and vasodilation. *Diabetologia* **2018**, *61*, 722–726. [CrossRef]
41. Aroor, A.R.; Das, N.A.; Carpenter, A.J.; Habibi, J.; Jia, G.; Ramirez-Perez, F.I.; Martinez-Lemus, L.; Manrique-Acevedo, C.M.; Hayden, M.R.; Duta, C.; et al. Glycemic control by the SGLT2 inhibitor empagliflozin decreases aortic stiffness, renal resistivity index and kidney injury. *Cardiovasc. Diabetol.* **2018**, *17*, 108. [CrossRef]
42. Sayour, A.A.; Korkmaz-Icöz, S.; Loganathan, S.; Ruppert, M.; Sayour, V.N.; Oláh, A.; Benke, K.; Brune, M.; Benkő, R.; Horváth, E.M.; et al. Acute canagliflozin treatment protects against in vivo myocardial ischemia-reperfusion injury in non-diabetic male rats and enhances endothelium-dependent vasorelaxation. *J. Trans. Med.* **2019**, *17*, 127. [CrossRef] [PubMed]

43. Uthman, L.; Homayr, A.; Juni, R.P.; Spin, E.L.; Kerindongo, R.; Boomsma, M.; Hollmann, M.W.; Preckel, B.; Koolwijk, P.; van Hinsbergh, V.W.M.; et al. Empagliflozin and Dapagliflozin Reduce ROS Generation and Restore NO Bioavailability in Tumor Necrosis Factor α-Stimulated Human Coronary Arterial Endothelial Cells. *Cell Physiol. Biochem.* **2019**, *53*, 865–886. [CrossRef]
44. Yang, X.; Li, Y.; Li, Y.; Ren, X.; Zhang, X.; Hu, D.; Gao, Y.; Xing, Y.; Shang, H. Oxidative Stress-Mediated Atherosclerosis: Mechanisms and Therapies. *Front. Physiol.* **2017**, *8*, 600. [CrossRef]
45. Rosenblat, M.; Volkova, N.; Paland, N.; Aviram, M. Triglyceride accumulation in macrophages upregulates paraoxonase 2 (PON2) expression via ROS-mediated JNK/c-Jun signaling pathway activation. *BioFactors* **2012**, *38*, 458–469. [CrossRef] [PubMed]
46. Schaffer, S.W.; Jong, C.J.; Mozaffari, M. Role of oxidative stress in diabetes-mediated vascular dysfunction: Unifying hypothesis of diabetes revisited. *Vasc. Pharmacol.* **2012**, *57*, 139–149. [CrossRef]
47. Furukawa, S.; Fujita, T.; Shimabukuro, M.; Iwaki, M.; Yamada, Y.; Nakajima, Y.; Nakayama, O.; Makishima, M.; Matsuda, M.; Shimomura, I. Increased oxidative stress in obesity and its impact on metabolic syndrome. *J. Clin. Investig.* **2004**, *114*, 1752–1761. [CrossRef] [PubMed]
48. Di Marco, E.; Gray, S.P.; Chew, P.; Koulis, C.; Ziegler, A.; Szyndralewiez, C.; Touyz, R.M.; Schmidt, H.H.; Cooper, M.E.; Slattery, R.; et al. Pharmacological inhibition of NOX reduces atherosclerotic lesions, vascular ROS and immune-inflammatory responses in diabetic Apoe$^{-/-}$ mice. *Diabetologia* **2014**, *57*, 633–642. [CrossRef]
49. Park, S.H.; Belcastro, E.; Hasan, H.; Matsushita, K.; Marchandot, B.; Abbas, M.; Toti, F.; Auger, C.; Jesel, L.; Ohlmann, P.; et al. Angiotensin II-induced upregulation of SGLT1 and 2 contributes to human microparticle-stimulated endothelial senescence and dysfunction: Protective effect of gliflozins. *Cardiovasc. Diabetol.* **2021**, *20*, 65. [CrossRef] [PubMed]
50. Rahadian, A.; Fukuda, D.; Salim, H.M.; Yagi, S.; Kusunose, K.; Yamada, H.; Soeki, T.; Sata, M. Canagliflozin Prevents Diabetes-Induced Vascular Dysfunction in ApoE-Deficient Mice. *J. Atherosc. Thrombosis* **2020**, *27*, 1141–1151. [CrossRef]
51. El-Daly, M.; Pulakazhi Venu, V.K.; Saifeddine, M.; Mihara, K.; Kang, S.; Fedak, P.W.M.; Alston, L.A.; Hirota, S.A.; Ding, H.; Triggle, C.R.; et al. Hyperglycaemic impairment of PAR2-mediated vasodilation: Prevention by inhibition of aortic endothelial sodium-glucose-co-Transporter-2 and minimizing oxidative stress. *Vasc. Pharmacol.* **2018**, *109*, 56–71. [CrossRef]
52. Nasiri-Ansari, N.; Dimitriadis, G.K.; Agrogiannis, G.; Perrea, D.; Kostakis, I.D.; Kaltsas, G.; Papavassiliou, A.G.; Randeva, H.S.; Kassi, E. Canagliflozin attenuates the progression of atherosclerosis and inflammation process in APOE knockout mice. *Cardiovasc. Diabetol.* **2018**, *17*, 106. [CrossRef]
53. Dimitriadis, G.K.; Nasiri-Ansari, N.; Agrogiannis, G.; Kostakis, I.D.; Randeva, M.S.; Nikiteas, N.; Patel, V.H.; Kaltsas, G.; Papavassiliou, A.G.; Randeva, H.S.; et al. Empagliflozin improves primary haemodynamic parameters and attenuates the development of atherosclerosis in high fat diet fed APOE knockout mice. *Mol. Cellul. Endoc.* **2019**, *494*, 110487. [CrossRef]
54. Gaspari, T.; Spizzo, I.; Liu, H.; Hu, Y.; Simpson, R.W.; Widdop, R.E.; Dear, A.E. Dapagliflozin attenuates human vascular endothelial cell activation and induces vasorelaxation: A potential mechanism for inhibition of atherogenesis. *Diab. Vasc. Dis. Res.* **2018**, *15*, 64–73. [CrossRef] [PubMed]
55. Mancini, S.J.; Boyd, D.; Katwan, O.J.; Strembitska, A.; Almabrouk, T.A.; Kennedy, S.; Palmer, T.M.; Salt, I.P. Canagliflozin inhibits interleukin-1β-stimulated cytokine and chemokine secretion in vascular endothelial cells by AMP-activated protein kinase-dependent and -independent mechanisms. *Sci. Rep.* **2018**, *8*, 5276. [CrossRef] [PubMed]
56. Duewell, P.; Kono, H.; Rayner, K.J.; Sirois, C.M.; Vladimer, G.; Bauernfeind, F.G.; Abela, G.S.; Franchi, L.; Nuñez, G.; Schnurr, M.; et al. NLRP3 inflammasomes are required for atherogenesis and activated by cholesterol crystals. *Nature* **2010**, *464*, 1357–1361. [CrossRef] [PubMed]
57. Razani, B.; Feng, C.; Coleman, T.; Emanuel, R.; Wen, H.; Hwang, S.; Ting, J.P.; Virgin, H.W.; Kastan, M.B.; Semenkovich, C.F. Autophagy links inflammasomes to atherosclerotic progression. *Cell Metab.* **2012**, *15*, 534–544. [CrossRef] [PubMed]
58. Satish, M.; Agrawal, D.K. Atherothrombosis and the NLRP3 inflammasome-endogenous mechanisms of inhibition. *Trans. Res. J. Lab. Clin. Med.* **2020**, *215*, 75–85. [CrossRef] [PubMed]
59. Qiu, Y.Y.; Tang, L.Q. Roles of the NLRP3 inflammasome in the pathogenesis of diabetic nephropathy. *Pharmacol. Res.* **2016**, *114*, 251–264. [CrossRef] [PubMed]
60. Luo, B.; Li, B.; Wang, W.; Liu, X.; Xia, Y.; Zhang, C.; Zhang, M.; Zhang, Y.; An, F. NLRP3 gene silencing ameliorates diabetic cardiomyopathy in a type 2 diabetes rat model. *PLoS ONE* **2014**, *9*, e104771. [CrossRef]
61. Bleda, S.; de Haro, J.; Varela, C.; Ferruelo, A.; Acin, F. Elevated levels of triglycerides and vldl-cholesterol provoke activation of nlrp1 inflammasome in endothelial cells. *Int. J. Cardiol.* **2016**, *220*, 52–55. [CrossRef]
62. Kim, S.R.; Lee, S.G.; Kim, S.H.; Kim, J.H.; Choi, E.; Cho, W.; Rim, J.H.; Hwang, I.; Lee, C.J.; Lee, M.; et al. SGLT2 inhibition modulates NLRP3 inflammasome activity via ketones and insulin in diabetes with cardiovascular disease. *Nat. Commun.* **2020**, *11*, 2127. [CrossRef]
63. Ye, Y.; Bajaj, M.; Yang, H.C.; Perez-Polo, J.R.; Birnbaum, Y. SGLT-2 Inhibition with Dapagliflozin Reduces the Activation of the Nlrp3/ASC Inflammasome and Attenuates the Development of Diabetic Cardiomyopathy in Mice with Type 2 Diabetes. Further Augmentation of the Effects with Saxagliptin, a DPP4 Inhibitor. *Cardiovasc. Drugs Therapy* **2017**, *31*, 119–132. [CrossRef] [PubMed]
64. Sukhanov, S.; Higashi, Y.; Yoshida, T.; Mummidi, S.; Aroor, A.R.; Jeffrey Russell, J.; Bender, S.B.; DeMarco, V.G.; Chandrasekar, B. The SGLT2 inhibitor Empagliflozin attenuates interleukin-17A-induced human aortic smooth muscle cell proliferation and migration by targeting TRAF3IP2/ROS/NLRP3/Caspase-1-dependent IL-1β and IL-18 secretion. *Cell. Signal.* **2021**, *77*, 109825. [CrossRef]

65. Martinet, W.; De Meyer, G.R. Autophagy in atherosclerosis: A cell survival and death phenomenon with therapeutic potential. *Circul. Res.* **2009**, *104*, 304–317. [CrossRef]
66. Kitada, M.; Ogura, Y.; Koya, D. The protective role of Sirt1 in vascular tissue: Its relationship to vascular aging and atherosclerosis. *Aging* **2016**, *8*, 2290–2307. [CrossRef] [PubMed]
67. Aragón-Herrera, A.; Feijóo-Bandín, S.; Otero Santiago, M.; Barral, L.; Campos-Toimil, M.; Gil-Longo, J.; Costa Pereira, T.M.; García-Caballero, T.; Rodríguez-Segade, S.; Rodríguez, J.; et al. Empagliflozin reduces the levels of CD36 and cardiotoxic lipids while improving autophagy in the hearts of Zucker diabetic fatty rats. *Biochem. Pharmacol.* **2019**, *170*, 113677. [CrossRef]
68. Jaikumkao, K.; Promsan, S.; Thongnak, L.; Swe, M.T.; Tapanya, M.; Htun, K.T.; Kothan, S.; Intachai, N.; Lungkaphin, A. Dapagliflozin ameliorates pancreatic injury and activates kidney autophagy by modulating the AMPK/mTOR signaling pathway in obese rats. *J. Cellul. Physiol.* **2021**, *236*, 6424–6440. [CrossRef]
69. Ren, C.; Sun, K.; Zhang, Y.; Hu, Y.; Hu, B.; Zhao, J.; He, Z.; Ding, R.; Wang, W.; Liang, C. Sodium-Glucose CoTransporter-2 Inhibitor Empagliflozin Ameliorates Sunitinib-Induced Cardiac Dysfunction via Regulation of AMPK-mTOR Signaling Pathway-Mediated Autophagy. *Front. Pharmacol.* **2021**, *12*, 664181. [CrossRef]
70. Xu, C.; Wang, W.; Zhong, J.; Lei, F.; Xu, N.; Zhang, Y.; Xie, W. Canagliflozin exerts anti-inflammatory effects by inhibiting intracellular glucose metabolism and promoting autophagy in immune cells. *Biochem. Pharmacol.* **2018**, *152*, 45–59. [CrossRef]
71. Xu, J.; Kitada, M.; Ogura, Y.; Liu, H.; Koya, D. Dapagliflozin Restores Impaired Autophagy and Suppresses Inflammation in High Glucose-Treated HK-2 Cells. *Cells* **2021**, *10*, 1457. [CrossRef] [PubMed]
72. Véniant, M.M.; Withycombe, S.; Young, S.G. Lipoprotein size and atherosclerosis susceptibility in Apoe$^{-/-}$ and Ldlr$^{-/-}$ mice. *Arteriosc. Thromb. Vasc. Biol.* **2001**, *21*, 1567–1570. [CrossRef]
73. Terasaki, M.; Hiromura, M.; Mori, Y.; Kohashi, K.; Nagashima, M.; Kushima, H.; Watanabe, T.; Hirano, T. Amelioration of Hyperglycemia with a Sodium-Glucose Cotransporter 2 Inhibitor Prevents Macrophage-Driven Atherosclerosis through Macrophage Foam Cell Formation Suppression in Type 1 and Type 2 Diabetic Mice. *PLoS ONE* **2015**, *10*, e0143396. [CrossRef]
74. Liu, Y.; Xu, J.; Wu, M.; Xu, B.; Kang, L. Empagliflozin protects against atherosclerosis progression by modulating lipid profiles and sympathetic activity. *Lipids. Health Dis.* **2021**, *20*, 5. [CrossRef] [PubMed]
75. Mori, Y.; Terasaki, M.; Hiromura, M.; Saito, T.; Kushima, H.; Koshibu, M.; Osaka, N.; Ohara, M.; Fukui, T.; Ohtaki, H.; et al. Luseogliflozin attenuates neointimal hyperplasia after wire injury in high-fat diet-fed mice via inhibition of perivascular adipose tissue remodeling. *Cardiovasc. Diabetol.* **2019**, *18*, 143. [CrossRef]
76. Mori, K.; Tsuchiya, K.; Nakamura, S.; Miyachi, Y.; Shiba, K.; Ogawa, Y.; Kitamura, K. Ipragliflozin-induced adipose expansion inhibits cuff-induced vascular remodeling in mice. *Cardiovasc. Diabetol.* **2019**, *18*, 83. [CrossRef]
77. Prattichizzo, F.; De Nigris, V.; Micheloni, S.; La Sala, L.; Ceriello, A. Increases in circulating levels of ketone bodies and cardiovascular protection with SGLT2 inhibitors: Is low-grade inflammation the neglected component? *Diabetes Obes. Metab.* **2018**, *20*, 2515–2522. [CrossRef]
78. Xu, L.; Ota, T. Emerging roles of SGLT2 inhibitors in obesity and insulin resistance: Focus on fat browning and macrophage polarization. *Adipocyte* **2018**, *7*, 121–128. [CrossRef]
79. Rosenstock, J.; Frias, J.; Páll, D.; Charbonnel, B.; Pascu, R.; Saur, D.; Darekar, A.; Huyck, S.; Shi, H.; Lauring, B.; et al. Effect of ertugliflozin on glucose control, body weight, blood pressure and bone density in type 2 diabetes mellitus inadequately controlled on metformin monotherapy (VERTIS MET). *Diabetes Obes. Metab.* **2018**, *20*, 520–529. [CrossRef]
80. Schork, A.; Saynisch, J.; Vosseler, A.; Jaghutriz, B.A.; Heyne, N.; Peter, A.; Häring, H.U.; Stefan, N.; Fritsche, A.; Artunc, F. Effect of SGLT2 inhibitors on body composition, fluid status and renin-angiotensin-aldosterone system in type 2 diabetes: A prospective study using bioimpedance spectroscopy. *Cardiovasc. Diabetol.* **2019**, *18*, 46. [CrossRef] [PubMed]
81. Sakai, S.; Kaku, K.; Seino, Y.; Inagaki, N.; Haneda, M.; Sasaki, T.; Fukatsu, A.; Kakiuchi, H.; Samukawa, Y. Efficacy and Safety of the SGLT2 Inhibitor Luseogliflozin in Japanese Patients With Type 2 Diabetes Mellitus Stratified According to Baseline Body Mass Index: Pooled Analysis of Data From 52-Week Phase III Trials. *Clin. Therap.* **2016**, *38*, 843–862.e849. [CrossRef]
82. Bode, B.; Stenlöf, K.; Harris, S.; Sullivan, D.; Fung, A.; Usiskin, K.; Meininger, G. Long-term efficacy and safety of canagliflozin over 104 weeks in patients aged 55–80 years with type 2 diabetes. *Diabetes Obes. Metab.* **2015**, *17*, 294–303. [CrossRef]
83. Mancia, G.; Cannon, C.P.; Tikkanen, I.; Zeller, C.; Ley, L.; Woerle, H.J.; Broedl, U.C.; Johansen, O.E. Impact of Empagliflozin on Blood Pressure in Patients With Type 2 Diabetes Mellitus and Hypertension by Background Antihypertensive Medication. *Hypertension* **2016**, *68*, 1355–1364. [CrossRef] [PubMed]
84. Chilton, R.; Tikkanen, I.; Hehnke, U.; Woerle, H.J.; Johansen, O.E. Impact of empagliflozin on blood pressure in dipper and non-dipper patients with type 2 diabetes mellitus and hypertension. *Diabetes Obes. Metab.* **2017**, *19*, 1620–1624. [CrossRef] [PubMed]
85. Kario, K.; Okada, K.; Kato, M.; Nishizawa, M.; Yoshida, T.; Asano, T.; Uchiyama, K.; Niijima, Y.; Katsuya, T.; Urata, H.; et al. Twenty-Four-Hour Blood Pressure-Lowering Effect of an SGLT-2 Inhibitor in Patients with Diabetes and Uncontrolled Nocturnal Hypertension: Results from the Randomized, Placebo-Controlled SACRA Study. *Circulation* **2018**, *139*, 2089–2097. [CrossRef] [PubMed]
86. Cefalu, W.T.; Stenlöf, K.; Leiter, L.A.; Wilding, J.P.; Blonde, L.; Polidori, D.; Xie, J.; Sullivan, D.; Usiskin, K.; Canovatchel, W.; et al. Effects of canagliflozin on body weight and relationship to HbA1c and blood pressure changes in patients with type 2 diabetes. *Diabetologia* **2015**, *58*, 1183–1187. [CrossRef] [PubMed]

87. Ramirez, A.J.; Sanchez, M.J.; Sanchez, R.A. Diabetic patients with essential hypertension treated with amlodipine: Blood pressure and arterial stiffness effects of canagliflozin or perindopril. *J. Hypertens.* **2019**, *37*, 636–642. [CrossRef]
88. Ye, N.; Jardine, M.J.; Oshima, M.; Hockham, C.; Heerspink, H.J.L.; Agarwal, R.; Bakris, G.; Schutte, A.E.; Arnott, C.; Chang, T.I.; et al. Blood Pressure Effects of Canagliflozin and Clinical Outcomes in Type 2 Diabetes and Chronic Kidney Disease: Insights From the CREDENCE Trial. *Circulation* **2021**, *143*, 1735–1749. [CrossRef]
89. Liu, J.; Pong, A.; Gallo, S.; Darekar, A.; Terra, S.G. Effect of ertugliflozin on blood pressure in patients with type 2 diabetes mellitus: A post hoc pooled analysis of randomized controlled trials. *Cardiovasc. Diabetol.* **2019**, *18*, 59. [CrossRef]
90. Briasoulis, A.; Al Dhaybi, O.; Bakris, G.L. SGLT2 Inhibitors and Mechanisms of Hypertension. *Curr. Cardiol. Rep.* **2018**, *20*, 1. [CrossRef]
91. Stenlöf, K.; Cefalu, W.T.; Kim, K.A.; Jodar, E.; Alba, M.; Edwards, R.; Tong, C.; Canovatchel, W.; Meininger, G. Long-term efficacy and safety of canagliflozin monotherapy in patients with type 2 diabetes inadequately controlled with diet and exercise: Findings from the 52-week CANTATA-M study. *Curr. Med. Res. Opin.* **2014**, *30*, 163–175. [CrossRef] [PubMed]
92. Cha, S.A.; Park, Y.M.; Yun, J.S.; Lim, T.S.; Song, K.H.; Yoo, K.D.; Ahn, Y.B.; Ko, S.H. A comparison of effects of DPP-4 inhibitor and SGLT2 inhibitor on lipid profile in patients with type 2 diabetes. *Lipids. Health Dis.* **2017**, *16*, 58. [CrossRef] [PubMed]
93. Jojima, T.; Sakurai, S.; Wakamatsu, S.; Iijima, T.; Saito, M.; Tomaru, T.; Kogai, T.; Usui, I.; Aso, Y. Empagliflozin increases plasma levels of campesterol, a marker of cholesterol absorption, in patients with type 2 diabetes: Association with a slight increase in high-density lipoprotein cholesterol. *Int. J. Cardiol.* **2021**, *331*, 243–248. [CrossRef]
94. Basu, D.; Huggins, L.A.; Scerbo, D.; Obunike, J.; Mullick, A.E.; Rothenberg, P.L.; Di Prospero, N.A.; Eckel, R.H.; Goldberg, I.J. Mechanism of Increased LDL (Low-Density Lipoprotein) and Decreased Triglycerides With SGLT2 (Sodium-Glucose Cotransporter 2) Inhibition. *Arteriosc. Thromb. Vasc. Biol.* **2018**, *38*, 2207–2216. [CrossRef] [PubMed]
95. Briand, F.; Mayoux, E.; Brousseau, E.; Burr, N.; Urbain, I.; Costard, C.; Mark, M.; Sulpice, T. Empagliflozin, via Switching Metabolism Toward Lipid Utilization, Moderately Increases LDL Cholesterol Levels Through Reduced LDL Catabolism. *Diabetes* **2016**, *65*, 2032–2038. [CrossRef] [PubMed]
96. Bailey, C.J. Uric acid and the cardio-renal effects of SGLT2 inhibitors. *Diabetes Obes. Metab.* **2019**, *21*, 1291–1298. [CrossRef]
97. Chino, Y.; Kuwabara, M.; Hisatome, I. Factors Influencing Change in Serum Uric Acid after Administration of the Sodium-Glucose Cotransporter 2 Inhibitor Luseogliflozin in Patients With Type 2 Diabetes Mellitus. *J. Clin. Pharmacol.* **2021**. [CrossRef]
98. Davies, M.J.; Trujillo, A.; Vijapurkar, U.; Damaraju, C.V.; Meininger, G. Effect of canagliflozin on serum uric acid in patients with type 2 diabetes mellitus. *Diabetes Obes. Metab.* **2015**, *17*, 426–429. [CrossRef]
99. McGuire, D.K.; Marx, N.; Johansen, O.E.; Inzucchi, S.E.; Rosenstock, J.; George, J.T. FDA guidance on antihyperglyacemic therapies for type 2 diabetes: One decade later. *Diabetes Obes. Metab.* **2019**, *21*, 1073–1078. [CrossRef]
100. Rangaswami, J.; Bhalla, V.; de Boer, I.H.; Staruschenko, A.; Sharp, J.A.; Singh, R.R.; Lo, K.B.; Tuttle, K.; Vaduganathan, M.; Ventura, H.; et al. Cardiorenal Protection With the Newer Antidiabetic Agents in Patients With Diabetes and Chronic Kidney Disease: A Scientific Statement From the American Heart Association. *Circulation* **2020**, *142*, e265–e286. [CrossRef]
101. Kosiborod, M.; Cavender, M.A.; Fu, A.Z.; Wilding, J.P.; Khunti, K.; Holl, R.W.; Norhammar, A.; Birkeland, K.I.; Jørgensen, M.E.; Thuresson, M.; et al. Lower Risk of Heart Failure and Death in Patients Initiated on Sodium-Glucose Cotransporter-2 Inhibitors Versus Other Glucose-Lowering Drugs: The CVD-REAL Study (Comparative Effectiveness of Cardiovascular Outcomes in New Users of Sodium-Glucose Cotransporter-2 Inhibitors). *Circulation* **2017**, *136*, 249–259. [CrossRef]
102. Kosiborod, M.; Birkeland, K.I.; Cavender, M.A.; Fu, A.Z.; Wilding, J.P.; Khunti, K.; Holl, R.W.; Norhammar, A.; Jørgensen, M.E.; Wittbrodt, E.T.; et al. Rates of myocardial infarction and stroke in patients initiating treatment with SGLT2-inhibitors versus other glucose-lowering agents in real-world clinical practice: Results from the CVD-REAL study. *Diabetes Obes. Metab.* **2018**, *20*, 1983–1987. [CrossRef] [PubMed]
103. Wu, J.H.; Foote, C.; Blomster, J.; Toyama, T.; Perkovic, V.; Sundström, J.; Neal, B. Effects of sodium-glucose cotransporter-2 inhibitors on cardiovascular events, death, and major safety outcomes in adults with type 2 diabetes: A systematic review and meta-analysis. *Lancet Diabetes Endocrinol.* **2016**, *4*, 411–419. [CrossRef]
104. Zinman, B.; Wanner, C.; Lachin, J.M.; Fitchett, D.; Bluhmki, E.; Hantel, S.; Mattheus, M.; Devins, T.; Johansen, O.E.; Woerle, H.J.; et al. Empagliflozin, Cardiovascular Outcomes, and Mortality in Type 2 Diabetes. *N. Engl. J. Med.* **2015**, *373*, 2117–2128. [CrossRef] [PubMed]
105. Anker, S.D.; Butler, J.; Filippatos, G.; Khan, M.S.; Marx, N.; Lam, C.S.P.; Schnaidt, S.; Ofstad, A.P.; Brueckmann, M.; Jamal, W.; et al. Effect of Empagliflozin on Cardiovascular and Renal Outcomes in Patients With Heart Failure by Baseline Diabetes Status: Results From the EMPEROR-Reduced Trial. *Circulation* **2021**, *143*, 337–349. [CrossRef] [PubMed]
106. Packer, M.; Anker, S.D.; Butler, J.; Filippatos, G.; Ferreira, J.P.; Pocock, S.J.; Carson, P.; Anand, I.; Doehner, W.; Haass, M.; et al. Effect of Empagliflozin on the Clinical Stability of Patients With Heart Failure and a Reduced Ejection Fraction: The EMPEROR-Reduced Trial. *Circulation* **2021**, *143*, 326–336. [CrossRef]
107. Anker, S.D.; Butler, J.; Filippatos, G.; Ferreira, J.P.; Bocchi, E.; Böhm, M.; Brunner-La Rocca, H.P.; Choi, D.J.; Chopra, V.; Chuquiure-Valenzuela, E.; et al. Empagliflozin in Heart Failure with a Preserved Ejection Fraction. *N. Engl. J. Med.* **2021**, *385*, 1451–1461. [CrossRef]
108. Wiviott, S.D.; Raz, I.; Bonaca, M.P.; Mosenzon, O.; Kato, E.T.; Cahn, A.; Silverman, M.G.; Zelniker, T.A.; Kuder, J.F.; Murphy, S.A.; et al. Dapagliflozin and Cardiovascular Outcomes in Type 2 Diabetes. *N. Engl. J. Med.* **2019**, *380*, 347–357. [CrossRef]

109. McMurray, J.J.V.; Solomon, S.D.; Inzucchi, S.E.; Køber, L.; Kosiborod, M.N.; Martinez, F.A.; Ponikowski, P.; Sabatine, M.S.; Anand, I.S.; Bělohlávek, J.; et al. Dapagliflozin in Patients with Heart Failure and Reduced Ejection Fraction. *N. Engl. J. Med.* **2019**, *381*, 1995–2008. [CrossRef] [PubMed]
110. Cannon, C.P.; Pratley, R.; Dagogo-Jack, S.; Mancuso, J.; Huyck, S.; Masiukiewicz, U.; Charbonnel, B.; Frederich, R.; Gallo, S.; Cosentino, F.; et al. Cardiovascular Outcomes with Ertugliflozin in Type 2 Diabetes. *N. Engl. J. Med.* **2020**, *383*, 1425–1435. [CrossRef]
111. Bhatt, D.L.; Szarek, M.; Steg, P.G.; Cannon, C.P.; Leiter, L.A.; McGuire, D.K.; Lewis, J.B.; Riddle, M.C.; Voors, A.A.; Metra, M.; et al. Sotagliflozin in Patients with Diabetes and Recent Worsening Heart Failure. *N. Engl. J. Med.* **2021**, *384*, 117–128. [CrossRef] [PubMed]
112. Bhatt, D.L.; Szarek, M.; Pitt, B.; Cannon, C.P.; Leiter, L.A.; McGuire, D.K.; Lewis, J.B.; Riddle, M.C.; Inzucchi, S.E.; Kosiborod, M.N.; et al. Sotagliflozin in Patients with Diabetes and Chronic Kidney Disease. *N. Engl. J. Med.* **2021**, *384*, 129–139. [CrossRef]
113. Hupfeld, C.; Mudaliar, S. Navigating the "MACE" in Cardiovascular Outcomes Trials and decoding the relevance of Atherosclerotic Cardiovascular Disease benefits versus Heart Failure benefits. *Diabetes Obes. Metab.* **2019**, *21*, 1780–1789. [CrossRef] [PubMed]
114. Natali, A.; Nesti, L.; Tricò, D.; Ferrannini, E. Effects of GLP-1 receptor agonists and SGLT-2 inhibitors on cardiac structure and function: A narrative review of clinical evidence. *Cardiovasc. Diabetol.* **2021**, *20*, 196. [CrossRef] [PubMed]
115. Shao, S.C.; Lin, Y.H.; Chang, K.C.; Chan, Y.Y.; Hung, M.J.; Kao Yang, Y.H.; Lai, E.C. Sodium glucose co-transporter 2 inhibitors and cardiovascular event protections: How applicable are clinical trials and observational studies to real-world patients? *BMJ Open Diabetes Res. Care* **2019**, *7*, e000742. [CrossRef]
116. Birkeland, K.I.; Bodegard, J.; Norhammar, A.; Kuiper, J.G.; Georgiado, E.; Beekman-Hendriks, W.L.; Thuresson, M.; Pignot, M.; Herings, R.M.C.; Kooy, A. How representative of a general type 2 diabetes population are patients included in cardiovascular outcome trials with SGLT2 inhibitors? A large European observational study. *Diabetes Obes. Metab.* **2019**, *21*, 968–974. [CrossRef]
117. Kosiborod, M.; Lam, C.S.P.; Kohsaka, S.; Kim, D.J.; Karasik, A.; Shaw, J.; Tangri, N.; Goh, S.Y.; Thuresson, M.; Chen, H.; et al. Cardiovascular Events Associated With SGLT-2 Inhibitors Versus Other Glucose-Lowering Drugs: The CVD-REAL 2 Study. *J. Am. College Cardiol.* **2018**, *71*, 2628–2639. [CrossRef]
118. Kohsaka, S.; Lam, C.S.P.; Kim, D.J.; Cavender, M.A.; Norhammar, A.; Jørgensen, M.E.; Birkeland, K.I.; Holl, R.W.; Franch-Nadal, J.; Tangri, N.; et al. Risk of cardiovascular events and death associated with initiation of SGLT2 inhibitors compared with DPP-4 inhibitors: An analysis from the CVD-REAL 2 multinational cohort study. *Lancet. Diabetes Endocrinol.* **2020**, *8*, 606–615. [CrossRef]
119. Lee, H.F.; Chen, S.W.; Liu, J.R.; Li, P.R.; Wu, L.S.; Chang, S.H.; Yeh, Y.H.; Kuo, C.T.; Chan, Y.H.; See, L.C. Major adverse cardiovascular and limb events in patients with diabetes and concomitant peripheral artery disease treated with sodium glucose cotransporter 2 inhibitor versus dipeptidyl peptidase-4 inhibitor. *Cardiovasc. Diabetol.* **2020**, *19*, 160. [CrossRef]
120. Paul, S.K.; Bhatt, D.L.; Montvida, O. The association of amputations and peripheral artery disease in patients with type 2 diabetes mellitus receiving sodium-glucose cotransporter type-2 inhibitors: Real-world study. *Eur. Heart J.* **2021**, *42*, 1728–1738. [CrossRef]
121. American Diabetes Association. Pharmacologic Approaches to Glycemic Treatment: Standards of Medical Care in Diabetes-2021. *Diabetes Care* **2021**, *44*, S111–S124. [CrossRef] [PubMed]

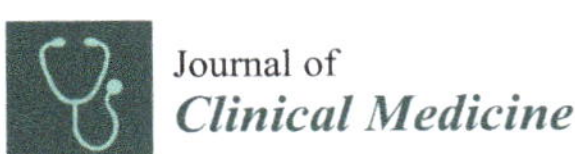
Journal of
Clinical Medicine

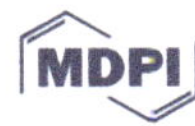

Review

Recent Advances on the Role and Therapeutic Potential of Regulatory T Cells in Atherosclerosis

Toru Tanaka [1], Naoto Sasaki [1,2,*] and Yoshiyuki Rikitake [1]

1 Laboratory of Medical Pharmaceutics, Kobe Pharmaceutical University, Kobe 658-8558, Japan; t-tanaka@kobepharma-u.ac.jp (T.T.); rikitake@kobepharma-u.ac.jp (Y.R.)
2 Division of Cardiovascular Medicine, Department of Internal Medicine, Kobe University Graduate School of Medicine, Kobe 658-8558, Japan
* Correspondence: n-sasaki@kobepharma-u.ac.jp; Tel./Fax: +81-78-441-7579

Abstract: Atherosclerotic diseases, including ischemic heart disease and stroke, are a main cause of mortality worldwide. Chronic vascular inflammation via immune dysregulation is critically involved in the pathogenesis of atherosclerosis. Accumulating evidence suggests that regulatory T cells (Tregs), responsible for maintaining immunological tolerance and suppressing excessive immune responses, play an important role in preventing the development and progression of atherosclerosis through the regulation of pathogenic immunoinflammatory responses. Several strategies to prevent and treat atherosclerosis through the promotion of regulatory immune responses have been developed, and could be clinically applied for the treatment of atherosclerotic cardiovascular disease. In this review, we summarize recent advances in our understanding of the protective role of Tregs in atherosclerosis and discuss attractive approaches to treat atherosclerotic disease by augmenting regulatory immune responses.

Keywords: atherosclerosis; immunology; inflammation; regulatory T cells

Citation: Tanaka, T.; Sasaki, N.; Rikitake, Y. Recent Advances on the Role and Therapeutic Potential of Regulatory T Cells in Atherosclerosis. *J. Clin. Med.* **2021**, *10*, 5907. https://doi.org/10.3390/jcm10245907

Academic Editor: Tomoaki Ishigami

Received: 3 December 2021
Accepted: 13 December 2021
Published: 16 December 2021

1. Introduction

Atherosclerosis provokes serious cardiovascular diseases (CVDs), such as ischemic heart disease and stroke, that are prominent causes of mortality worldwide. Although patients at high risk of atherosclerotic CVD usually receive state-of-the-art intensive treatment, there remains much residual risk of this disease. Experimental and clinical studies have provided firm evidence that innate and adaptive immune responses are critical factors for provoking vascular inflammation and atherosclerosis [1,2]. Although accumulating evidence suggests that vascular inflammatory responses could be responsible for the residual risk of atherosclerotic disease, we have no clinical therapies aimed to directly suppress inflammatory reactions in atherosclerotic lesions [3].

The first clinical evidence to prove the involvement of inflammation in atherosclerotic disease was provided by the Canakinumab Anti-inflammatory Thrombosis Outcomes Study (CANTOS) trial, clearly showing that treatment with a fully human monoclonal antibody targeting interleukin (IL)-1β reduced the cardiovascular disease risk in patients with old myocardial infarction (MI) [4]. Other evidence has been provided by recent clinical trials, the Colchicine Cardiovascular Outcomes Trial (COLCOT) [5] and low-dose colchicine (LoDoCo2) [6], demonstrating that treatment with colchicine, an anti-inflammatory drug indicated for the treatment of gout, familial Mediterranean fever, and pericarditis, resulted in a significantly lower risk of cardiovascular events in patients with recent MI or chronic coronary disease. These clinical trials highlight the efficacy of anti-inflammatory therapies as potentially feasible strategies to treat CVD at least in patients with past disease history.

Experimental and clinical data suggest that in addition to innate immune responses, adaptive immune responses, particularly T cell-mediated immune responses, have detrimental or protective roles in atherosclerosis depending on the cell types or experimental conditions [7]. Firm evidence indicates that regulatory T cells (Tregs), responsible for maintaining immunological tolerance and suppressing excessive immune responses [8], play an important role in preventing the development and progression of atherosclerotic disease through the regulation of pathogenic effector T cell (Teff) immune responses [9]. Several strategies to prevent and treat atherosclerosis via promoting regulatory immune responses have been developed [10]. Tuning the balance between proatherogenic Teffs and atheroprotective Tregs could be an effective therapeutic strategy for atherosclerotic disease.

In this review, we summarize recent advances in our understanding of the protective role of Tregs in atherosclerosis, and discuss attractive approaches to treat atherosclerotic disease by augmenting regulatory immune responses.

2. Role of the Immune System in Atherosclerotic Disease

Immune dysregulation causes chronic inflammation in the arterial wall, which is a key feature of atherosclerosis [11] (Figure 1). It has been suggested that the dysregulated arterial immunoinflammatory responses could induce atherosclerotic plaque instability and eventually lead to severe clinical events, including acute coronary syndrome (ACS) and stroke. It is believed that as the initial inflammatory response in atherosclerosis, accumulation and retention of low-density lipoprotein (LDL) in the arterial intima could occur. Upon endothelial activation, inflammatory monocytes enter the subendothelial space or the intima of the arterial wall, differentiate into macrophages, and form lipid-laden foam cells via uptake of modified LDL particles, leading to the promotion of arterial immunoinflammatory responses including proatherogenic Teff immune responses. A large number of experimental and clinical studies have revealed that various immune cells that mediate innate and adaptive immunity are deeply involved in the pathogenesis of atherosclerosis [1]. In particular, genetically altered mouse models of atherosclerosis including the apolipoprotein E-deficient (*Apoe*$^{-/-}$) [12] and low-density lipoprotein receptor-deficient (*Ldlr*$^{-/-}$) mice [13] have substantially contributed to the development of the atherosclerosis research field.

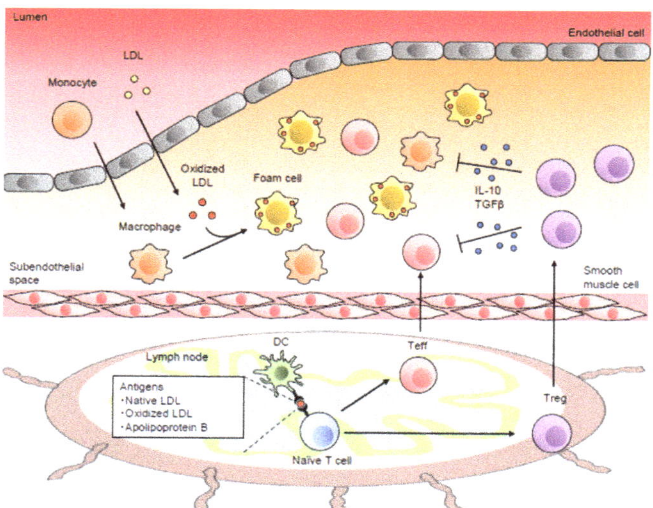

Figure 1. Role of the immune system in atherosclerosis. Chronic vascular inflammation via immune dysregulation is critically involved in the pathogenesis of atherogenesis. Regulatory T cells (Tregs) protect against atherosclerosis by suppressing activation of various immune cells. DC, dendritic cell; IL, interleukin; LDL, low-density lipoprotein; Teff, effector T cell; TGF, transforming growth factor.

Naïve T cells are presented with some atherosclerosis-associated antigens by antigen-presenting cells (APCs), and differentiate into activated Teffs, including CD4$^+$ or CD8$^+$ T cells that accumulate into atherosclerotic lesions of atherosclerosis-prone *Apoe*$^{-/-}$ or *Ldlr*$^{-/-}$ mice and humans. Dendritic cells (DCs) have a capacity to present antigens and play complex roles in atherosclerosis. Various subsets of DCs have been shown to play protective or detrimental roles in atherosclerosis, depending on their subsets [14]. The finding of oligoclonal expansion of T cells in mouse atherosclerotic lesions indicates that T cells may expand in an antigen-specific manner within atherosclerotic plaques [15]. Several self-antigens, native LDL, oxidized LDL, and the major component of LDL, such as apolipoprotein B (ApoB), could provoke autoimmune responses in atherosclerotic lesions and be involved in the pathogenesis of atherosclerosis [16]. However, the role of these atherosclerosis-specific antigens in the development of atherosclerosis remains obscure, and a detailed analysis is needed. With the help of T cells and antigenic stimulation, B cell differentiation and activation occur. Recent experimental studies have revealed that several subsets of B cells play differential and complex roles in atherosclerosis [17]. Conventional B2 cells contribute to proatherogenic immune responses, while B1 cells or regulatory B cells protect against atherosclerosis by secreting natural IgM antibodies against oxidation-specific epitopes or IL-10, respectively.

Depending on the expression of specific transcriptional factors or variations in the local cytokine milieu along with antigen presentation, naïve CD4$^+$ T cells differentiate into different Teff lineages, including T helper type 1 (Th1), T helper type 2 (Th2), and T helper type 17 (Th17) lineages, which have critical roles in the development of atherosclerosis in mice and humans [1]. Recent experimental and clinical studies using sophisticated methodologies, such as single-cell RNA sequencing and mass cytometry revealed that a distinct subset of T cells is the major cellular component in atherosclerotic plaques of mice [18] and humans [19]. Th1 cells specifically express the transcription factor T-box expressed in T cells (T-bet) and secrete pro-inflammatory cytokines, interferon (IFN)-γ, IL-2, and tumor necrosis factor (TNF)-α. Among these cytokines, the major Th1 cytokine, IFN-γ, has been shown to have potent pro-atherogenic effects [20,21]. Th1 cells predominantly exist in mouse [22] and human [23] atherosclerotic plaques and promote atherosclerosis. Th2 cells specifically expressing the transcription factor GATA3 secrete IL-4, IL-5, IL-10, and IL-13, and its major cytokine is IL-4. The genetic deletion of IL-4 in *Ldlr*$^{-/-}$ mice reduces atherosclerosis [24], while exogenous administration of IL-4 did not affect atherosclerosis in *Apoe*$^{-/-}$ mice [25], producing discrepant results. The role of Th2-mediated immune responses in atherosclerosis is heavily influenced by the secreted specific cytokines or animal models and remains controversial. Th17 cells specifically expressing the transcription factor RAR-related orphan receptor (ROR)-γt produce pro-inflammatory cytokine IL-17, and have been shown to substantially contribute to the development of several autoimmune diseases [26]. However, pharmacological inhibition of IL-17 function or its genetic inactivation yielded discrepant outcomes in atherosclerosis [27–29]. The role of Th17 cells in atherosclerosis may vary depending on animal models or experimental conditions, and further investigations are required. CD8$^+$ T cells also infiltrate into atherosclerotic lesions, and their numbers are higher than CD4$^+$ T cells in advanced human atherosclerotic lesions [19]. Experiments performing CD8α or CD8β monoclonal antibody-mediated depletion of CD8$^+$ T cells in *Apoe*$^{-/-}$ mice or their transfer into lymphocyte-deficient *Apoe*$^{-/-}$ mice revealed that CD8$^+$ T cells promote the development of atherosclerotic lesions with an unstable plaque phenotype [30]. On the other hand, depletion of CD8$^+$ T cells by injecting CD8α-depleting antibodies in *Ldlr*$^{-/-}$ mice resulted in less stable plaques characterized by reduced collagen content and increased macrophage content and necrosis, though that did not affect atherosclerotic lesion size [31]. Thus, CD8$^+$ T cells have pro- and anti-atherogenic actions depending on experimental models.

T cell activation occurs after receiving two signals from APCs that involve interaction of the T cell receptor (TCR) with antigenic peptide/major histocompatibility complex (MHC) ligand and costimulation. The costimulatory signals promote or inhibit the

TCR-MHC signal, depending on the type of costimulation. The T cell costimulatory and coinhibitory pathways play crucial roles in modulating functions of Teffs and Tregs and their balance, and these pathways have been shown to be involved in the pathogenesis of atherosclerosis in recent animal studies using genetically modified mice or neutralizing antibodies [32]. Activated T cells and forkhead box P3 (Foxp3)$^+$ Tregs highly express the coinhibitory molecule cytotoxic T-lymphocyte-associated antigen-4 (CTLA-4) that binds to B7 family molecules, B7-1 (CD80) and B7-2 (CD86), on APCs and interrupts the interaction of these molecules with CD28 on T cells, resulting in potent suppression of T cell activation [33]. Our recent studies using CTLA-4 transgenic mice on an *Apoe*$^{-/-}$ background in which T cells constitutively express CTLA-4 demonstrated that CTLA-4 overexpression protected against the development of atherosclerosis [34], abdominal aortic aneurysm (AAA) [35], and kidney disease [36] by suppressing maturation of DCs and proinflammatory Teff immune responses. CTLA-4-Ig that binds to CD80 and CD86 and has an inhibitory effect on the CD80/CD86–CD28 costimulation pathway is clinically effective in treating rheumatoid arthritis [37], and has also been shown to protect against experimental atherosclerosis [38]. These reports suggest that CTLA-4 could be a possible therapeutic target for atherosclerosis. Another important coinhibitory pathway is the interactions between programmed cell death protein 1 (PD-1) and programmed cell death ligand 1 (PD-L1)/PD-L2. Genetic deletion of both PD-L1 and PD-L2 [39] or of their receptor PD-1 [40] in *Ldlr*$^{-/-}$ mice led to accelerated development of atherosclerotic lesions with increased accumulation of intraplaque CD4$^+$ and CD8$^+$ T cells, indicating an atheroprotective role of the PD-1–PD-L1/PD-L2 pathway.

In recent years, the new field termed immuno-oncology has emerged, and immunotherapies for various types of cancer have attained great success. Monoclonal antibodies to block PD-1, PD-L1, or CTLA-4, called immune checkpoint inhibitors (ICIs), have been developed. Recent experimental and clinical evidence suggests that stimulation of the antitumor functions of T cells with these ICIs is quite effective for the treatment of cancer, and has become a major treatment for advanced unresectable cancer [41]. In consideration of findings obtained from animal studies showing that these inhibitory molecules are negative regulators of atherosclerosis [34,38–40], treatment with ICIs have the potential to accelerate atherosclerosis in cancer patients who could have a higher risk of CVD. Importantly, a recent clinical trial has demonstrated that treatment with ICIs was associated with a higher risk of atherosclerosis-related cardiovascular events in patients with various types of cancer, providing evidence that T cell activation is critically involved in the development of atherosclerotic disease in humans [42]. Careful management is required for the use of ICIs for treating cancer patients with cardiovascular risk factors.

3. Protective Role of Tregs in Atherosclerotic Disease

Thymus-derived natural Tregs were discovered by Sakaguchi et al. in 1995 [43]. Tregs constitutively express high levels of CD25 (IL-2 receptor α-chain) molecule [43] and the transcription factor Foxp3, an essential factor for their differentiation and function [44,45]. Impaired Treg function has been shown to be a primary cause of several autoimmune diseases in mice [46] and humans [47], indicating that this cell population plays an indispensable role in the dominant suppression of autoimmune responses and the maintenance of immune homeostasis. Tregs have multiple inhibitory actions, including suppression of autoimmune T cell proliferation and its differentiation into Th1, Th2, and Th17 lineage, and the inactivation of various immune cells, including B cells, DCs, and macrophages [48]. Several lines of evidence indicate that Tregs protect against atherosclerosis by regulating pathogenic immunoinflammatory responses (Figure 1 and Table 1). Foxp3$^+$ Tregs could also be generated from naïve T cells in the periphery, such as gut-associated lymphoid tissue (GALT), which are called peripherally derived Tregs (pTregs) that maintain mucosal immune tolerance and suppress autoimmune responses [49]. However, the differences in their characteristics between thymus-derived natural Tregs and pTregs remain obscure, and further investigation will be needed. For more detailed information about the diverse role of Tregs in immunology, the reader is referred to a recent review [8].

3.1. Protective Role of Tregs in Experimental Atherosclerosis

The costimulatory pathway CD80/CD86–CD28 plays a role in the generation and homeostasis of Tregs [50]. Genetic deficiency of this costimulatory signaling exacerbated atherosclerosis in *Ldlr*$^{-/-}$ or *Apoe*$^{-/-}$ mice, and was associated with a significant decrease in $CD4^{+}CD25^{+}$ Treg numbers in lymphoid tissues [51]. Notably, adoptive transfer of $CD4^{+}CD25^{+}$ Tregs abrogated the detrimental effects on atherosclerosis observed in *Apoe*$^{-/-}$ mice with the CD80/CD86–CD28 pathway deficiency [51]. In line with this, another research group reported that adoptive transfer of $CD4^{+}CD25^{+}$ Tregs attenuated the development of atherosclerosis in Treg-competent *Apoe*$^{-/-}$ mice [52]. These findings provided the novel concept that $CD4^{+}CD25^{+}$ Tregs protect against atherosclerosis in mice under hypercholesterolemia. A recent study investigated the role of another costimulatory pathway, CD27–CD70, in atherosclerosis by inducing bone marrow-derived and systemic CD27 deficiency in *Apoe*$^{-/-}$ mice, and showed that CD27 deficiency exacerbated early stages of atherosclerosis, along with reduced Treg numbers in various lymphoid organs and the aorta [53]. Interestingly, this study also demonstrated that adoptive transfer of wild-type $CD4^{+}CD25^{+}$ Tregs expressing folate receptor 4 into CD27-deficient *Apoe*$^{-/-}$ mice reversed the phenotype of atherosclerosis, indicating a causative role of decreased Treg frequency in CD27-deficiency-dependent atherosclerosis progression [53].

An important issue for the definition of Tregs is that CD25-expressing $CD4^{+}$ T cell population may contain activated conventional T cells. Firm experimental evidence supports that Foxp3 is the most reliable molecular marker for Tregs in mice [48]. To investigate the precise role of Tregs in atherosclerosis, Klingenberg et al. utilized the DEREG (depletion of regulatory T cells) mice, in which $Foxp3^{+}$ Tregs faithfully express a diphtheria toxin receptor and can be specifically depleted by diphtheria toxin administration [54]. Treg deficiency by transplanting DEREG bone marrow into lethally irradiated *Ldlr*$^{-/-}$ mice accelerated atherosclerosis development without affecting aortic inflammatory responses [55]. This pro-atherogenic effect caused by Treg depletion was associated with markedly elevated plasma cholesterol levels in the very low-density lipoprotein and chylomicron remnant fractions [55]. This study identified for the first time the role of $Foxp3^{+}$ Tregs in atherosclerosis and demonstrated a novel suppressive mechanism that modulates lipid metabolism other than the well-recognized inflammation regulation.

3.2. Possible Protective Role of Tregs in Human Atherosclerosis

In addition to the strong experimental evidence for atheroprotective actions of Tregs, accumulating evidence highlights their importance in human atherosclerotic disease. Low numbers of $FOXP3^{+}$ Tregs were detected in all the progression stages of human atherosclerotic plaques [56]. Single-cell RNA sequencing of a broad cohort of human carotid plaques identified a small sized cluster, showing Tregs detected by the expression of *FOXP3*, *CD25*, and *CTLA4* [57]. Although the number and phenotype of Tregs in human atherosclerotic lesions have not been extensively explored, there are a number of studies that examined the correlation between circulating Treg levels and coronary artery disease (CAD) [58–62], showing reduced peripheral Treg numbers in ACS patients compared with healthy controls or stable angina patients [58,61]. A recent large and long follow-up study showed an association between low levels of baseline $CD4^{+}FOXP3^{+}$ Tregs and an increased risk of acute coronary events, but not stroke [63]. The $CD4^{+}CD25^{+}CD127^{low}$ Treg counts in coronary thrombi were significantly increased compared with peripheral blood in patients with ST elevation or non-ST elevation ACS, indicating that peripheral Tregs might decrease due to their accumulation in ACS lesions in the acute phase of MI [64]. Together, these results suggest that decreased numbers of Tregs may be responsible for the pathogenic inflammation in ACS.

Several markers, such as CD25, CD127, and FOXP3 have been used to define Tregs in previous clinical studies. The strategy of staining the FOXP3 molecule can discriminate Tregs from Teffs more precisely than by the combination of CD25 and CD127 molecules. However, as opposed to murine CD4$^+$Foxp3$^+$ T cells, FOXP3 expression is induced in human CD4$^+$FOXP3$^-$ T cells upon TCR stimulation, which do not exhibit suppressive functions, and therefore such a population may contain some Teffs [8]. Miyara et al. proposed a new strategy to define human Tregs, demonstrating that Tregs are separated into two subsets (CD4$^+$CD45RA$^+$FOXP3^{low} resting Tregs and CD4$^+$CD45RA$^-$FOXP3^{high} activated Tregs) and that activated Teffs are defined as CD4$^+$CD45RA$^-$FOXP3^{low} T cells or CD4$^+$CD45RA$^-$FOXP3$^-$ T cells [65]. The combination of CD45RA and FOXP3 staining of CD4$^+$ T cells may identify Tregs in human peripheral blood more precisely than previous methods. Using this strategy to accurately define human Tregs, we reported that both resting Treg and activated Treg levels were decreased, whereas the CD4$^+$CD45RA$^-$FOXP3$^-$ fraction of activated Teffs was increased in the peripheral blood of patients with stable angina pectoris and old MI compared with healthy controls [66]. These results imply that dysregulated Treg responses might promote atherosclerosis in humans, though it remains unclear whether the imbalance between proatherogenic Teffs and atheroprotective Tregs is a cause or result of CAD. Another important issue regarding the difference in FOXP3 expression between mice and humans is that there are several different isoforms for FOXP3, including FOXP3 lacking the region encoded by exon 2 (FOXP3Δ2). A recent clinical study revealed that not total FOXP3 levels but the proportion of FOXP3Δ2 expression was associated with symptomatic atherosclerotic disease, and that Treg activation led to the induction of FOXP3Δ2 isoform expression that plays an important role in the regulation of its effector functions [67]. Collectively, these reports highlight the possible role of Tregs in the protection against human atherosclerotic disease.

3.3. Protective Role of Tregs in AAA

AAA characterized by dilation of the abdominal aorta is a lethal aortic disease and associated with atherosclerosis. Importantly, there are no effective pharmacological therapies against this disease, and surgical treatment is performed if the risk of rupture is higher than that of the procedure. Therefore, it is important to elucidate the detailed mechanisms underlying AAA development and develop noninvasive therapies for this disease. Clinical and experimental evidence suggests that inflammation caused by accumulation of Teffs and macrophages in aneurysmal lesions contributes to the development of AAA, and that Tregs protect against AAA formation [68]. Genetic deficiency of CD4$^+$CD25$^+$ Tregs promotes the development and rupture of angiotensin II-induced AAA in normocholesterolemic mice [69]. Adoptive transfer of CD4$^+$CD25$^+$ Tregs prevents angiotensin II-induced AAA formation in atherosclerosis-prone *Apoe*$^{-/-}$ mice [70]. Using hypercholesterolemic DEREG mice, we demonstrated that genetic depletion of CD4$^+$Foxp3$^+$ Tregs aggravates AAA formation and rupture in angiotensin II-infused *Apoe*$^{-/-}$ mice by upregulating immunoinflammatory responses in the aneurysmal lesions, providing direct evidence for a protective role of CD4$^+$Foxp3$^+$ Tregs in the development of AAA [71]. In patients with AAA, decreased numbers of CD4$^+$CD25$^+$FOXP3$^+$ Tregs were observed, and Foxp3 expression in peripheral CD4$^+$CD25$^+$ cells was decreased compared with healthy control subjects [72]. FOXP3 expression levels in human aneurysmal tissues are significantly lower than in normal thoracic aortic tissues [70]. These reports suggest that impaired immunoregulation by Tregs may be involved in the development of AAA, and that promotion of endogenous regulatory immune responses may represent an attractive therapeutic approach to AAA.

3.4. Mechanisms of Treg-Mediated Atheroprotection

A large number of studies in immunology fields have elucidated the mechanisms by which Tregs control pathogenic immune responses, leading to the development of effective approaches to prevent and treat inflammatory diseases based on the modulation of their functions. Tregs exert suppressive functions via multiple mechanisms, including cell contact-dependent suppression, secretion of immunosuppressive factors including IL-10, IL-35, and transforming growth factor (TGF)-β, intracellular molecule (granzyme, cyclic adenosine monophosphate, and indoleamine 2,3-dioxygenase)-dependent suppression, and IL-2 deprivation from responder T cells, which could operate in a synergistical or complementary manner [8]. Although it remains obscure which mechanism is dominant for the Treg-mediated regulation of pathogenic immune responses, core suppressive pathways may depend on the type and stage of disease, or subsets of Tregs.

Among cytokines secreted from T cells, IL-10 and TGF-β have potent anti-inflammatory actions and have attracted much attention as potent anti-atherosclerotic cytokines [73]. Regarding the suppressive actions of Tregs in atherosclerosis, IL-10 and TGF-β production might be involved in this process. In *Ldlr*$^{-/-}$ mice fed a high-cholesterol diet, overexpression of IL-10 in T cells inhibited the development of advanced atherosclerotic lesions by shifting the Th1/Th2 balance toward Th2 phenotype [74]. Genetic deletion of TGF-β signaling in T cells led to a dramatic increase in atherosclerotic lesion development with an unstable plaque phenotype in *Apoe*$^{-/-}$ mice [75]. As described above, our recent study demonstrated that overexpression of CTLA-4 in T cells inhibited atherosclerosis development in *Apoe*$^{-/-}$ mice by downregulating the CD80 and CD86 expression on DCs and limiting the CD80/CD86–CD28-dependent activation of Teffs [34]. CTLA-4-dependent suppression of DC function by Tregs may also be involved in the reduction in atherosclerosis. However, it remains to be determined whether these suppressive mechanisms depend on Tregs or other subsets of T cells. Tregs contribute to the promotion of inflammation resolution by enhancing apoptotic cell clearance (efferocytosis) by macrophages, which could contribute to the prevention of atherosclerosis development [76]. The identification of dominant atheroprotective mechanisms mediated by Tregs would lead to the establishment of novel Treg-based therapies for atherosclerotic disease.

3.5. *Treg Immune Responses under Hypercholesterolemia*

Several experimental reports have shown the close link between hypercholesterolemia and Treg number and function (Table 1). The proportion of Foxp3$^+$ Tregs within the splenic CD4$^+$ T cell population was markedly increased in *Ldlr*$^{-/-}$ mice fed a cholesterol-rich diet, whereas their accumulation in atherosclerotic plaques was impaired in association with decreased expression of their surface molecules related to migratory function, which was prevented by reversal of hypercholesterolemia [77]. The in vitro suppressive function of Tregs was maintained under hypercholesterolemia, although their expression of various selectin ligands and binding capacity to aortic endothelium were decreased and apoptosis of intraplaque Tregs was promoted under such conditions [77]. Another experimental study in wild-type mice fed a cholesterol-rich diet demonstrated that diet-induced hypercholesterolemia rather increased an in vitro Treg suppressive activity [78]. In *Ldlr*$^{-/-}$ mice fed a high-cholesterol diet exhibiting mild hypercholesterolemia, Treg differentiation was promoted in the liver [79]. However, under severe hypercholesterolemia, disrupted homeostasis in the liver promoted Th1 cell differentiation and CD11b$^+$CD11c$^+$ leukocyte accumulation, resulting in the abrogation of Treg responses and the promotion of atherosclerosis [79]. A recent study in *Ldlr*$^{-/-}$ mice fed a high-cholesterol diet has shown that diet-induced hypercholesterolemia modulated the intracellular metabolism of Tregs and the expression of several molecules involved in their migration, which led to the conversion of Tregs to an effector-like migratory phenotype and the promotion of their migration towards atherosclerotic aortas [80]. These results imply that decreased Treg migratory capacity due to hypercholesterolemia may not be responsible for the dysfunction of their ability to control atherosclerosis. Thus, accumulating experimental evidence indicates that hypercholesterolemia affects the number, function, migratory capacity, and intracellular metabolism in Tregs. Further studies are needed to better understand these mechanisms.

It is supposed that Tregs in circulation enter the lymphoid tissues surrounding atherosclerotic arteries where they may be presented with some atherosclerosis-associated antigens by DCs, become activated, and migrate into atherosclerotic aortas to mitigate lesional inflammation and plaque development. This implies that the expansion of Tregs in atherosclerotic lesions could lead to reduced plaque inflammation and lesion development. The chemokine system plays an important role in the recruitment of T cells and monocytes to atherosclerotic lesions [81]. Several chemokine receptors are specifically expressed on each Th subset, whereas Treg-specific chemokine receptors have not been identified. An experimental report demonstrated that the expression of the chemokine CX3CL1 was selectively upregulated in the aorta of *Ldlr*$^{-/-}$ mice fed a high-cholesterol diet compared with other lymphoid tissues, and that the adoptive transfer of its counterreceptor CX3CR1-transduced Tregs promoted their migration to the atherosclerotic lesions and reduced atherosclerosis development, although CX3CR1 is mainly expressed on Ly6C^{+} monocytes and its endogenous expression on Tregs is relatively low [82]. The role of chemokine–chemokine receptor interactions in Treg recruitment to atherosclerotic lesions remains largely unknown. Importantly, it remains unclear whether lesional Tregs suppress inflammatory reactions responsible for atherosclerotic lesion development, and further extensive experiments are required to identify the exact role of lesional Tregs in atherosclerosis.

3.6. Stability, Plasticity, and Antigen-Specificity of Tregs in Atherosclerosis

Tregs may stably exert suppressive activities for a long time under physiological conditions, while they have been reported to lose inhibitory functions (instability) and show an effector-like phenotype (plasticity) under inflammatory conditions (Table 1) [83]. Similar phenomena are observed under the conditions of prolonged hypercholesterolemia [84]. In *Apoe*$^{-/-}$ mice, CD4^{+}Foxp3^{+} Tregs could differentiate into proinflammatory Th1-like cells in the aorta and secondary lymphoid tissues and become dysfunctional, leading to the exacerbation of arterial inflammation and lesion development [85]. CD4^{+}Foxp3^{+}CCR5^{+}CD25^{-} Tregs found exclusively in the aorta and draining lymph nodes of *Apoe*$^{-/-}$ mice fed a high-cholesterol diet for a long period exhibit impaired suppressive activities and exacerbate atherosclerosis, although it remains unclear whether this cell population is derived from bona fide Tregs [86].

Table 1. Role of Tregs in atherosclerotic disease.

	Possible Protective Role of Tregs in Atherosclerosis	
	Description	**References**
Mouse	Genetic deficiency of the CD80/CD86–CD28 signaling decreases CD4^{+}CD25^{+} Tregs in lymphoid tissues and exacerbates atherosclerosis in *Apoe*$^{-/-}$ or *Ldlr*$^{-/-}$ mice.	[51]
	Adoptive transfer of CD4^{+}CD25^{+} Tregs attenuates the development of atherosclerosis in Treg-competent *Apoe*$^{-/-}$ mice.	[52]
	Genetic deletion of Foxp3^{+} Tregs accelerates atherosclerosis development in *Ldlr*$^{-/-}$ mice.	[55]
Human	Low numbers of FOXP3^{+} Tregs are detected in all the progression stages of atherosclerotic plaques.	[56,57]
	Peripheral Treg numbers are reduced in CAD patients	[58,61,66]

Table 1. *Cont.*

Possible mechanisms of Treg-mediated atheroprotection		
	Description	**References**
Cytokine secretion	Overexpression of IL-10 in T cells inhibits the development of atherosclerosis.	[74]
	Genetic deletion of TGF-β signaling in T cells dramatically accelerates atherosclerotic lesion development with unstable plaque phenotype.	[75]
Cell–cell contact	Overexpression of CTLA-4 in T cells inhibits atherosclerosis development by downregulating the CD80 and CD86 expression on DCs.	[34]
Efferocytosis	Tregs enhance apoptotic cell clearance by macrophages.	[76]
Treg immune responses under hypercholesterolemia		
Cell number	The proportion of splenic $CD4^+Foxp3^+$ Tregs is markedly increased.	[77]
	Treg differentiation is promoted in the liver under mild hypercholesterolemia.	[79]
Function	The expression of Treg surface molecules related to migratory function is decreased.	[77]
	Hypercholesterolemia increases in vitro Treg suppressive activity.	[78]
	Hypercholesterolemia modulates the intracellular metabolism of Tregs and promotes their migration towards atherosclerotic aortas.	[80]
	$CD4^+Foxp3^+$ Tregs differentiate into Th1-like cells in the aorta and secondary lymphoid tissues and become dysfunctional.	[85]

Apoe$^{-/-}$, apolipoprotein E-deficient; CAD, coronary artery disease; CTLA-4, cytotoxic T-lymphocyte-associated antigen-4; DC, dendritic cell; Foxp3, forkhead box P3; IL, interleukin; *Ldlr*$^{-/-}$, low-density lipoprotein receptor-deficient; TGF, transforming growth factor; Th1, T helper type 1; Treg, regulatory T cell.

As the disruption of immunologic tolerance against modified lipoproteins may be responsible for the pathogenesis of atherosclerosis, it could be considered as an autoimmune disease. T cells including Tregs respond to some antigens derived from components of LDL particles [7]. MHC class II-deficient *Apoe*$^{-/-}$ mice had greater atherosclerotic lesions and reduced numbers of Tregs, implying that MHC class II-mediated generation and activation of antigen-specific Tregs would have a protective role in the development of atherosclerosis [87]. However, due to technical limitations, the role of antigen-specific T cells in atherosclerosis has not been elucidated in most experimental or clinical studies. A recent study using newly designed tetramers to detect human T cells specific for ApoB-derived peptides $ApoB_{3036–3050}$, possible atherosclerosis-related antigens, has shown that healthy subjects have ApoB-specific $Foxp3^+$ Tregs, and that these Tregs coexpress other CD4 lineage transcription factors, such as ROR-γt, in patients with subclinical cardiovascular disease [88]. Another study by the same group using a tetramer to detect $ApoB_{978–993}$-specific T cells has revealed that ApoB-specific T cells in *Apoe*$^{-/-}$ mice convert from mixed Th17/Treg cells with a regulatory anti-inflammatory transcriptome into proinflammatory Th1/Th17-like cells that secrete inflammatory cytokines, and that these ApoB-specific $CD4^+$ T cells with a predominant Th1/Th17 phenotype were detected in the blood of patients with CAD [89]. Many questions remain to be answered regarding the role of stability, plasticity, and antigen specificity of Tregs in atherosclerosis [7]. Further studies should address these issues to translate findings obtained by experimental studies to the clinical settings.

4. Therapeutic Approaches for Atherosclerotic Disease by Promoting Regulatory Immune Responses

The balance between Teffs and Tregs is critical for the control of atherosclerotic disease. Based on recent experimental and clinical evidence, we expect that improving this balance, by enhancing Treg responses or dampening Teff responses, could be an effective therapy for atherosclerotic disease [9,10] (Figure 2). A large number of experimental studies have shown that the activation and expansion of antigen-specific or non-specific Tregs protect against atherosclerosis by suppressing pathogenic immune responses (Table 2). This may be supported by the fact that upon antigen presentation, Tregs also exert suppressive functions in an antigen-non-specific manner [48].

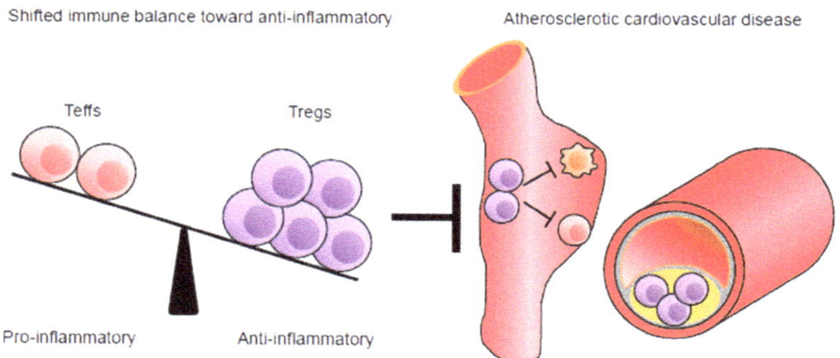

Figure 2. The balance between proatherogenic effector T cells (Teffs) and atheroprotective regulatory T cells (Tregs) is critical for the control of atherosclerosis.

4.1. Vaccination Strategies

Experimental studies in atherosclerosis-prone mice have demonstrated that immunization with several atherosclerosis-related antigens, native LDL, oxidized LDL, or ApoB-derived peptides, induces antigen-specific Tregs and attenuates atherosclerotic lesion development [16]. The induction of antigen-specific immunological tolerance could be an attractive therapeutic strategy for atherosclerosis, because this approach can dampen pathogenic immune responses against atherosclerosis-related antigens and avoid general immunosuppression. The identification of atherosclerosis-related antigens and the development of effective immunization methods would advance the field in designing a novel approach to prevent human atherosclerosis. For more in-depth information on vaccination strategies in atherosclerosis, the reader is referred to a recent review [16].

4.2. Modulation of DC Functions

The interaction between Tregs and some DC subsets play a protective role in atherosclerosis [9]. DC maturation mediated by MyD88, a key Toll-like receptor adaptor, is atheroprotective through controlling Treg responses in Western-type diet-fed *Ldlr*$^{-/-}$ mice [90]. Flt3 signaling-dependent CD11c^{hi}MHC-II^{hi}CD11b^{-}CD103^{+} DCs in aortic tissue promote accumulation of CD4^{+}Foxp3^{+} Tregs and protect against atherosclerosis in *Ldlr*$^{-/-}$ mice fed a high-fat diet [91]. Immature tolerogenic DCs, characterized by low expression levels of MHC class II molecule and costimulatory molecules, expand CD4^{+}Foxp3^{+} Tregs and inhibit Teff responses, contributing to the maintenance of immune tolerance and regulation of atherosclerosis [92]. Adoptive transfer of ApoB100-pulsed tolerogenic DCs prevented atherosclerosis development in hypercholesterolemic mice by diminishing pathogenic T cell responses to ApoB100 and promoting antigen-specific CD4^{+}Foxp3^{+} Treg responses [93]. Our study showed that oral administration of the active form of vitamin D_3 (calcitriol) attenuated atherosclerosis development in *Apoe*$^{-/-}$ mice by expanding tolerogenic DCs and CD4^{+}Foxp3^{+} Tregs systemically and locally in atherosclerotic lesions, which might interact with each other and efficiently regulate aortic inflammatory responses associated with atherosclerosis [94]. This study provided direct evidence for a possible anti-atherogenic role of vitamin D reported in an epidemiological study showing the association between vitamin D deficiency and increased cardiovascular events and mortality [95]. Collectively, strategies to expand and activate several types of atheroprotective DCs could be possible therapies for the prevention of atherosclerosis [92].

4.3. Modulation of Intestinal Immunity

As described above, Foxp3$^+$ Tregs (known as pTregs) differentiate from naïve T cells not only in the thymus but also in GALT, where multiple stimuli such as commensal microbiota and food antigens could effectively promote their induction [49,96]. T regulatory type 1 (Tr1) or T helper type 3 (Th3) cells that do not express Foxp3 are induced in GALT and produce immunomodulatory cytokines IL-10 or TGF-β, respectively [96]. The development of atherosclerosis was attenuated by in vivo induction of Tr1 cells in atherosclerosis-prone mice, which was associated with increased production of IL-10 [97,98]. Experimental evidence indicates that induction of mucosal (oral or nasal) tolerance may be an effective way to prevent and treat various autoimmune diseases, including atherosclerosis, and has attracted much interest, although clinical trials to examine the preventive effect of this approach on some autoimmune diseases were unsuccessful [96]. One of the critical mechanisms for mucosal tolerance induction is supposed to be induction of several types of self-antigen-specific Tregs described above [96]. Oral tolerance induction to oxidized LDL [98] or heat shock protein 60 [99] reduced the development of atherosclerosis in *Ldlr*$^{-/-}$ mice, in association with increased proportion of CD4$^+$CD25$^+$Foxp3$^+$ Tregs in several lymphoid organs and promoted the production of TGF-β or IL-10 in mesenteric lymph nodes upon each antigen stimulation, respectively. However, antigen-specificity of expanded Tregs was not clearly determined in these studies.

Gut microbiota are highly associated with the intestinal immunity and systemic metabolic disorders. Recent experimental and clinical studies have provided evidence for an association between gut microbiota composition and development of CVD [100]. By performing 16S ribosomal RNA gene sequencing in fecal samples from CAD patients and mechanistic studies with *Apoe*$^{-/-}$ mice, we have recently demonstrated that the relative abundance of *Bacteroides vulgatus* and *Bacteroides dorei* was lower in patients with CAD compared with controls, and that this microbiota protects against atherosclerosis by ameliorating endotoxemia and systemic inflammation [101]. CD4$^+$Foxp3$^+$ Tregs were expanded in the colon lamina propria by oral administration of mouse [102] and human [103] *Clostridium* species, the spore-forming component of indigenous intestinal microbiota, and this Treg induction resulted in attenuation of experimental colitis. As the mechanisms for induction of colonic Tregs, butyrate, one of commensal bacteria-derived short-chain fatty acids, was shown to regulate the differentiation of Tregs and ameliorate the development of experimental colitis [104]. Although no prior reports investigated the role of *Clostridium* species or microbial-derived butyrate in atherosclerosis, a recent experimental study using hypertensive mice with or without atherosclerosis has reported that treatment with another short-chain fatty acid propionate prevents cardiac damage and atherosclerosis by regulating inflammatory responses, which was mainly dependent on Tregs [105]. Collectively, recent experimental and clinical data suggest that some specific gut microbiota and microbial-derived metabolites may modulate atherosclerosis. Further investigation will contribute to the development of novel therapies to prevent atherosclerotic disease through modulation of intestinal immune system.

4.4. Treatment with Antibodies and Cytokines

Intravenously administered anti-CD3 monoclonal antibodies, effective in treating autoimmune diabetes in mice [106] and humans [107], also improve atherosclerosis in mice [108] by regulating Teff immune responses and expanding CD4$^+$CD25$^+$ Tregs. Oral or nasal anti-CD3 antibody administration can induce CD4$^+$LAP (latency-associated peptide)$^+$ Tregs that suppress experimental autoimmune diseases in a TGF-β-dependent manner [109,110]. We orally treated $Apoe^{-/-}$ mice with anti-CD3 antibodies and observed significantly reduced plaque formation and inflammation, associated with the expansion of $CD4^+LAP^+$ Tregs and $CD4^+Foxp3^+$ Tregs in mesenteric lymph nodes [111]. As a mechanism of this suppression, we speculate that expanded Tregs may move to other lymphoid organs or atherosclerotic lesions and suppress proatherogenic immune responses. We propose the novel idea that oral immune modulation could serve as an attractive therapeutic approach to atherosclerotic disease.

$CD4^+Foxp3^+$ Tregs highly express CD25, a component of the high-affinity IL-2 receptor, and vigorously proliferate in the presence of IL-2. Recombinant mouse IL-2/anti-IL-2 monoclonal antibody complexes (IL-2 complexes) efficiently and selectively expand $CD4^+CD25^+Foxp3^+$ Tregs and attenuate atherosclerosis in $Ldlr^{-/-}$ [112] or $Apoe^{-/-}$ mice [113]. Induction of $CD4^+Foxp3^+$ Tregs by IL-2 complex treatment also provides protection against angiotensin II-induced AAA formation in $Apoe^{-/-}$ mice [71]. These reports suggest that IL-2 complex treatment could be a possible strategy to prevent both atherosclerosis and AAA. Considering that suppressive functions of Tregs can be impaired under inflammatory conditions [114], we speculate that both Treg expansion and inhibition of Teff responses could be necessary to potently suppress atherosclerosis. In line with this idea, we found that the combination treatment with anti-CD3 antibodies and IL-2 complexes was effective in expanding Treg with activated phenotype and preventing atherosclerosis development in $Apoe^{-/-}$ mice [115].

Interestingly, a recent observational cohort study in patients with chronic graft-versus-host disease demonstrated that low-dose IL-2 was safely administered in these patients, which was associated with marked and sustained expansion of Tregs and improvement of the disease manifestations in a substantial proportion of treated patients [116]. Another clinical study in patients with vasculitis induced by the hepatitis C virus showed that the administration of low-dose IL-2 increased the percentage of Tregs without adverse effects in all subjects and led to the improvement of vasculitis in most patients [117]. Based on the data obtained from experimental and clinical studies described above, a randomized, double-blind, placebo-controlled, phase I/II clinical trial in patients with stable ischemic heart disease and ACS (LILACS), has begun to assess the safety and efficacy of low-dose IL-2 in patients with CAD [118,119]. It is expected that interesting results of this trial will be reported in the future.

4.5. Ultraviolet B (UVB)-Based Phototherapy

It is historically clear that sunlight exposure is indispensable for the maintenance of our health. UV is categorized into UVA (320–400 nm), UVB (280–320 nm), and UVC (100–280 nm). As UVC is blocked by the atmosphere and the ozone layer, we receive UVA and UVB wavelengths from natural sunlight in daily life. UVB irradiation is known to have beneficial effects on the immune system due to its anti-inflammatory and immunosuppressive actions, although chronic excessive UVB exposure could cause skin cancer or infectious diseases [120]. Based on this, UVB-based phototherapy is an established treatment for various human skin diseases without severe adverse effects [121].

Our recent work revealed that broad-band UVB (a continuous spectrum from 280 to 320 nm with a peak around 313 nm) exposure attenuates the development and progression of atherosclerosis in $Apoe^{-/-}$ mice, associated with a systemic increase in $CD4^+Foxp3^+$ Tregs with higher suppressive capacity and a decrease in proinflammatory IFN-γ production from T cells [122]. Langerhans cells (LCs), epidermal $Langerin^+$ DCs having an important role in presenting antigens to T cells, are reported to regulate immunoinflammatory reactions following their activation by various environmental stimuli, such as UVB [123,124]. Using LC-depleted mice on an $Apoe^{-/-}$ background, we clearly showed that LCs play an indispensable role in the systemic expansion of Tregs and attenuation of atherosclerosis development and progression, suggesting the skin immune system as a novel therapeutic target for atherosclerosis. We also investigated the effect of UVB irradiation on the development of atherosclerosis-related vascular disease, such as AAA, and found that UVB irradiation attenuated the development of angiotensin II-induced AAA under hypercholesterolemia and prevented death due to its rupture [125]. Further analysis using hypercholesterolemic DEREG mice revealed that genetic depletion of CD4$^+$Foxp3$^+$ Tregs abrogated the protective effect of UVB treatment, indicating an indispensable role of Tregs for UVB-mediated prevention of AAA formation.

Clinical studies in patients with skin autoimmune disease demonstrated that bath-psoralen UVA or narrow-band UVB (a narrow peak around 311 nm) therapy expanded CD4$^+$CD25$^+$Foxp3$^+$ Tregs in the periphery and improved disease state [126,127]. The efficacy of UVB therapy may vary depending on its wavelengths, although the detailed mechanisms of UVB-mediated protective effects on skin diseases remain obscure. Within the UVB spectrum, narrow-band UVB is the most effective wavelength for treating psoriasis [121]. Likewise, there might be some specific UVB wavelengths that are effective in preventing atherosclerosis, although we have no information about this so far. If the issues regarding the efficacy and safety of UVB therapy are overcome, UVB phototherapy could be an attractive immunomodulatory strategy for preventing atherosclerotic CVD.

4.6. Approaches to Regress Atherosclerosis

A great number of human and animal studies have revealed mechanisms of atherosclerotic plaque development, whereas mechanisms that reverse the disease remain obscure. In a clinical study, very intensive statin therapy lowered LDL cholesterol levels and increased high-density lipoprotein cholesterol levels, resulting in atherosclerosis regression, indicating the importance of lipid control for regressing established plaques [128]. In addition, experimental studies using several mouse models of atherosclerosis regression have highlighted the involvement of immunoinflammatory reactions in the process of atherosclerosis regression [129–131], although the precise mechanisms underlying this process have not been completely elucidated. Using a new mouse model of atherosclerosis regression in *Ldlr*$^{-/-}$, we found that Eicosapentaenoic acid induced atherosclerosis regression by modulating DC functions and reducing CD4$^+$ T cell numbers without increasing CD4$^+$CD25$^+$Foxp3$^+$ Tregs [132], supporting the clinical benefits of this drug for the treatment of CVD in Japanese hypercholesterolemic patients [133]. Using the same mouse model, we also reported that intravenous injection of anti-CD3 antibodies induced rapid regression of established atherosclerotic lesions, associated with increased proportion of CD4$^+$CD25$^+$Foxp3$^+$ Tregs in the regressing plaques as well as in the lymphoid organs [134]. This study for the first time suggested the possibility that the expansion of Tregs might contribute to regressing atherosclerotic plaques in mice. In line with this, a recent experimental study using various mouse models of atherosclerosis regression has demonstrated that CD4$^+$CD25$^+$Foxp3$^+$ Tregs accumulated in the regressing plaques, and played an indispensable role for inflammation resolution in the artery wall by regulating macrophage- and T cell-mediated pro-inflammatory responses [135]. Collectively, these reports imply that in addition to intensive lipid-lowering therapies, the promotion of Treg immune responses may represent an effective therapeutic approach for atherosclerosis regression.

Table 2. Strategies to prevent or treat atherosclerosis by promoting regulatory immune responses.

Strategies	Treatment	Immune Effects	References
Vaccination	Treatment with native LDL, oxidized LDL, or ApoB-derived peptides	Induction of antigen-specific Tregs	[16]
Modulation of DC functions	Transfer of ApoB100-plused tolerogenic DCs	Promoted antigen-specific $CD4^+Foxp3^+$ Treg responses and suppressed pathogenic T cell responses to ApoB100	[93]
	Oral administration of active form of vitaminD_3 (calcitriol)	Increased tolerogenic DCs and $CD4^+Foxp3^+$ Tregs	[94]
Modulation of intestinal immunity	Oral tolerance induction to oxidized LDL or heat shock protein 60	Increased $CD4^+CD25^+Foxp3^+$ Tregs and promoted production of TGF-β or IL-10 in mesenteric lymph nodes	[98,99]
	Oral administration of short-chain fatty acid propionate	Suppressed inflammatory responses mainly dependent on Tregs	[105]
Treatment with antibodies and cytokines	Intravenous administration of anti-CD3 monoclonal antibodies	Increased $CD4^+CD25^+Foxp3^+$ Tregs and suppressed Teff immune responses	[108,134]
	Oral administration of anti-CD3 monoclonal antibodies	Increased $CD4^+LAP^+$ or $CD4^+Foxp3^+$ Tregs in mesenteric lymph nodes and suppressed Teff immune responses	[111]
	Treatment with recombinant mouse IL-2/anti-IL-2 monoclonal antibody complexes	Increased $CD4^+CD25^+Foxp3^+$ Tregs and suppressed Teff immune responses	[112,113]
	Combination treatment with anti-CD3 monoclonal antibodies and IL-2 complexes	Increased $CD4^+Foxp3^+$ Tregs with activated phenotype	[115]
UVB-based phototherapy	UVB irradiation to the skin	Increased $CD4^+Foxp3^+$ Tregs and decreased IFN-γ production from T cells	[122]

ApoB, apolipoprotein B; DC, dendritic cell; Foxp3, forkhead box P3; IFN, interferon; IL, interleukin; LAP, latency-associated peptide; LDL, low-density lipoprotein; Teff, effector T cell; TGF, transforming growth factor; Treg, regulatory T cell; UVB, ultraviolet B.

5. Conclusions

It has now become evident that arterial inflammation caused by immune dysregulation critically contributes to the development of atherosclerotic CVD. Recent clinical studies have confirmed that an anti-inflammatory therapy could be a possible strategy to prevent atherosclerotic CVD in patients with past cardiovascular disease history [4–6]. Although anti-inflammatory pharmacological therapies seem to be safe and effective in treating experimental atherosclerosis in mice, general immunosuppression caused by such therapies would cause adverse immune responses in humans [3]. Moreover, it will take much cost to prescribe expensive drugs for a long time. Therefore, other strategies to dampen inflammatory responses in atherosclerosis should be considered.

Notably, firm evidence indicating the involvement of the adaptive immunity including Teff and Treg immune responses in atherosclerosis has accumulated [7]. Pharmacological approaches, vaccination strategies, and cell transfer of Tregs have been shown to reduce atherosclerosis development in mice [9,10]. Strategies to prevent atherosclerosis through boosting regulatory immune responses seem to be attractive and could be clinically applied for the treatment of atherosclerotic disease. However, despite accumulated knowledge about the role of protective Tregs in experimental atherosclerosis, we still lack direct clinical evidence to support this idea. To translate a large number of important findings obtained by animal experiments to clinical settings, extensive clinical studies will be required.

Author Contributions: T.T. and N.S. wrote the manuscript and contributed equally to this work. Y.R. critically revised the manuscript. All authors have read and agreed to the published version of the manuscript.

Funding: This work was supported by JSPS KAKENHI Grant Numbers 23790849, 25860601, 15K09156, and 18K08088.

Acknowledgments: We would like to thank our laboratory members for helpful discussions.

Conflicts of Interest: The authors declare no conflict of interest.

References

1. Hansson, G.K.; Hermansson, A. The immune system in atherosclerosis. *Nat. Immunol.* **2011**, *12*, 204–212. [CrossRef]
2. Tabas, I.; Lichtman, A.H. Monocyte-macrophages and T cells in atherosclerosis. *Immunity* **2017**, *47*, 621–634. [CrossRef]
3. Lutgens, E.; Atzler, D.; Doring, Y.; Duchene, J.; Steffens, S.; Weber, C. Immunotherapy for cardiovascular disease. *Eur. Heart J.* **2019**, *40*, 3937–3946. [CrossRef] [PubMed]
4. Ridker, P.M.; Everett, B.M.; Thuren, T.; MacFadyen, J.G.; Chang, W.H.; Ballantyne, C.; Fonseca, F.; Nicolau, J.; Koenig, W.; Anker, S.D.; et al. Antiinflammatory therapy with canakinumab for atherosclerotic disease. *N. Engl. J. Med.* **2017**, *377*, 1119–1131. [CrossRef] [PubMed]
5. Tardif, J.C.; Kouz, S.; Waters, D.D.; Bertrand, O.F.; Diaz, R.; Maggioni, A.P.; Pinto, F.J.; Ibrahim, R.; Gamra, H.; Kiwan, G.S.; et al. Efficacy and safety of low-dose colchicine after myocardial infarction. *N. Engl. J. Med.* **2019**, *381*, 2497–2505. [CrossRef]
6. Nidorf, S.M.; Fiolet, A.T.L.; Mosterd, A.; Eikelboom, J.W.; Schut, A.; Opstal, T.S.J.; The, S.H.K.; Xu, X.F.; Ireland, M.A.; Lenderink, T.; et al. Colchicine in patients with chronic coronary disease. *N. Engl. J. Med.* **2020**, *383*, 1838–1847. [CrossRef] [PubMed]
7. Saigusa, R.; Winkels, H.; Ley, K. T cell subsets and functions in atherosclerosis. *Nat. Rev. Cardiol.* **2020**, *17*, 387–401.
8. Sakaguchi, S.; Mikami, N.; Wing, J.B.; Tanaka, A.; Ichiyama, K.; Ohkura, N. Regulatory T cells and human disease. *Annu. Rev. Immunol.* **2020**, *38*, 541–566. [CrossRef]
9. Sasaki, N.; Yamashita, T.; Kasahara, K.; Takeda, M.; Hirata, K. Regulatory T cells and tolerogenic dendritic cells as critical immune modulators in atherogenesis. *Curr. Pharm. Des.* **2015**, *21*, 1107–1117. [CrossRef] [PubMed]
10. Ait-Oufella, H.; Lavillegrand, J.R.; Tedgui, A. Regulatory T cell-enhancing therapies to treat atherosclerosis. *Cells* **2021**, *10*, 723.
11. Ross, R. Atherosclerosis—An inflammatory disease. *N. Engl. J. Med.* **1999**, *340*, 115–126. [CrossRef] [PubMed]
12. Zhang, S.H.; Reddick, R.L.; Piedrahita, J.A.; Maeda, N. Spontaneous hypercholesterolemia and arterial lesions in mice lacking apolipoprotein E. *Science* **1992**, *258*, 468–471. [CrossRef]
13. Ishibashi, S.; Brown, M.S.; Goldstein, J.L.; Gerard, R.D.; Hammer, R.E.; Herz, J. Hypercholesterolemia in low density lipoprotein receptor knockout mice and its reversal by adenovirus-mediated gene delivery. *J. Clin. Investig.* **1993**, *92*, 883–893. [CrossRef]
14. Ait-Oufella, H.; Sage, A.P.; Mallat, Z.; Tedgui, A. Adaptive (T and B cells) immunity and control by dendritic cells in atherosclerosis. *Circ. Res.* **2014**, *114*, 1640–1660. [CrossRef]
15. Paulsson, G.; Zhou, X.; Tornquist, E.; Hansson, G.K. Oligoclonal T cell expansions in atherosclerotic lesions of apolipoprotein E-deficient mice. *Arterioscler. Thromb. Vasc. Biol.* **2000**, *20*, 10–17. [CrossRef]
16. Nilsson, J.; Hansson, G.K. Vaccination strategies and immune modulation of atherosclerosis. *Circ. Res.* **2020**, *126*, 1281–1296.
17. Sage, A.P.; Tsiantoulas, D.; Binder, C.J.; Mallat, Z. The role of B cells in atherosclerosis. *Nat. Rev. Cardiol.* **2019**, *16*, 180–196. [CrossRef] [PubMed]
18. Winkels, H.; Ehinger, E.; Vassallo, M.; Buscher, K.; Dinh, H.Q.; Kobiyama, K.; Hamers, A.A.J.; Cochain, C.; Vafadarnejad, E.; Saliba, A.E.; et al. Atlas of the immune cell repertoire in mouse atherosclerosis defined by single-cell RNA-sequencing and mass cytometry. *Circ. Res.* **2018**, *122*, 1675–1688. [CrossRef] [PubMed]

19. Fernandez, D.M.; Rahman, A.H.; Fernandez, N.F.; Chudnovskiy, A.; Amir, E.D.; Amadori, L.; Khan, N.S.; Wong, C.K.; Shamailova, R.; Hill, C.A.; et al. Single-cell immune landscape of human atherosclerotic plaques. *Nat. Med.* **2019**, *25*, 1576–1588. [CrossRef] [PubMed]
20. Gupta, S.; Pablo, A.M.; Jiang, X.; Wang, N.; Tall, A.R.; Schindler, C. IFN-gamma potentiates atherosclerosis in ApoE knock-out mice. *J. Clin. Investig.* **1997**, *99*, 2752–2761. [CrossRef]
21. Whitman, S.C.; Ravisankar, P.; Elam, H.; Daugherty, A. Exogenous interferon-gamma enhances atherosclerosis in apolipoprotein $E^{-/-}$ mice. *Am. J. Pathol.* **2000**, *157*, 1819–1824. [CrossRef]
22. Buono, C.; Binder, C.J.; Stavrakis, G.; Witztum, J.L.; Glimcher, L.H.; Lichtman, A.H. T-bet deficiency reduces atherosclerosis and alters plaque antigen-specific immune responses. *Proc. Natl. Acad. Sci. USA* **2005**, *102*, 1596–1601. [CrossRef] [PubMed]
23. Frostegard, J.; Ulfgren, A.K.; Nyberg, P.; Hedin, U.; Swedenborg, J.; Andersson, U.; Hansson, G.K. Cytokine expression in advanced human atherosclerotic plaques: Dominance of pro-inflammatory (Th1) and macrophage-stimulating cytokines. *Atherosclerosis* **1999**, *145*, 33–43. [CrossRef]
24. King, V.L.; Szilvassy, S.J.; Daugherty, A. Interleukin-4 deficiency decreases atherosclerotic lesion formation in a site-specific manner in female LDL receptor$^{-/-}$ mice. *Arterioscler. Thromb. Vasc. Biol.* **2002**, *22*, 456–461. [CrossRef]
25. King, V.L.; Cassis, L.A.; Daugherty, A. Interleukin-4 does not influence development of hypercholesterolemia or angiotensin II-induced atherosclerotic lesions in mice. *Am. J. Pathol.* **2007**, *171*, 2040–2047. [CrossRef] [PubMed]
26. Littman, D.R.; Rudensky, A.Y. Th17 and regulatory T cells in mediating and restraining inflammation. *Cell* **2010**, *140*, 845–858. [CrossRef]
27. Erbel, C.; Chen, L.; Bea, F.; Wangler, S.; Celik, S.; Lasitschka, F.; Wang, Y.; Bockler, D.; Katus, H.A.; Dengler, T.J. Inhibition of IL-17A attenuates atherosclerotic lesion development in apoE-deficient mice. *J. Immunol.* **2009**, *183*, 8167–8175. [CrossRef]
28. Smith, E.; Prasad, K.M.; Butcher, M.; Dobrian, A.; Kolls, J.K.; Ley, K.; Galkina, E. Blockade of interleukin-17A results in reduced atherosclerosis in apolipoprotein E-deficient mice. *Circulation* **2010**, *121*, 1746–1755. [CrossRef] [PubMed]
29. Danzaki, K.; Matsui, Y.; Ikesue, M.; Ohta, D.; Ito, K.; Kanayama, M.; Kurotaki, D.; Morimoto, J.; Iwakura, Y.; Yagita, H.; et al. Interleukin-17A deficiency accelerates unstable atherosclerotic plaque formation in apolipoprotein E-deficient mice. *Arterioscler. Thromb. Vasc. Biol.* **2012**, *32*, 273–280. [CrossRef]
30. Kyaw, T.; Winship, A.; Tay, C.; Kanellakis, P.; Hosseini, H.; Cao, A.; Li, P.; Tipping, P.; Bobik, A.; Toh, B.H. Cytotoxic and proinflammatory CD8+ T lymphocytes promote development of vulnerable atherosclerotic plaques in ApoE-deficient mice. *Circulation* **2013**, *127*, 1028–1039. [CrossRef]
31. van Duijn, J.; Kritikou, E.; Benne, N.; van der Heijden, T.; van Puijvelde, G.H.; Kroner, M.J.; Schaftenaar, F.H.; Foks, A.C.; Wezel, A.; Smeets, H.; et al. CD8+ T-cells contribute to lesion stabilization in advanced atherosclerosis by limiting macrophage content and CD4+ T-cell responses. *Cardiovasc. Res.* **2019**, *115*, 729–738. [CrossRef]
32. Ley, K.; Gerdes, N.; Winkels, H. ATVB distinguished scientist award: How costimulatory and coinhibitory pathways shape atherosclerosis. *Arterioscler. Thromb. Vasc. Biol.* **2017**, *37*, 764–777. [CrossRef] [PubMed]
33. Wing, K.; Yamaguchi, T.; Sakaguchi, S. Cell-autonomous and -non-autonomous roles of CTLA-4 in immune regulation. *Trends Immunol.* **2011**, *32*, 428–433. [CrossRef]
34. Matsumoto, T.; Sasaki, N.; Yamashita, T.; Emoto, T.; Kasahara, K.; Mizoguchi, T.; Hayashi, T.; Yodoi, K.; Kitano, N.; Saito, T.; et al. Overexpression of cytotoxic T-lymphocyte-associated antigen-4 prevents atherosclerosis in mice. *Arterioscler. Thromb. Vasc. Biol.* **2016**, *36*, 1141–1151. [CrossRef]
35. Amin, H.Z.; Sasaki, N.; Yamashita, T.; Mizoguchi, T.; Hayashi, T.; Emoto, T.; Matsumoto, T.; Yoshida, N.; Tabata, T.; Horibe, S.; et al. CTLA-4 protects against angiotensin II-induced abdominal aortic aneurysm formation in mice. *Sci. Rep.* **2019**, *9*, 8065. [CrossRef] [PubMed]
36. Amin, H.Z.; Sasaki, N.; Hirata, K.I.; Rikitake, Y. Cytotoxic T lymphocyte-associated antigen-4 protects against angiotensin II-induced kidney injury in mice. *Circ. Rep.* **2020**, *2*, 339–342. [CrossRef] [PubMed]
37. Linsley, P.S.; Nadler, S.G. The clinical utility of inhibiting CD28-mediated costimulation. *Immunol. Rev.* **2009**, *229*, 307–321. [CrossRef]
38. Ma, K.; Lv, S.; Liu, B.; Liu, Z.; Luo, Y.; Kong, W.; Xu, Q.; Feng, J.; Wang, X. CTLA4-IgG ameliorates homocysteine-accelerated atherosclerosis by inhibiting T-cell overactivation in apo$E^{-/-}$ mice. *Cardiovasc. Res.* **2013**, *97*, 349–359. [CrossRef]
39. Gotsman, I.; Grabie, N.; Dacosta, R.; Sukhova, G.; Sharpe, A.; Lichtman, A.H. Proatherogenic immune responses are regulated by the PD-1/PD-L pathway in mice. *J. Clin. Investig.* **2007**, *117*, 2974–2982. [CrossRef]
40. Bu, D.X.; Tarrio, M.; Maganto-Garcia, E.; Stavrakis, G.; Tajima, G.; Lederer, J.; Jarolim, P.; Freeman, G.J.; Sharpe, A.H.; Lichtman, A.H. Impairment of the programmed cell death-1 pathway increases atherosclerotic lesion development and inflammation. *Arterioscler. Thromb. Vasc. Biol.* **2011**, *31*, 1100–1107.
41. Ribas, A.; Wolchok, J.D. Cancer immunotherapy using checkpoInt blockade. *Science* **2018**, *359*, 1350–1355. [CrossRef] [PubMed]
42. Drobni, Z.D.; Alvi, R.M.; Taron, J.; Zafar, A.; Murphy, S.P.; Rambarat, P.K.; Mosarla, R.C.; Lee, C.; Zlotoff, D.A.; Raghu, V.K.; et al. Association between immune checkpoInt. inhibitors with cardiovascular events and atherosclerotic plaque. *Circulation* **2020**, *142*, 2299–2311. [CrossRef] [PubMed]
43. Sakaguchi, S.; Sakaguchi, N.; Asano, M.; Itoh, M.; Toda, M. Immunologic self-tolerance maintained by activated T cells expressing IL-2 receptor alpha-chains (CD25). Breakdown of a single mechanism of self-tolerance causes various autoimmune diseases. *J. Immunol.* **1995**, *155*, 1151–1164. [PubMed]

44. Hori, S.; Nomura, T.; Sakaguchi, S. Control of regulatory T cell development by the transcription factor Foxp3. *Science* **2003**, *299*, 1057–1061. [CrossRef]
45. Fontenot, J.D.; Gavin, M.A.; Rudensky, A.Y. Foxp3 programs the development and function of CD4+CD25+ regulatory T cells. *Nat. Immunol.* **2003**, *4*, 330–336. [CrossRef]
46. Brunkow, M.E.; Jeffery, E.W.; Hjerrild, K.A.; Paeper, B.; Clark, L.B.; Yasayko, S.A.; Wilkinson, J.E.; Galas, D.; Ziegler, S.F.; Ramsdell, F. Disruption of a new forkhead/winged-helix protein, scurfin, results in the fatal lymphoproliferative disorder of the scurfy mouse. *Nat. Genet.* **2001**, *27*, 68–73. [CrossRef]
47. Bennett, C.L.; Christie, J.; Ramsdell, F.; Brunkow, M.E.; Ferguson, P.J.; Whitesell, L.; Kelly, T.E.; Saulsbury, F.T.; Chance, P.F.; Ochs, H.D. The immune dysregulation, polyendocrinopathy, enteropathy, X-linked syndrome (IPEX) is caused by mutations of FOXP3. *Nat. Genet.* **2001**, *27*, 20–21. [CrossRef]
48. Sakaguchi, S.; Yamaguchi, T.; Nomura, T.; Ono, M. Regulatory T cells and immune tolerance. *Cell* **2008**, *133*, 775–787. [CrossRef]
49. Shevach, E.M.; Thornton, A.M. tTregs, pTregs, and iTregs: Similarities and differences. *Immunol. Rev.* **2014**, *259*, 88–102. [CrossRef]
50. Greenwald, R.J.; Freeman, G.J.; Sharpe, A.H. The B7 family revisited. *Annu. Rev. Immunol.* **2005**, *23*, 515–548. [CrossRef] [PubMed]
51. Ait-Oufella, H.; Salomon, B.L.; Potteaux, S.; Robertson, A.K.; Gourdy, P.; Zoll, J.; Merval, R.; Esposito, B.; Cohen, J.L.; Fisson, S.; et al. Natural regulatory T cells control the development of atherosclerosis in mice. *Nat. Med.* **2006**, *12*, 178–180. [CrossRef] [PubMed]
52. Mor, A.; Planer, D.; Luboshits, G.; Afek, A.; Metzger, S.; Chajek-Shaul, T.; Keren, G.; George, J. Role of naturally occurring CD4+ CD25+ regulatory T cells in experimental atherosclerosis. *Arterioscler. Thromb. Vasc. Biol.* **2007**, *27*, 893–900. [CrossRef] [PubMed]
53. Winkels, H.; Meiler, S.; Lievens, D.; Engel, D.; Spitz, C.; Burger, C.; Beckers, L.; Dandl, A.; Reim, S.; Ahmadsei, M.; et al. CD27 co-stimulation increases the abundance of regulatory T cells and reduces atherosclerosis in hyperlipidaemic mice. *Eur. Heart J.* **2017**, *38*, 3590–3599. [CrossRef] [PubMed]
54. Lahl, K.; Loddenkemper, C.; Drouin, C.; Freyer, J.; Arnason, J.; Eberl, G.; Hamann, A.; Wagner, H.; Huehn, J.; Sparwasser, T. Selective depletion of Foxp3+ regulatory T cells induces a scurfy-like disease. *J. Exp. Med.* **2007**, *204*, 57–63. [CrossRef] [PubMed]
55. Klingenberg, R.; Gerdes, N.; Badeau, R.M.; Gistera, A.; Strodthoff, D.; Ketelhuth, D.F.; Lundberg, A.M.; Rudling, M.; Nilsson, S.K.; Olivecrona, G.; et al. Depletion of FOXP3+ regulatory T cells promotes hypercholesterolemia and atherosclerosis. *J. Clin. Investig.* **2013**, *123*, 1323–1334. [CrossRef]
56. De Boer, O.J.; van der Meer, J.J.; Teeling, P.; van der Loos, C.M.; van der Wal, A.C. Low numbers of FOXP3 positive regulatory T cells are present in all developmental stages of human atherosclerotic lesions. *PLoS ONE* **2007**, *2*, e779. [CrossRef] [PubMed]
57. Depuydt, M.A.C.; Prange, K.H.M.; Slenders, L.; Ord, T.; Elbersen, D.; Boltjes, A.; de Jager, S.C.A.; Asselbergs, F.W.; de Borst, G.J.; Aavik, E.; et al. Microanatomy of the human atherosclerotic plaque by single-cell transcriptomics. *Circ. Res.* **2020**, *127*, 1437–1455. [CrossRef]
58. Mor, A.; Luboshits, G.; Planer, D.; Keren, G.; George, J. Altered status of CD4(+)CD25(+) regulatory T cells in patients with acute coronary syndromes. *Eur. Heart J.* **2006**, *27*, 2530–2537. [CrossRef] [PubMed]
59. Ammirati, E.; Cianflone, D.; Banfi, M.; Vecchio, V.; Palini, A.; De Metrio, M.; Marenzi, G.; Panciroli, C.; Tumminello, G.; Anzuini, A.; et al. Circulating CD4+CD25hiCD127lo regulatory T-Cell levels do not reflect the extent or severity of carotid and coronary atherosclerosis. *Arterioscler. Thromb. Vasc. Biol.* **2010**, *30*, 1832–1841. [CrossRef]
60. George, J.; Schwartzenberg, S.; Medvedovsky, D.; Jonas, M.; Charach, G.; Afek, A.; Shamiss, A. Regulatory T cells and IL-10 levels are reduced in patients with vulnerable coronary plaques. *Atherosclerosis* **2012**, *222*, 519–523. [CrossRef]
61. Zhang, W.C.; Wang, J.; Shu, Y.W.; Tang, T.T.; Zhu, Z.F.; Xia, N.; Nie, S.F.; Liu, J.; Zhou, S.F.; Li, J.J.; et al. Impaired thymic export and increased apoptosis account for regulatory T cell defects in patients with non-ST segment elevation acute coronary syndrome. *J. Biol. Chem.* **2012**, *287*, 34157–34166. [CrossRef] [PubMed]
62. Potekhina, A.V.; Pylaeva, E.; Provatorov, S.; Ruleva, N.; Masenko, V.; Noeva, E.; Krasnikova, T.; Arefieva, T. Treg/Th17 balance in stable CAD patients with different stages of coronary atherosclerosis. *Atherosclerosis* **2015**, *238*, 17–21. [CrossRef] [PubMed]
63. Wigren, M.; Bjorkbacka, H.; Andersson, L.; Ljungcrantz, I.; Fredrikson, G.N.; Persson, M.; Bryngelsson, C.; Hedblad, B.; Nilsson, J. Low levels of circulating CD4+FoxP3+ T cells are associated with an increased risk for development of myocardial infarction but not for stroke. *Arterioscler. Thromb. Vasc. Biol.* **2012**, *32*, 2000–2004. [CrossRef] [PubMed]
64. Klingenberg, R.; Brokopp, C.E.; Grives, A.; Courtier, A.; Jaguszewski, M.; Pasqual, N.; Vlaskou Badra, E.; Lewandowski, A.; Gaemperli, O.; Hoerstrup, S.P.; et al. Clonal restriction and predominance of regulatory T cells in coronary thrombi of patients with acute coronary syndromes. *Eur. Heart J.* **2015**, *36*, 1041–1048. [CrossRef] [PubMed]
65. Miyara, M.; Yoshioka, Y.; Kitoh, A.; Shima, T.; Wing, K.; Niwa, A.; Parizot, C.; Taflin, C.; Heike, T.; Valeyre, D.; et al. Functional delineation and differentiation dynamics of human CD4+ T cells expressing the FoxP3 transcription factor. *Immunity* **2009**, *30*, 899–911. [CrossRef]
66. Emoto, T.; Sasaki, N.; Yamashita, T.; Kasahara, K.; Yodoi, K.; Sasaki, Y.; Matsumoto, T.; Mizoguchi, T.; Hirata, K. Regulatory/effector T-cell ratio is reduced in coronary artery disease. *Circ. J.* **2014**, *78*, 2935–2941. [CrossRef]
67. Joly, A.L.; Seitz, C.; Liu, S.; Kuznetsov, N.V.; Gertow, K.; Westerberg, L.S.; Paulsson-Berne, G.; Hansson, G.K.; Andersson, J. Alternative splicing of FOXP3 controls regulatory T cell effector functions and is associated with human atherosclerotic plaque stability. *Circ. Res.* **2018**, *122*, 1385–1394. [CrossRef]
68. Dale, M.A.; Ruhlman, M.K.; Baxter, B.T. Inflammatory cell phenotypes in AAAs: Their role and potential as targets for therapy. *Arterioscler. Thromb. Vasc. Biol.* **2015**, *35*, 1746–1755. [CrossRef]

69. Ait-Oufella, H.; Wang, Y.; Herbin, O.; Bourcier, S.; Potteaux, S.; Joffre, J.; Loyer, X.; Ponnuswamy, P.; Esposito, B.; Dalloz, M.; et al. Natural regulatory T cells limit angiotensin II-induced aneurysm formation and rupture in mice. *Arterioscler. Thromb. Vasc. Biol.* **2013**, *33*, 2374–2379. [CrossRef]
70. Meng, X.; Yang, J.; Zhang, K.; An, G.; Kong, J.; Jiang, F.; Zhang, Y.; Zhang, C. Regulatory T cells prevent angiotensin II-induced abdominal aortic aneurysm in apolipoprotein E knockout mice. *Hypertension* **2014**, *64*, 875–882. [CrossRef]
71. Yodoi, K.; Yamashita, T.; Sasaki, N.; Kasahara, K.; Emoto, T.; Matsumoto, T.; Kita, T.; Sasaki, Y.; Mizoguchi, T.; Sparwasser, T.; et al. Foxp3+ regulatory T cells play a protective role in angiotensin II-induced aortic aneurysm formation in mice. *Hypertension* **2015**, *65*, 889–895. [CrossRef]
72. Yin, M.; Zhang, J.; Wang, Y.; Wang, S.; Bockler, D.; Duan, Z.; Xin, S. Deficient CD4+CD25+ T regulatory cell function in patients with abdominal aortic aneurysms. *Arterioscler. Thromb. Vasc. Biol.* **2010**, *30*, 1825–1831. [CrossRef]
73. Ait-Oufella, H.; Taleb, S.; Mallat, Z.; Tedgui, A. Recent advances on the role of cytokines in atherosclerosis. *Arterioscler. Thromb. Vasc. Biol.* **2011**, *31*, 969–979. [CrossRef] [PubMed]
74. Pinderski, L.J.; Fischbein, M.P.; Subbanagounder, G.; Fishbein, M.C.; Kubo, N.; Cheroutre, H.; Curtiss, L.K.; Berliner, J.A.; Boisvert, W.A. Overexpression of interleukin-10 by activated T lymphocytes inhibits atherosclerosis in LDL receptor-deficient Mice by altering lymphocyte and macrophage phenotypes. *Circ. Res.* **2002**, *90*, 1064–1071. [CrossRef]
75. Robertson, A.K.; Rudling, M.; Zhou, X.; Gorelik, L.; Flavell, R.A.; Hansson, G.K. Disruption of TGF-beta signaling in T cells accelerates atherosclerosis. *J. Clin. Investig.* **2003**, *112*, 1342–1350. [CrossRef] [PubMed]
76. Proto, J.D.; Doran, A.C.; Gusarova, G.; Yurdagul, A., Jr.; Sozen, E.; Subramanian, M.; Islam, M.N.; Rymond, C.C.; Du, J.; Hook, J.; et al. Regulatory T cells promote macrophage efferocytosis during inflammation resolution. *Immunity* **2018**, *49*, 666–677. [CrossRef] [PubMed]
77. Maganto-Garcia, E.; Tarrio, M.L.; Grabie, N.; Bu, D.X.; Lichtman, A.H. Dynamic changes in regulatory T cells are linked to levels of diet-induced hypercholesterolemia. *Circulation* **2011**, *124*, 185–195. [CrossRef] [PubMed]
78. Mailer, R.K.W.; Gistera, A.; Polyzos, K.A.; Ketelhuth, D.F.J.; Hansson, G.K. Hypercholesterolemia enhances T cell receptor signaling and increases the regulatory T cell population. *Sci. Rep.* **2017**, *7*, 15655. [CrossRef] [PubMed]
79. Mailer, R.K.W.; Gistera, A.; Polyzos, K.A.; Ketelhuth, D.F.J.; Hansson, G.K. Hypercholesterolemia induces differentiation of regulatory T cells in the liver. *Circ. Res.* **2017**, *120*, 1740–1753. [CrossRef]
80. Amersfoort, J.; Schaftenaar, F.H.; Douna, H.; van Santbrink, P.J.; van Puijvelde, G.H.M.; Slutter, B.; Foks, A.C.; Harms, A.; Moreno-Gordaliza, E.; Wang, Y.; et al. Diet-induced dyslipidemia induces metabolic and migratory adaptations in regulatory T cells. *Cardiovasc. Res.* **2021**, *117*, 1309–1324. [CrossRef] [PubMed]
81. Noels, H.; Weber, C.; Koenen, R.R. Chemokines as therapeutic targets in cardiovascular disease. *Arterioscler. Thromb. Vasc. Biol.* **2019**, *39*, 583–592. [CrossRef] [PubMed]
82. Bonacina, F.; Martini, E.; Svecla, M.; Nour, J.; Cremonesi, M.; Beretta, G.; Moregola, A.; Pellegatta, F.; Zampoleri, V.; Catapano, A.L.; et al. Adoptive transfer of CX3CR1 transduced-T regulatory cells improves homing to the atherosclerotic plaques and dampens atherosclerosis progression. *Cardiovasc. Res.* **2021**, *117*, 2069–2082. [CrossRef]
83. Sakaguchi, S.; Vignali, D.A.; Rudensky, A.Y.; Niec, R.E.; Waldmann, H. The plasticity and stability of regulatory T cells. *Nat. Rev. Immunol.* **2013**, *13*, 461–467. [CrossRef]
84. Ali, A.J.; Makings, J.; Ley, K. Regulatory T cell stability and plasticity in atherosclerosis. *Cells* **2020**, *9*, 2665. [CrossRef] [PubMed]
85. Butcher, M.J.; Filipowicz, A.R.; Waseem, T.C.; McGary, C.M.; Crow, K.J.; Magilnick, N.; Boldin, M.; Lundberg, P.S.; Galkina, E.V. Atherosclerosis-driven treg plasticity results in formation of a dysfunctional subset of plastic IFNgamma+ Th1/tregs. *Circ. Res.* **2016**, *119*, 1190–1203. [CrossRef] [PubMed]
86. Li, J.; McArdle, S.; Gholami, A.; Kimura, T.; Wolf, D.; Gerhardt, T.; Miller, J.; Weber, C.; Ley, K. CCR5+T-bet+FoxP3+ effector CD4 T cells drive atherosclerosis. *Circ. Res.* **2016**, *118*, 1540–1552. [CrossRef]
87. Wigren, M.; Rattik, S.; Yao Mattisson, I.; Tomas, L.; Gronberg, C.; Soderberg, I.; Alm, R.; Sundius, L.; Ljungcrantz, I.; Bjorkbacka, H.; et al. Lack of ability to present antigens on major histocompatibility complex class II molecules aggravates atherosclerosis in ApoE$^{-/-}$ mice. *Circulation* **2019**, *139*, 2554–2566. [CrossRef] [PubMed]
88. Kimura, T.; Kobiyama, K.; Winkels, H.; Tse, K.; Miller, J.; Vassallo, M.; Wolf, D.; Ryden, C.; Orecchioni, M.; Dileepan, T.; et al. Regulatory CD4(+) T cells recognize MHC-II-restricted peptide epitopes of apolipoprotein B. *Circulation* **2018**, *138*, 1130–1143. [CrossRef]
89. Wolf, D.; Gerhardt, T.; Winkels, H.; Michel, N.A.; Pramod, A.B.; Ghosheh, Y.; Brunel, S.; Buscher, K.; Miller, J.; McArdle, S.; et al. Pathogenic autoimmunity in atherosclerosis evolves from initially protective apolipoprotein B100-reactive CD4(+) T-regulatory cells. *Circulation* **2020**, *142*, 1279–1293. [CrossRef]
90. Subramanian, M.; Thorp, E.; Hansson, G.K.; Tabas, I. Treg-mediated suppression of atherosclerosis requires MYD88 signaling in DCs. *J. Clin. Investig.* **2013**, *123*, 179–188. [CrossRef]
91. Choi, J.H.; Cheong, C.; Dandamudi, D.B.; Park, C.G.; Rodriguez, A.; Mehandru, S.; Velinzon, K.; Jung, I.H.; Yoo, J.Y.; Oh, G.T.; et al. Flt3 signaling-dependent dendritic cells protect against atherosclerosis. *Immunity* **2011**, *35*, 819–831. [CrossRef] [PubMed]
92. Takeda, M.; Yamashita, T.; Sasaki, N.; Hirata, K. Dendritic cells in atherogenesis: Possible novel targets for prevention of atherosclerosis. *J. Atheroscler. Thromb.* **2012**, *19*, 953–961. [CrossRef]

93. Hermansson, A.; Johansson, D.K.; Ketelhuth, D.F.; Andersson, J.; Zhou, X.; Hansson, G.K. Immunotherapy with tolerogenic apolipoprotein B-100-loaded dendritic cells attenuates atherosclerosis in hypercholesterolemic mice. *Circulation* **2011**, *123*, 1083–1091. [CrossRef]
94. Takeda, M.; Yamashita, T.; Sasaki, N.; Nakajima, K.; Kita, T.; Shinohara, M.; Ishida, T.; Hirata, K. Oral administration of an active form of vitamin D3 (calcitriol) decreases atherosclerosis in mice by inducing regulatory T cells and immature dendritic cells with tolerogenic functions. *Arterioscler. Thromb. Vasc. Biol.* **2010**, *30*, 2495–2503. [CrossRef]
95. Wang, T.J.; Pencina, M.J.; Booth, S.L.; Jacques, P.F.; Ingelsson, E.; Lanier, K.; Benjamin, E.J.; D'Agostino, R.B.; Wolf, M.; Vasan, R.S. Vitamin D deficiency and risk of cardiovascular disease. *Circulation* **2008**, *117*, 503–511. [CrossRef] [PubMed]
96. Weiner, H.L.; da Cunha, A.P.; Quintana, F.; Wu, H. Oral tolerance. *Immunol. Rev.* **2011**, *241*, 241–259. [CrossRef] [PubMed]
97. Mallat, Z.; Gojova, A.; Brun, V.; Esposito, B.; Fournier, N.; Cottrez, F.; Tedgui, A.; Groux, H. Induction of a regulatory T cell type 1 response reduces the development of atherosclerosis in apolipoprotein E-knockout mice. *Circulation* **2003**, *108*, 1232–1237.
98. van Puijvelde, G.H.; Hauer, A.D.; de Vos, P.; van den Heuvel, R.; van Herwijnen, M.J.; van der Zee, R.; van Eden, W.; van Berkel, T.J.; Kuiper, J. Induction of oral tolerance to oxidized low-density lipoprotein ameliorates atherosclerosis. *Circulation* **2006**, *114*, 1968–1976. [CrossRef]
99. van Puijvelde, G.H.; van Es, T.; van Wanrooij, E.J.; Habets, K.L.; de Vos, P.; van der Zee, R.; van Eden, W.; van Berkel, T.J.; Kuiper, J. Induction of oral tolerance to HSP60 or an HSP60-peptide activates T cell regulation and reduces atherosclerosis. *Arterioscler. Thromb. Vasc. Biol.* **2007**, *27*, 2677–2683. [CrossRef]
100. Yamashita, T.; Kasahara, K.; Emoto, T.; Matsumoto, T.; Mizoguchi, T.; Kitano, N.; Sasaki, N.; Hirata, K. Intestinal immunity and gut microbiota as therapeutic targets for preventing atherosclerotic cardiovascular diseases. *Circ. J.* **2015**, *79*, 1882–1890. [CrossRef]
101. Yoshida, N.; Emoto, T.; Yamashita, T.; Watanabe, H.; Hayashi, T.; Tabata, T.; Hoshi, N.; Hatano, N.; Ozawa, G.; Sasaki, N.; et al. *Bacteroides vulgatus* and *Bacteroides dorei* reduce gut microbial lipopolysaccharide production and inhibit atherosclerosis. *Circulation* **2018**, *138*, 2486–2498. [CrossRef] [PubMed]
102. Atarashi, K.; Tanoue, T.; Shima, T.; Imaoka, A.; Kuwahara, T.; Momose, Y.; Cheng, G.; Yamasaki, S.; Saito, T.; Ohba, Y.; et al. Induction of colonic regulatory T cells by indigenous Clostridium species. *Science* **2011**, *331*, 337–341. [CrossRef]
103. Atarashi, K.; Tanoue, T.; Oshima, K.; Suda, W.; Nagano, Y.; Nishikawa, H.; Fukuda, S.; Saito, T.; Narushima, S.; Hase, K.; et al. Treg induction by a rationally selected mixture of Clostridia strains from the human microbiota. *Nature* **2013**, *500*, 232–236. [CrossRef]
104. Furusawa, Y.; Obata, Y.; Fukuda, S.; Endo, T.A.; Nakato, G.; Takahashi, D.; Nakanishi, Y.; Uetake, C.; Kato, K.; Kato, T.; et al. Commensal microbe-derived butyrate induces the differentiation of colonic regulatory T cells. *Nature* **2013**, *504*, 446–450. [CrossRef] [PubMed]
105. Bartolomaeus, H.; Balogh, A.; Yakoub, M.; Homann, S.; Marko, L.; Hoges, S.; Tsvetkov, D.; Krannich, A.; Wundersitz, S.; Avery, E.G.; et al. Short-chain fatty acid propionate protects from hypertensive cardiovascular damage. *Circulation* **2019**, *139*, 1407–1421. [CrossRef]
106. Belghith, M.; Bluestone, J.A.; Barriot, S.; Megret, J.; Bach, J.F.; Chatenoud, L. TGF-beta-dependent mechanisms mediate restoration of self-tolerance induced by antibodies to CD3 in overt autoimmune diabetes. *Nat. Med.* **2003**, *9*, 1202–1208. [CrossRef] [PubMed]
107. Herold, K.C.; Hagopian, W.; Auger, J.A.; Poumian-Ruiz, E.; Taylor, L.; Donaldson, D.; Gitelman, S.E.; Harlan, D.M.; Xu, D.; Zivin, R.A.; et al. Anti-CD3 monoclonal antibody in new-onset type 1 diabetes mellitus. *N. Engl. J. Med.* **2002**, *346*, 1692–1698. [CrossRef]
108. Steffens, S.; Burger, F.; Pelli, G.; Dean, Y.; Elson, G.; Kosco-Vilbois, M.; Chatenoud, L.; Mach, F. Short-term treatment with anti-CD3 antibody reduces the development and progression of atherosclerosis in mice. *Circulation* **2006**, *114*, 1977–1984. [CrossRef]
109. Ochi, H.; Abraham, M.; Ishikawa, H.; Frenkel, D.; Yang, K.; Basso, A.S.; Wu, H.; Chen, M.L.; Gandhi, R.; Miller, A.; et al. Oral CD3-specific antibody suppresses autoimmune encephalomyelitis by inducing CD4+ CD25− LAP+ T cells. *Nat. Med.* **2006**, *12*, 627–635. [CrossRef] [PubMed]
110. Ishikawa, H.; Ochi, H.; Chen, M.L.; Frenkel, D.; Maron, R.; Weiner, H.L. Inhibition of autoimmune diabetes by oral administration of anti-CD3 monoclonal antibody. *Diabetes* **2007**, *56*, 2103–2109. [CrossRef]
111. Sasaki, N.; Yamashita, T.; Takeda, M.; Shinohara, M.; Nakajima, K.; Tawa, H.; Usui, T.; Hirata, K. Oral anti-CD3 antibody treatment induces regulatory T cells and inhibits the development of atherosclerosis in mice. *Circulation* **2009**, *120*, 1996–2005. [CrossRef] [PubMed]
112. Foks, A.C.; Frodermann, V.; ter Borg, M.; Habets, K.L.; Bot, I.; Zhao, Y.; van Eck, M.; van Berkel, T.J.; Kuiper, J.; van Puijvelde, G.H. Differential effects of regulatory T cells on the initiation and regression of atherosclerosis. *Atherosclerosis* **2011**, *218*, 53–60. [CrossRef] [PubMed]
113. Dinh, T.N.; Kyaw, T.S.; Kanellakis, P.; To, K.; Tipping, P.; Toh, B.H.; Bobik, A.; Agrotis, A. Cytokine therapy with interleukin-2/anti-interleukin-2 monoclonal antibody complexes expands CD4+CD25+Foxp3+ regulatory T cells and attenuates development and progression of atherosclerosis. *Circulation* **2012**, *126*, 1256–1266. [CrossRef]
114. Korn, T.; Reddy, J.; Gao, W.; Bettelli, E.; Awasthi, A.; Petersen, T.R.; Backstrom, B.T.; Sobel, R.A.; Wucherpfennig, K.W.; Strom, T.B.; et al. Myelin-specific regulatory T cells accumulate in the CNS but fail to control autoimmune inflammation. *Nat. Med.* **2007**, *13*, 423–431. [CrossRef] [PubMed]

115. Kasahara, K.; Sasaki, N.; Yamashita, T.; Kita, T.; Yodoi, K.; Sasaki, Y.; Takeda, M.; Hirata, K. CD3 antibody and IL-2 complex combination therapy inhibits atherosclerosis by augmenting a regulatory immune response. *J. Am. Heart Assoc.* **2014**, *3*, e000719. [CrossRef]
116. Koreth, J.; Matsuoka, K.; Kim, H.T.; McDonough, S.M.; Bindra, B.; Alyea, E.P., 3rd; Armand, P.; Cutler, C.; Ho, V.T.; Treister, N.S.; et al. Interleukin-2 and regulatory T cells in graft-versus-host disease. *N. Engl. J. Med.* **2011**, *365*, 2055–2066. [CrossRef]
117. Saadoun, D.; Rosenzwajg, M.; Joly, F.; Six, A.; Carrat, F.; Thibault, V.; Sene, D.; Cacoub, P.; Klatzmann, D. Regulatory T-cell responses to low-dose interleukin-2 in HCV-induced vasculitis. *N. Engl. J. Med.* **2011**, *365*, 2067–2077. [CrossRef]
118. Zhao, T.X.; Kostapanos, M.; Griffiths, C.; Arbon, E.L.; Hubsch, A.; Kaloyirou, F.; Helmy, J.; Hoole, S.P.; Rudd, J.H.F.; Wood, G.; et al. Low-dose interleukin-2 in patients with stable ischaemic heart disease and acute coronary syndromes (LILACS): Protocol and study rationale for a randomised, double-blind, placebo-controlled, phase I/II clinical trial. *BMJ. Open* **2018**, *8*, e022452. [CrossRef]
119. Zhao, T.X.; Newland, S.A.; Mallat, Z. 2019 ATVB Plenary Lecture: Interleukin-2 Therapy in Cardiovascular Disease: The Potential to Regulate Innate and Adaptive Immunity. *Arterioscler. Thromb. Vasc. Biol.* **2020**, *40*, 853–864. [CrossRef]
120. Schwarz, T. Mechanisms of UV-induced immunosuppression. *Keio J. Med.* **2005**, *54*, 165–171. [CrossRef]
121. Morita, A. Current developments in phototherapy for psoriasis. *J. Dermatol.* **2018**, *45*, 287–292. [CrossRef] [PubMed]
122. Sasaki, N.; Yamashita, T.; Kasahara, K.; Fukunaga, A.; Yamaguchi, T.; Emoto, T.; Yodoi, K.; Matsumoto, T.; Nakajima, K.; Kita, T.; et al. UVB exposure prevents atherosclerosis by regulating immunoinflammatory responses. *Arterioscler. Thromb. Vasc. Biol.* **2017**, *37*, 66–74. [CrossRef] [PubMed]
123. Fukunaga, A.; Khaskhely, N.M.; Ma, Y.; Sreevidya, C.S.; Taguchi, K.; Nishigori, C.; Ullrich, S.E. Langerhans cells serve as immunoregulatory cells by activating NKT cells. *J. Immunol.* **2010**, *185*, 4633–4640. [CrossRef] [PubMed]
124. Schwarz, A.; Noordegraaf, M.; Maeda, A.; Torii, K.; Clausen, B.E.; Schwarz, T. Langerhans cells are required for UVR-induced immunosuppression. *J. Investig. Dermatol.* **2010**, *130*, 1419–1427. [CrossRef]
125. Hayashi, T.; Sasaki, N.; Yamashita, T.; Mizoguchi, T.; Emoto, T.; Amin, H.Z.; Yodoi, K.; Matsumoto, T.; Kasahara, K.; Yoshida, N.; et al. Ultraviolet B exposure inhibits angiotensin II-induced abdominal aortic aneurysm formation in mice by expanding CD4+Foxp3+ regulatory T cells. *J. Am. Heart Assoc.* **2017**, *6*, 007024. [CrossRef]
126. Furuhashi, T.; Saito, C.; Torii, K.; Nishida, E.; Yamazaki, S.; Morita, A. Photo(chemo)therapy reduces circulating Th17 cells and restores circulating regulatory T cells in psoriasis. *PLoS ONE* **2013**, *8*, e54895. [CrossRef] [PubMed]
127. Iyama, S.; Murase, K.; Sato, T.; Hashimoto, A.; Tatekoshi, A.; Horiguchi, H.; Kamihara, Y.; Ono, K.; Kikuchi, S.; Takada, K.; et al. Narrowband ultraviolet B phototherapy ameliorates acute graft-versus-host disease by a mechanism involving in vivo expansion of CD4+CD25+Foxp3+ regulatory T cells. *Int. J. Hematol.* **2014**, *99*, 471–476. [CrossRef]
128. Nissen, S.E.; Nicholls, S.J.; Sipahi, I.; Libby, P.; Raichlen, J.S.; Ballantyne, C.M.; Davignon, J.; Erbel, R.; Fruchart, J.C.; Tardif, J.C.; et al. Effect of very high-intensity statin therapy on regression of coronary atherosclerosis: The ASTEROID trial. *JAMA* **2006**, *295*, 1556–1565. [CrossRef] [PubMed]
129. Trogan, E.; Feig, J.E.; Dogan, S.; Rothblat, G.H.; Angeli, V.; Tacke, F.; Randolph, G.J.; Fisher, E.A. Gene expression changes in foam cells and the role of chemokine receptor CCR7 during atherosclerosis regression in ApoE-deficient mice. *Proc. Natl. Acad. Sci. USA* **2006**, *103*, 3781–3786. [CrossRef]
130. Feig, J.E.; Parathath, S.; Rong, J.X.; Mick, S.L.; Vengrenyuk, Y.; Grauer, L.; Young, S.G.; Fisher, E.A. Reversal of hyperlipidemia with a genetic switch favorably affects the content and inflammatory state of macrophages in atherosclerotic plaques. *Circulation* **2011**, *123*, 989–998. [CrossRef]
131. Rayner, K.J.; Sheedy, F.J.; Esau, C.C.; Hussain, F.N.; Temel, R.E.; Parathath, S.; van Gils, J.M.; Rayner, A.J.; Chang, A.N.; Suarez, Y.; et al. Antagonism of miR-33 in mice promotes reverse cholesterol transport and regression of atherosclerosis. *J. Clin. Investig.* **2011**, *121*, 2921–2931. [CrossRef]
132. Nakajima, K.; Yamashita, T.; Kita, T.; Takeda, M.; Sasaki, N.; Kasahara, K.; Shinohara, M.; Rikitake, Y.; Ishida, T.; Yokoyama, M.; et al. Orally administered eicosapentaenoic acid induces rapid regression of atherosclerosis via modulating the phenotype of dendritic cells in LDL receptor-deficient mice. *Arterioscler. Thromb. Vasc. Biol.* **2011**, *31*, 1963–1972. [CrossRef] [PubMed]
133. Yokoyama, M.; Origasa, H.; Matsuzaki, M.; Matsuzawa, Y.; Saito, Y.; Ishikawa, Y.; Oikawa, S.; Sasaki, J.; Hishida, H.; Itakura, H.; et al. Effects of eicosapentaenoic acid on major coronary events in hypercholesterolaemic patients (JELIS): A randomised open-label, blinded endpoInt. analysis. *Lancet* **2007**, *369*, 1090–1098. [CrossRef]
134. Kita, T.; Yamashita, T.; Sasaki, N.; Kasahara, K.; Sasaki, Y.; Yodoi, K.; Takeda, M.; Nakajima, K.; Hirata, K. Regression of atherosclerosis with anti-CD3 antibody via augmenting a regulatory T-cell response in mice. *Cardiovasc. Res.* **2014**, *102*, 107–117. [CrossRef] [PubMed]
135. Sharma, M.; Schlegel, M.P.; Afonso, M.S.; Brown, E.J.; Rahman, K.; Weinstock, A.; Sansbury, B.E.; Corr, E.M.; van Solingen, C.; Koelwyn, G.J.; et al. Regulatory T cells license macrophage pro-resolving functions during atherosclerosis regression. *Circ. Res.* **2020**, *127*, 335–353. [CrossRef]

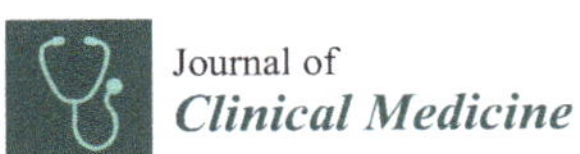
Journal of
Clinical Medicine

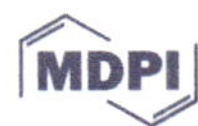

Systematic Review

Optimal Anticoagulant Strategy for Periprocedural Management of Atrial Fibrillation Ablation: A Systematic Review and Network Meta-Analysis

Tabito Kino [1], Minako Kagimoto [2], Takayuki Yamada [3], Satoshi Ishii [2], Masanari Asai [4], Shunichi Asano [5], Hideto Yano [6], Toshiyuki Ishikawa [7] and Tomoaki Ishigami [7,*]

1 Cardiovascular Research Center, Lewis Katz School of Medicine, Temple University, Philadelphia, PA 19140, USA; tabito.kino@temple.edu
2 Department of Cardiology, Kanagawa Cardiovascular and Respiratory Center, Yokohama 236-0051, Japan; minako.kagimoto@gmail.com (M.K.); e103004g@yokohama-cu.ac.jp (S.I.)
3 Department of Medicine, University of Pittsburgh, Pittsburgh, PA 15261, USA; yamadat@upmc.edu
4 Department of Cardiology, Saiseikai Yokohamashi Nanbu Hospital, Yokohama 234-0054, Japan; masanari@yokohama-cu.ac.jp
5 Department of Cardiology, Yokohama Rosai Hospital, Yokohama 222-0036, Japan; shunasncirc@gmail.com
6 Department of Cardiology, Gyotoku General Hospital, Ichikawa 272-0103, Japan; yanohi@juno.dti.ne.jp
7 Department of Medical Science and Cardiorenal Medicine, Yokohama City University Graduate School of Medicine, Yokohama 236-0004, Japan; tishika@yokohama-cu.ac.jp
* Correspondence: tommmish@hotmail.com; Tel.: +81-45-787-2635

Abstract: This network meta-analysis was performed to rank the safety and efficacy of periprocedural anticoagulant strategies in patients undergoing atrial fibrillation ablation. MEDLINE, EMBASE, CENTRAL, and Web of Science were searched to identify randomized controlled trials comparing anticoagulant regimens in patients undergoing atrial fibrillation ablation up to July 1, 2021. The primary efficacy and safety outcomes were thromboembolic and major bleeding events, respectively, and the net clinical benefit was investigated as the primary-outcome composite. Seventeen studies were included (n = 6950). The mean age ranged from 59 to 70 years; 74% of patients were men and 55% had paroxysmal atrial fibrillation. Compared with the uninterrupted vitamin-K antagonist strategy, the odds ratios for the composite of primary safety and efficacy outcomes were 0.61 (95%CI: 0.31–1.17) with uninterrupted direct oral anticoagulants, 0.63 (95%CI: 0.26–1.54) with interrupted direct oral anticoagulants, and 8.02 (95%CI: 2.35–27.45) with interrupted vitamin-K antagonists. Uninterrupted dabigatran significantly reduced the risk of the composite of primary safety and efficacy outcomes (odds ratio, 0.21; 95%CI, 0.08–0.55). Uninterrupted direct oral anticoagulants are preferred alternatives to uninterrupted vitamin-K antagonists. Interrupted direct oral anticoagulants may be feasible as alternatives. Our results support the use of uninterrupted direct oral anticoagulants as the optimal periprocedural anticoagulant strategy for patients undergoing atrial fibrillation ablation.

Keywords: periprocedural anticoagulant management; atrial fibrillation ablation; direct oral anticoagulant; vitamin-K antagonist; network meta-analysis

Citation: Kino, T.; Kagimoto, M.; Yamada, T.; Ishii, S.; Asai, M.; Asano, S.; Yano, H.; Ishikawa, T.; Ishigami, T. Optimal Anticoagulant Strategy for Periprocedural Management of Atrial Fibrillation Ablation: A Systematic Review and Network Meta-Analysis. *J. Clin. Med.* **2022**, *11*, 1872. https://doi.org/10.3390/jcm11071872

Academic Editor: Gani Bajraktari

Received: 2 February 2022
Accepted: 25 March 2022
Published: 28 March 2022

1. Introduction

Atrial fibrillation (AF) is a cardiac arrhythmia common worldwide [1]. Catheter ablation (CA) is the most effective treatment to prevent AF recurrence [2], and over the last decade, it has resulted in dramatic improvements in safety and efficacy [3–7]. However, periprocedural complications occur in approximately 4–14% of patients undergoing AF ablation, 2–3% of which are potentially life-threatening [8]. Periprocedural stroke or transient ischemic attack (TIA) and cardiac tamponade are the most notable complications [9,10]. As these adverse events are affected by periprocedural anticoagulant management, an optimal anticoagulant strategy is essential for the prevention of thromboembolic and bleeding complications.

Compared with vitamin-K antagonists (VKAs), direct oral anticoagulants (DOACs) have been shown to have a favorable risk-benefit profile, as they significantly reduce the incidence of stroke and also carry a similar bleeding risk in the long-term treatment of patients with AF [11]. With respect to CA, many studies have found that DOACs have similar efficacy and safety compared with VKAs [12–19]. These results led to the guideline recommendation of uninterrupted anticoagulants for the perioperative management of patients undergoing AF ablation [8,9]. Conversely, a German survey reported that interrupted and minimally interrupted DOAC was used more frequently than truly uninterrupted DOAC to avoid bleeding complications [20]. Moreover, some meta-analyses including randomized controlled trials (RCTs) have revealed that interrupted DOAC was not inferior to uninterrupted DOAC administration and was preferable to uninterrupted VKA administration [21,22]. Currently, guidelines lack indications based on these RCTs regarding which strategy is preferable for periprocedural anticoagulant management. This was the first study comparing each strategy and regimen with network meta-analysis (NMA) to simultaneously compare multiple treatments in a single analysis by combining direct and indirect evidence within a network of RCTs [23].

This study aimed to synthesize the available evidence from RCTs using NMA to: (1) assess the relative effects of different uninterrupted or interrupted anticoagulant strategies between DOACs and VKAs for reducing thromboembolic or bleeding events in patients undergoing AF ablation; and (2) to rank regimens, uninterrupted or interrupted, and DOAC or VKA administration for effectiveness in preventing thromboembolic or bleeding complications.

2. Materials and Methods

2.1. Protocol and Registration

Our report follows the preferred reporting items for systematic reviews and meta-analyses (PRISMA)-NMA extension (Table S1) [24]. The study protocol was registered at PROSPERO (CRD42021268787).

2.2. Eligibility Criteria

Only studies that met the eligibility criteria were included. The criteria were: (1) only RCTs; (2) uninterrupted or interrupted anticoagulant strategy in the periprocedural period; (3) patients undergoing AF ablation; and (4) publication of efficacy (stroke, TIA, or systemic embolism) and safety (major bleeding) outcomes. We excluded duplicate studies. There were no language or publication date restrictions.

2.3. Search Strategy

We performed a systematic search of the MEDLINE, EMBASE, Cochrane Central Register of Controlled Trials, and Web of Science databases up to July 1, 2021. The search used the Population, Intervention, Comparators, Outcomes, and Study design format and included the following terms: atrial fibrillation, ablation, periprocedural anticoagulation, and randomized controlled trial (Table S2). Three independent and blinded reviewers (SI, MA, and SA) separately assessed the search results to select studies based on the eligibility criteria. When a consensus was not reached by the three reviewers, a fourth author (TI) was consulted to reach a decision.

2.4. Outcomes

The primary efficacy outcome was thromboembolic events, including stroke, TIA, or systemic embolism. The primary safety outcome was major bleeding as defined by the Bleeding Academic Research Consortium (BARC) [25] or the International Society on Thrombosis and Hemostasis (ISTH) [26]. The secondary safety outcome was minor bleeding, and the secondary efficacy outcome was asymptomatic cerebral embolism (ACE).

ACE was diagnosed using diffusion-weighted magnetic resonance imaging (MRI). Minor bleeding was defined as any bleeding that did not fulfil the BARC or ISTH criteria. The net clinical benefit was investigated as a composite of the primary safety and efficacy outcomes.

2.5. Data Extraction and Synthesis

We extracted the following data from the studies: study name, baseline characteristics, anticoagulant regimens, and outcomes. Two reviewers (MK and TY) independently extracted the data. When disagreements between reviewers occurred, a third author (TI) was consulted to reach a decision.

All study regimens were synthesized as follows: uninterrupted DOAC (UI-DOAC), interrupted DOAC (I-DOAC), uninterrupted VKA (UI-VKA), and interrupted VKA (I-VKA) administration. The number of thromboembolic events, major bleeding, composite of primary outcomes, minor bleeding, and ACE were synthesized, and odds ratios (ORs) were estimated. Additionally, all strategies were synthesized per anticoagulant (apixaban, dabigatran, edoxaban, rivaroxaban, and warfarin), and the ORs of the composite of the primary outcomes were estimated in subgroup analyses. The geometry of the network was illustrated using direct comparative treatments.

2.6. Risk of Bias Assessment

We evaluated the risk of bias using the revised Cochrane risk-of-bias tool for randomized trials (RoB2) [27]. Two reviewers (MK and TY) were involved in the quality assessment; if disagreements occurred, a third author (TI) was consulted to reach a consensus.

2.7. Statistical Analysis

NMA statistical analyses were performed with frequentist methods using *Netmeta* (version 1.5-0) in R 4.1.0 (R Foundation for Statistical Computing, Vienna, Austria). The ORs and 95% confidence intervals (CIs) were estimated based on a random effects model. Additionally, we calculated the P-score and the surface under the cumulative ranking (SUCRA) to evaluate and rank the anticoagulant strategies and regimens [28,29]. Both rankings are measured on a scale from 0 (worst) to 1 (best). Common network heterogeneity was evaluated using the I^2 measure to locate the source of heterogeneity [30]. Heterogeneity was defined as low, moderate, or high when I^2 was 25%, 50%, or 75%, respectively [31]. Inconsistency between direct and indirect evidence was examined globally and locally [32,33]. Begg's rank correlation and Egger's linear regression were performed to assess publication bias among the studies [34,35]. We conducted sensitivity analyses by excluding one study at a time for the four different strategies of the network. Subgroup analysis was performed to evaluate each anticoagulant regimen for the composite of the primary outcomes.

3. Results

3.1. Study Identification and Study Population Characteristics

We initially identified 124 studies via the electronic databases, and four additional studies were identified through references. Fifty duplicate studies were removed and 78 were screened. We excluded 57 studies after screening the titles and abstracts, and 21 were retrieved for detailed evaluation, from which four studies were subsequently excluded from the analysis because they did not meet the eligibility criteria (Figure 1). Finally, our meta-analysis included 17 RCTs with 6950 patients undergoing AF ablation [36–52]. They were allocated to I-VKA (n = 835) [36,37], UI-VKA (n = 2097) [36,38–44], I-DOAC (n = 1465) [37,38,45–51], and UI-DOAC (n = 2553) groups [39–52]. All approved DOACs (apixaban [40,43,45–51], dabigatran [37,38,41,47,48,51], edoxaban [44,48,49,51,52], and rivaroxaban [39,42,45,47–49,51,52]) were included.

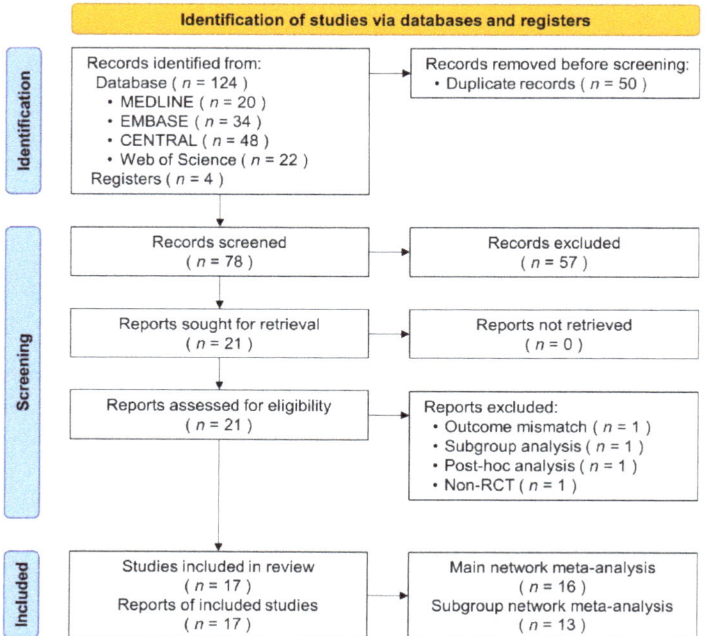

Figure 1. Flow diagram of the included studies. The PRISMA flow diagram depicts the phases of the systematic review and shows the number of records identified, screened, included, and excluded. RCT, randomized controlled trial.

The age of the participants ranged from 59 to 70 years (median = 62 years); 74% were men and 55% had paroxysmal AF. Twelve studies (71%) reported mean CHA_2DS_2-VASc scores ranging from 1.5 to 2.8 (median 2.0). In 15 studies (88%), the median follow-up duration was 30 days (range: 2–90 days). The detailed clinical characteristics of the included studies are summarized in Tables 1 and S3.

Table 1. Baseline characteristics in the included studies.

Study	Year	Regimen	n	Age (years)	Male Sex	Paroxysmal AF	CHA_2DS_2-VASc	HAS-BLED	Mean ACT	Target ACT	Total UFH Dose	Protamine	ICE	Ablation Technology	Follow-Up Period
COMPARE [36] (International)	2014	UI-Warfarin I-Warfarin	794 790	59 59	230 (73%) 245 (77%)	200 (63%) 229 (72%)	NR	NR	NR	>300 >350	NR	Used †	794 (100%) 790 (100%)	RF	48 h
Nin [37] (Japan)	2013	I-Dabigatran 110 mg BID I-Warfarin	45 45	61 61	38 (84%) 36 (80%)	34 (76%) 32 (71%)	NR	NR	NR	300–400	NR	Used †	NR	RF	14 days
ABRIDGE-J [38] (Japan)	2019	I-Dabigatran 150/110 mg BID UI-Warfarin	220 222	65 66	171 (78%) 160 (72%)	138 (63%) 138 (62%)	2.0 * 2.0 *	1.0 * 1.0 *	NR	300–400	14,000 9000	Used †	52 (24%) 58 (26%)	RF/Cryo	3 months
VENTURE-AF [39] (International)	2015	UI-Rivaroxaban 20 mg OD UI-Warfarin	114 107	59 61	86 (75%) 90 (84%)	95 (83%) 87 (81%)	1.5 1.7	NR	302 332	300–400	13,871 10,964	32 (28%) 27 (25%)	Used †	Unclear	30 days
Kuwahara [40] (Japan)	2016	UI-Apixaban 5/2.5 mg BID UI-Warfarin	100 100	65 66	75 (75%) 72 (72%)	59 (59%) 60 (60%)	2.1 2.4	NR	322 357	>300	14,000 9000	Used †	NR	RF	7 days
RE-CIRCUIT [41] (International)	2017	UI-Dabigatran 150 mg BID UI-Warfarin	317 318	59 59	230 (73%) 245 (77%)	213 (67%) 219 (69%)	2.0 2.2	NR	330 342	>300	12,402 11,910	Used †	NR	Mixed	56 days
ASCERTAIN [42] (Japan)	2018	UI-Rivaroxaban 15/10 mg OD UI-Warfarin	64 63	59 62	53 (83%) 53 (84%)	40 (63%) 42 (67%)	NR	NR	299 341	300–350	12,500 9000	Used †	NR	RF	30 days
AXAFA-AFNET 5 [43] (International)	2018	UI-Apixaban 5/2.5 mg BID UI-Warfarin	318 315	64 64	218 (69%) 206 (65%)	189 (59%) 178 (57%)	2.4 2.4	NR	310 349	>300	NR	Used †	Used †	Mixed	3 months
ELIMINATE-AF [44] (International)	2019	UI-Edoxaban 60 mg OD UI-Warfarin	375 178	60 61	290 (77%) 149 (84%)	284 (76%) 131 (74%)	1.8 1.7	NR	303 338	300–400	14,261 11,473	NR	92 (25%) 42 (24%)	RF/Cryo	90 days
Yoshimura [45] (Japan)	2017	UI-Rivaroxaban 15/10 mg OD I-Apixaban 5/2.5 mg BID	55 50	59 59	45 (82%) 41 (82%)	33 (60%) 31 (62%)	1.7 1.7	NR	275 286	>300	15,745 14,240	NR	NR	RF	Unclear
AEIOU [46] (USA)	2018	UI-Apixaban 5 mg BID I-Apixaban 5/2.5 mg BID	150 145	63 64	101 (67%) 97 (67%)	100 (67%) 91 (63%)	2.2 2.4	1.0 1.1	NR	>300	17,800 19,700	137 (91%) 128 (88%)	NR	RF/Cryo	30 days
Yu [47] (Korea)	2019	UI-DOAC (Api/Dab/Riv) I-DOAC (Api/Dab/Riv)	106 110	59 58	81 (76%) 79 (72%)	67 (63%) 74 (67%)	1.6 1.7	NR	352 348	350–400	18,740 20,136	NR	Used †	RF	1 month
Nakamura [48] (Japan)	2019	UI-DOAC (Api/Dab/Edo/Riv) I-DOAC (Api/Dab/Edo/Riv)	421 423	65 65	298 (71%) 298 (70%)	222 (53%) 236 (58%)	2.0 2.1	1.3 1.4	358 330	300–400	12,936 13,830	405 (96%) 371 (88%)	NR	RF	30 days

Table 1. *Cont.*

Study	Year	Regimen	*n*	Age (years)	Male Sex	Paroxysmal AF	CHA_2DS_2-VASc	HAS-BLED	Mean ACT	Target ACT	Total UFH Dose	Protamine	ICE	Ablation Technology	Follow-Up Period
Nagao [49] (Japan)	2019	UI-DOAC (Api/Edo/Riv)	100	70	64 (64%)	57 (57%)	2.8	NR	285	>300	8704	Used †	Used †	RF	1 month
		I-DOAC (Api/Edo/Riv)	100	70	62 (62%)	59 (59%)	2.6		280		9945				
Ando [50] (Japan)	2019	UI-Apixaban 5 mg BID	32	67	26 (81%)	32 (100%)	NR	NR	NR	300–350	NR	Used †	NR	Cryo	30 days
		I-Apixaban 5 mg BID	65	66	49 (75%)	65 (100%)									
Yamaji [51] (Japan)	2019	UI-DOAC (Api/Dab/Edo/Riv)	277	66	211 (76%)	171 (62%)	1.9	1.4	NR	300–400	NR	Used †	NR	RF	90 days
		I-DOAC (Api/Dab/Edo/Riv)	307	65	212 (69%)	199 (65%)	1.9	1.4							
Yoshimoto [52] (Japan)	2021	UI-Edoxaban 60/30 mg OD	61	62	43 (70%)	38 (62%)	1.7	1.1	300	>300	7333	NR	NR	RF	Unclear
		UI-Rivaroxaban 15/10 mg OD	63	62	46 (73%)	45 (71%)	1.8	1.2	298		7865				

CHA_2DS_2-VASc and HAS-BLED scores are the risk prediction scores of stroke and major bleeding, respectively. AF, atrial fibrillation; ACT, activated coagulation time; UFH, unfractionated heparin; ICE, intracardiac echocardiography; UI, uninterrupted; I, interrupted; DOAC, direct anticoagulant; Api, apixaban; Dab, dabigatran; Edo, edoxaban; Riv, rivaroxaban; OD, omni die (once a day); BID, bis in die (twice a day); NR, not reported; RF, radiofrequency ablation; Cryo, cryoballoon ablation. * Median. † Numbers were unclear.

All studies reported primary efficacy (thromboembolic events) and safety (major bleeding) outcomes, while 14 and 8 studies (82% and 47%, respectively) reported minor bleeding [36–44,46,48–51] and ACE [40,42–45,48,49,52], respectively.

3.2. Risk of Bias Assessment

We evaluated all studies in five dimensions (Table S4). Concerns were noted for 14 RCTs (82%). All protocols were composed of two interventions after randomization: anticoagulant initiation and AF ablation. Since some deviations occurred before CA, outcomes were analyzed as a modified intention-to-treat population who underwent AF ablation. Some small RCTs did not mention the concealment method. However, none of the studies were classified as having a high bias risk. Therefore, we included all studies in the NMA.

3.3. Structure of the Network

Figure 2 shows the network of anticoagulant strategies used in the main analysis. We compared four strategies: UI-DOAC, I-DOAC, UI-VKA, and I-VKA, and set UI-VKA as a reference. All direct comparative studies were included, except UI-DOAC vs. I-VKA.

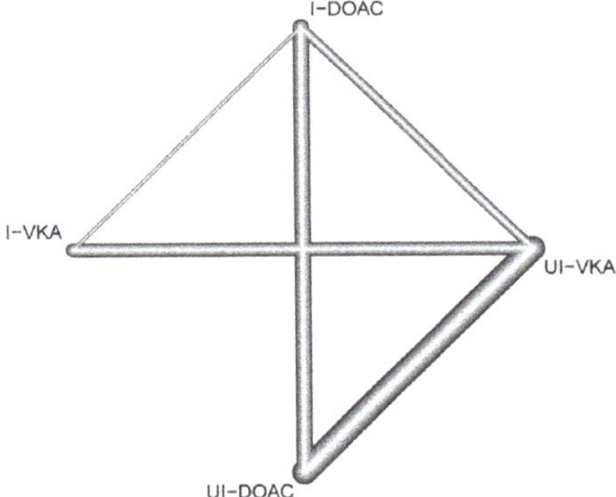

Figure 2. Network of treatment comparisons for the overall primary efficacy and safety outcomes. Directly comparable treatments are linked to lines. The nodes are placed and labelled according to the treatments. The thickness of the edges is proportional to the inverse standard error of the treatment effects, aggregated over all studies, including the two respective treatments. The network includes 16 two-armed studies. UI, uninterrupted; I, interrupted; DOAC, direct oral anticoagulant; VKA, vitamin-K antagonist.

3.4. NMA Results for the Primary and Secondary Outcomes

The results of the NMA for thromboembolic events, major bleeding, and the composite of primary outcomes are presented as forest plots (Figure 3a–c). I-VKA was associated with an increased risk of thromboembolic events compared to UI-VKA (OR [95% CI]: 15.77 [4.16–59.70]), whereas there was no significant difference between UI-DOAC and I-DOAC (OR: 0.97 [0.24–3.87] and OR: 1.31 [0.25–6.86]). Compared to UI-VKA, UI-DOAC significantly decreased the risk of major bleeding (OR: 0.55 [0.31–0.97]). However, I-DOAC and I-VKA did not have a significant effect (OR: 0.53 [0.22–1.23] and OR: 2.70 [0.65–11.18]). In the composite of thromboembolic events and major bleeding, UI-DOAC and I-DOAC were not inferior to UI-VKA (OR: 0.61 [0.31–1.17] and OR: 0.63 [0.26–1.54]), while I-VKA significantly increased the risk of thromboembolic events and major bleeding (OR: 8.02 [2.35–27.45]). Heterogeneity was low for primary outcomes (thromboembolic events, $I^2 = 0.0\%$; major bleeding, $I^2 = 7.8\%$; and the composite of primary outcomes, $I^2 = 23.4\%$).

(a) **Thromboembolic events (Stroke, TIA, or systemic embolism)**

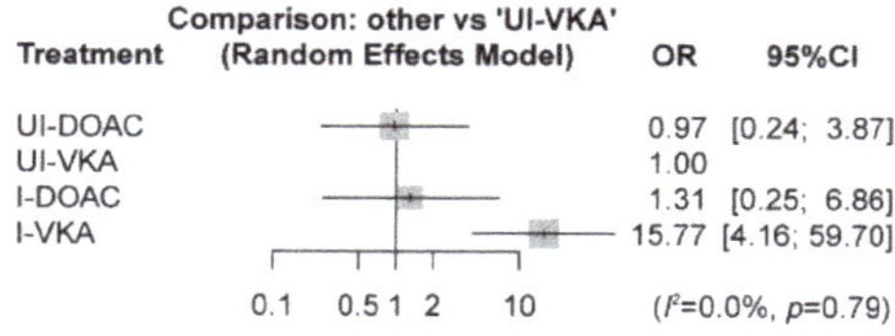

(b) **Major bleeding**

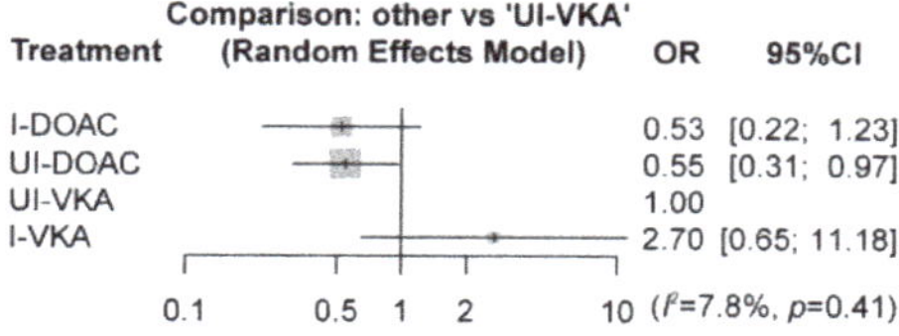

(c) **Composite of primary outcomes (Thromboembolic events and major bleeding)**

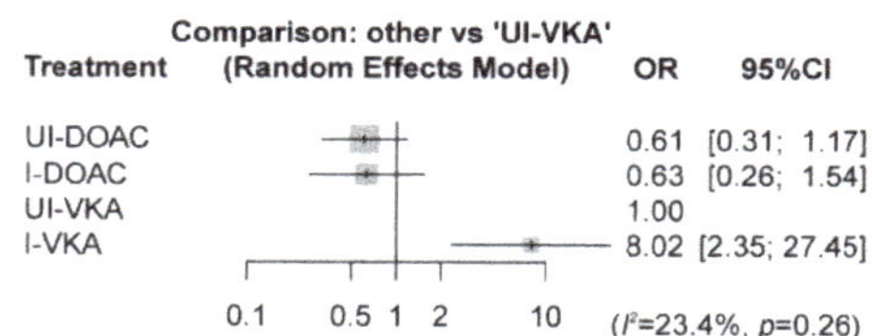

(d) **Minor bleeding**

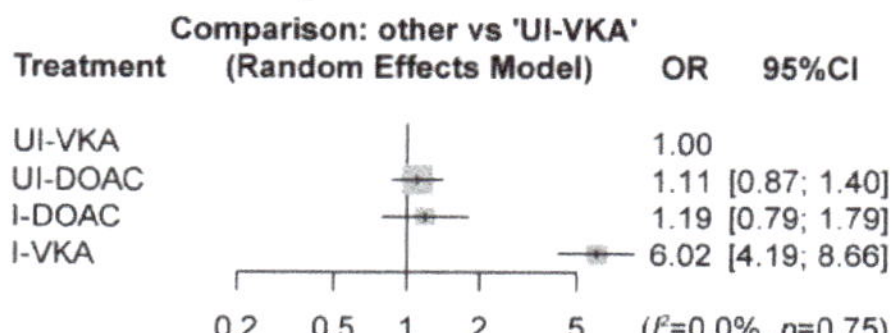

(e) **Asymptomatic cerebral embolism**

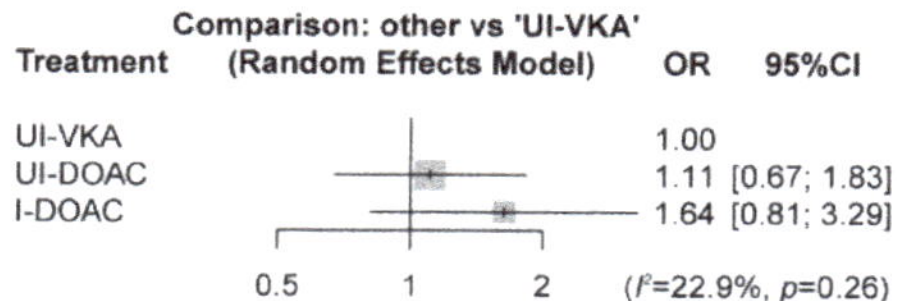

Figure 3. Forest plots for efficacy and safety of anticoagulant strategies compared with UI-VKA. (**a**) The efficacy of thromboembolic events (stroke, TIA, or systemic embolism); (**b**) the safety of major bleeding; (**c**) the efficacy and safety of the composite of the primary outcomes (stroke, TIA, or systemic embolism and major bleeding); (**d**) the safety of minor bleeding; and (**e**) the efficacy of asymptomatic cerebral embolism. TIA, transient ischemic attack; OR, odds ratio; CI, confidence interval; UI, uninterrupted; I, interrupted; DOAC, direct oral anticoagulant; VKA, vitamin-K antagonist.

Regarding the secondary outcomes, the NMA results for minor bleeding and ACE are presented in Figure 3d,e. Both UI-DOAC and I-DOAC carried comparable risks of minor bleeding with UI-VKA (OR: 1.11 [0.87–1.40] and OR: 1.19 [0.79–1.79]), but I-VKA significantly increased the risk (OR: 6.02 [4.19–8.66]). UI-DOAC and I-DOAC were also similar to UI-VKA for the risk of ACE (OR: 1.11 [0.67–1.83] and OR: 1.64 [0.81–3.29]). Heterogeneity was low for secondary outcomes (minor bleeding, I^2 = 0.0%; and ACE, I^2 = 22.9%).

Table 2 displays the P-score and SUCRA values for the primary and secondary outcomes. There were no ranking mismatches between the P-score and SUCRA. The SUCRA value of DOACs was nearly twice that of UI-VKA in the composite of the primary outcomes (UI-DOAC, 0.82; I-DOAC, 0.77; and UI-VKA, 0.40). In contrast, the secondary outcome SUCRA values were higher for UI-VKA than for DOACs; particularly, the ACE value for I-DOAC was markedly low (UI-DOAC, 0.60; I-DOAC, 0.09; and UI-VKA, 0.82).

Table 2. P-score and the SUCRA values for each strategy and outcome.

Strategy	Thromboembolic Events		Major Bleeding		Composite of Primary Outcomes		Minor Bleeding		Asymptomatic Cerebral Embolism	
	P-Score	SUCRA	P-Score	SUCRA	P-Score	SUCRA	P-Score	SUCRA	P-Score	SUCRA
UI-DOAC	0.72	0.73	0.81	0.76	0.82	0.82	0.62	0.65	0.64	0.60
I-DOAC	0.68	0.70	0.82	0.85	0.77	0.77	0.52	0.49	0.07	0.09
UI-VKA	0.60	0.57	0.33	0.34	0.41	0.40	0.87	0.86	0.79	0.82
I-VKA	0.00	0.00	0.04	0.05	0.00	0.00	0.00	0.00	-	-

SUCRA, surface under the cumulative ranking; UI, uninterrupted; I, interrupted; DOAC, direct oral anticoagulant; VKA, vitamin-K antagonist.

Overall, the UI-DOAC strategy was favorable and the I-DOAC strategy was feasible compared with the UI-VKA strategy for the primary and secondary outcomes. However, the I-VKA strategy significantly increased the risk of thromboembolic and bleeding events compared to the UI-VKA strategy.

3.5. Sensitivity Analyses

We performed sensitivity analyses for the composite of the primary outcomes (Table S5). RE-CIRCUIT and ELIMINATE-AF were the main sources of heterogeneity [41,44]. Moreover, UI-DOAC was associated with a significant reduction in major bleeding; however, this finding was not robust because it was no longer significant when 10 studies were excluded. Overall, this analysis did not suggest that the excluded studies would affect the relative effects and rankings of the anticoagulant strategies.

3.6. Assessment of Inconsistency and Publication Bias

The inconsistency test did not suggest the presence of inconsistency in the network (Figure S1). Begg's and Egger's tests did not reveal significant publication bias among the included studies (Figure S2).

3.7. Subgroup Analysis

We conducted a subgroup analysis based on each anticoagulant regimen. The composite of thromboembolic and major bleeding events was analyzed and displayed in a forest plot (Figure 4) and a league table (Table S6); we also calculated the P-score and SUCRA values (Table 3). Four studies were excluded because they had no randomized regimens for each DOAC [47–49,51], and one study included both UI-DOAC arms [52]. The structure of the subgroup network is shown in Figure S3. UI-dabigatran significantly decreased the risk of the composite of the primary outcomes compared with UI-VKA (OR: 0.21 [0.08–0.55]), whereas I-VKA significantly increased the risk (OR: 8.39 [3.43–20.56]). Other anticoagulants had a comparable risk to that of UI-VKA. The P-score and SUCRA values were notably higher for UI-dabigatran and I-dabigatran than for the other anticoagulant regimens (UI-dabigatran, 0.95; and I-dabigatran, 0.82 in SUCRA).

Table 3. P-score and the SUCRA values for each strategy and composite of primary outcome.

Strategy	Composite of Primary Outcomes	
	P-Score	SUCRA
UI-dabigatran	0.93	0.95
I-dabigatran	0.89	0.82
UI-apixaban	0.52	0.53
I-apixaban	0.51	0.52
UI-VKA	0.46	0.47
UI-rivaroxaban	0.36	0.41
UI-edoxaban	0.33	0.30
I-VKA	0.00	0.00

SUCRA, surface under the cumulative ranking; UI, uninterrupted; I, interrupted; VKA, vitamin-K antagonist.

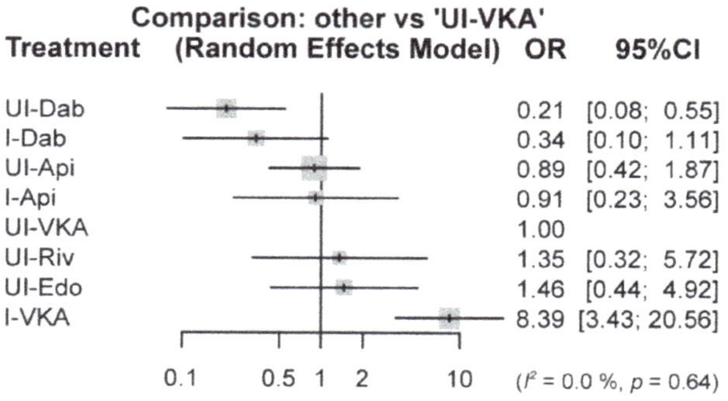

Comparison: other vs 'UI-VKA'

Treatment (Random Effects Model)	OR	95%CI
UI-Dab	0.21	[0.08; 0.55]
I-Dab	0.34	[0.10; 1.11]
UI-Api	0.89	[0.42; 1.87]
I-Api	0.91	[0.23; 3.56]
UI-VKA	1.00	
UI-Riv	1.35	[0.32; 5.72]
UI-Edo	1.46	[0.44; 4.92]
I-VKA	8.39	[3.43; 20.56]

0.1 0.5 1 2 10 (I^2 = 0.0 %, p = 0.64)

Figure 4. Forest plot for the composite of primary outcomes for each anticoagulant regimen. OR, odds ratio; CI, confidence interval; VKA, vitamin-K antagonist; UI, uninterrupted; I, interrupted; Dab, dabigatran; Api, apixaban; Riv, rivaroxaban; Edo, edoxaban.

4. Discussion

In this study, we compared uninterrupted or interrupted DOAC administration with uninterrupted or interrupted VKA administration as periprocedural anticoagulant strategies for patients undergoing AF ablation. The main findings were as follows: (1) the risk of thromboembolic events among the strategies was exceedingly rare (UI-DOAC: 0.20%, I-DOAC: 0.20%, and UI-VKA: 0.24%) and not significantly different within strategies, except for the I-VKA strategy (4.79%); (2) ACE occurred with an incidence of 15–21%; (3) major bleeding tended to be halved by DOAC compared with UI-VKA administration; (4) minor bleeding did not differ between DOACs and VKAs, except for I-VKA; and (5) UI-dabigatran significantly reduced the composite of thromboembolic and major bleeding events.

After the COMPARE trial [36], the UI-VKA strategy has been widely adopted as a periprocedural anticoagulant strategy for patients undergoing AF ablation. Meanwhile, there is growing evidence regarding the efficacy and safety of DOACs in patients with AF [53–56]. Recently, worldwide RCTs have revealed that UI-DOAC may be equivalent to UI-VKA [39,41,43,44]. Therefore, the latest guidelines classify the UI-DOAC strategy as a class I recommendation [8,9]. However, I-DOAC is also used as a periprocedural anticoagulant strategy in clinical practice owing to concerns regarding bleeding complications [20]. Although the HRS/EHRA/ECAS/APHRS/SOLAECE 2017 expert consensus statement on CA of AF classified the I-DOAC strategy as a class IIa recommendation [9], RCTs published after 2017 have demonstrated that there were no significant differences between the UI-DOAC and I-DOAC for the prevention of thromboembolic and major bleeding complications [46–51].

Thromboembolism is the most notable complication of CA for AF. The occurrence of periprocedural stroke or TIA was reported to be 0.1–0.6% in the latest guidelines [8]. Herein, both the DOAC and UI-VKA strategies revealed comparable efficacy in preventing thromboembolic events compared with I-VKA, and there were no significant differences among them. Therefore, an uninterrupted anticoagulant strategy is usually favorable, but an interrupted DOAC administration is feasible for the prevention of thromboembolism.

The safety of anticoagulants during periprocedural management must be carefully considered. Our NMA revealed a significant reduction in major bleeding complications with UI-DOAC compared with UI-VKA, consistent with the results of a previous meta-analysis [18]. The mechanism of reduction may be related to the type of anticoagulant (thrombin or factor Xa inhibitor) and a shorter half-life than warfarin. However, a recent meta-analysis showed no significant differences between UI-DOAC and UI-VKA [19]. In the sensitivity analysis, which excluded individual studies, we could not identify the robustness of UI-DOAC for significant reduction of major bleeding without each of the

10 studies in Table S5b. However, the estimated ORs with both DOAC strategies tended to carry a lower risk of major bleeding; thus, they may be safer alternatives to UI-VKA.

The ACE associated with CA for AF is relatively common and reported in 0–12.5% of UI-DOAC, 15.0–35.7% of I-DOAC, and 8.7–18.6% of UI-VKA cases [57–59]. In a previous meta-analysis, UI-DOAC significantly reduced the occurrence of ACE compared to I-DOAC [60]. In our review, similar ACE incidence rates were observed (UI-DOAC, 16.0%; I-DOAC, 20.7%; and UI-VKA, 15.4%), but we were unable to identify a significant reduction with UI-DOAC. Although ACE is classified as a complication of unknown significance in the current guidelines [8], it may be associated with the risk of dementia, cognitive impairment, and future stroke [61,62]. Nakamura et al. reported ACE detected post CA on follow-up MRI disappeared in 79.8% of cases [48]. The remaining 20.2% may develop chronic infarcts due to debris dislodging, air embolism, or small thrombosis [63,64]. The significance of ACE remains unclear, but a continuous anticoagulant strategy is feasible as a periprocedural treatment for ACE prevention.

We set another network with each anticoagulant regimen as a subgroup analysis and found that UI-dabigatran could significantly reduce the composite of the primary outcomes. Since UI-dabigatran did not influence significantly for thromboembolic events in Table S6b, the reduction of major bleeding complications can lead to this result. Although the DOACs included apixaban, dabigatran, edoxaban, and rivaroxaban, dabigatran is a thrombin inhibitor, while the others are factor Xa inhibitors. Dabigatran can extend the activated thromboplastin time, activated coagulation time (ACT), and thrombin time to a greater extent than factor Xa inhibitors [8]. Recent RCTs that compared UI-DOAC and UI-VKA revealed that the total amount of unfractionated heparin (UFH) during AF ablation increased, owing to the use of factor Xa inhibitors (apixaban, 156% [40]; edoxaban, 124% [44]; and rivaroxaban, 133% [39,42]) compared with thrombin inhibitors (dabigatran, 104% [41]), and the mean ACT was lower with factor Xa inhibitors than with thrombin inhibitors (307 vs. 330 s). This previously reported finding [65] may contribute to the increased risk of major bleeding. Martin et al. reported that ACT was strongly correlated with the prothrombin time-international normalized ratio and dabigatran concentration, but not with factor Xa inhibitor concentration [66]. Moreover, only dabigatran was parallel with VKA in the UFH dose–response curves. In contrast, factor Xa inhibitors had a smaller effect on ACT prolongation in response to heparin. The target ACT at 300 s is supported by robust evidence for controlling the thromboembolic and bleeding risks, but this evidence depends on VKA and UFH management [67]. Consequently, dabigatran is the optimal periprocedural anticoagulant for ACT monitoring during AF ablation.

As DOACs have become the practical standard for periprocedural anticoagulant strategies, the management of major bleeding is more important. Idarucizumab, a specific reversal agent for dabigatran, is now available worldwide [68]. In contrast, andexanet alfa, a specific reversal agent for factor Xa inhibitors, is only available in some countries [69]. Therefore, UI-dabigatran allows an option to manage complications if emergency bleeding occurs anywhere in the world.

Although NMA can assess the relative effectiveness of different strategies, our study has limitations. A primary limitation is that this NMA was based on study-level rather than patient-level data, which would considerably weaken the comparison validity. Second, differentiations of bleeding criteria, the usage of protamine and intracardiac echocardiography (ICE), lengths of follow-up, and methods of measuring ACE with MRI may contribute to heterogeneity and potentially affect the interpretation of the results. In particular, the number of participants who underwent MRI was limited in three RCTs. Further studies are needed to determine the significance of the optimal anticoagulant strategy for ACE. Additionally, the usage of protamine after the ablation procedure, and ICE during transseptal puncture, can prevent bleeding events. However, there were few studies to report those applications, and this can influence bleeding outcomes. Since four studies that investigated DOACs were not randomized into individual anticoagulants, a pooled comparison of a specific regimen in NMA could not be performed, and this weakened the interpretation of the results. Moreover, some regimens lacked data and were dependent on one study because of the limited number of RCTs. As RCTs of I-DOAC were mainly conducted in Japan, their results may involve regional bias.

5. Conclusions

In patients undergoing AF ablation, both DOAC strategies were associated with a lower incidence of major bleeding and had a similar effect on the prevention of thromboembolic events and minor bleeding compared with the UI-VKA strategy, whereas the I-VKA strategy should generally be avoided. Continuous DOAC and VKA administration was associated with a lower incidence of ACE. Therefore, UI-DOAC is the preferable alternative to UI-VKA. Although further data on the outcomes of patients receiving UI-dabigatran are needed for definitive conclusions, our results support the use of UI-dabigatran as the optimal periprocedural anticoagulant for ACT monitoring during AF ablation.

Supplementary Materials: The following supporting information can be downloaded at: https://www.mdpi.com/article/10.3390/jcm11071872/s1, Figure S1: Inconsistency analysis; Figure S2: Comparison adjusted funnel plot; Figure S3: Network of anticoagulant comparisons for the composite of primary outcomes; Table S1: PRISMA network meta-analysis checklist; Table S2: PICOS format and detailed search code; Table S3: Efficacy and safety outcomes in the included studies; Table S4: Assessment of bias in the randomized clinical trials; Table S5: Sensitivity analysis; Table S6: Summary estimates for outcomes with each anticoagulant regimen from network meta-analysis.

Author Contributions: Conceptualization, T.K.; methodology, T.Y.; software, T.K.; validation, H.Y. and T.I. (Tomoaki Ishigami); formal analysis, T.K.; investigation, S.I., M.A. and S.A.; resources, T.K.; data curation, M.K. and T.Y.; writing—original draft preparation, T.K.; writing—review and editing, M.K., T.Y., H.Y. and T.I. (Tomoaki Ishigami); visualization, T.K.; supervision, T.I. (Toshiyuki Ishikawa); project administration, T.K. All authors have read and agreed to the published version of the manuscript.

Funding: This research received no external funding.

Institutional Review Board Statement: Not applicable.

Informed Consent Statement: Not applicable.

Data Availability Statement: All data are incorporated into the article and its online supplementary material.

Conflicts of Interest: The authors declare no conflict of interest.

References

1. Benjamin, E.J.; Muntner, P.; Alonso, A.; Bittencourt, M.S.; Callaway, C.W.; Carson, A.P.; Chamberlain, A.M.; Chang, A.R.; Cheng, S.; Das, S.R.; et al. Heart Disease and Stroke Statistics-2019 Update: A Report From the American Heart Association. *Circulation* **2019**, *139*, e56–e528. [CrossRef] [PubMed]
2. Arbelo, E.; Brugada, J.; Hindricks, G.; Maggioni, A.; Tavazzi, L.; Vardas, P.; Anselme, F.; Inama, G.; Jais, P.; Kalarus, Z.; et al. ESC-EURObservational Research Programme: The Atrial Fibrillation Ablation Pilot Study, conducted by the European Heart Rhythm Association. *Europace* **2012**, *14*, 1094–1103. [CrossRef] [PubMed]
3. Reddy, V.Y.; Dukkipati, S.R.; Neuzil, P.; Natale, A.; Albenque, J.P.; Kautzner, J.; Shah, D.; Michaud, G.; Wharton, M.; Harari, D.; et al. Randomized, Controlled Trial of the Safety and Effectiveness of a Contact Force-Sensing Irrigated Catheter for Ablation of Paroxysmal Atrial Fibrillation: Results of the TactiCath Contact Force Ablation Catheter Study for Atrial Fibrillation (TOCCASTAR) Study. *Circulation* **2015**, *132*, 907–915. [CrossRef]
4. Stabile, G.; Scaglione, M.; del Greco, M.; De Ponti, R.; Bongiorni, M.G.; Zoppo, F.; Soldati, E.; Marazzi, R.; Marini, M.; Gaita, F.; et al. Reduced fluoroscopy exposure during ablation of atrial fibrillation using a novel electroanatomical navigation system: A multicentre experience. *Europace* **2012**, *14*, 60–65. [CrossRef] [PubMed]
5. McLellan, A.J.; Ling, L.H.; Azzopardi, S.; Lee, G.A.; Lee, G.; Kumar, S.; Wong, M.C.; Walters, T.E.; Lee, J.M.; Looi, K.L.; et al. A minimal or maximal ablation strategy to achieve pulmonary vein isolation for paroxysmal atrial fibrillation: A prospective multi-centre randomized controlled trial (the Minimax study). *Eur. Heart J.* **2015**, *36*, 1812–1821. [CrossRef] [PubMed]
6. Verma, A.; Jiang, C.Y.; Betts, T.R.; Chen, J.; Deisenhofer, I.; Mantovan, R.; Macle, L.; Morillo, C.A.; Haverkamp, W.; Weerasooriya, R.; et al. Approaches to catheter ablation for persistent atrial fibrillation. *N. Engl. J. Med.* **2015**, *372*, 1812–1822. [CrossRef]

7. Nery, P.B.; Belliveau, D.; Nair, G.M.; Bernick, J.; Redpath, C.J.; Szczotka, A.; Sadek, M.M.; Green, M.S.; Wells, G.; Birnie, D.H. Relationship Between Pulmonary Vein Reconnection and Atrial Fibrillation Recurrence: A Systematic Review and Meta-Analysis. *JACC Clin. Electrophysiol.* **2016**, *2*, 474–483. [CrossRef]
8. Hindricks, G.; Potpara, T.; Dagres, N.; Arbelo, E.; Bax, J.J.; Blomström-Lundqvist, C.; Boriani, G.; Castella, M.; Dan, G.A.; Dilaveris, P.E.; et al. 2020 ESC Guidelines for the diagnosis and management of atrial fibrillation developed in collaboration with the European Association for Cardio-Thoracic Surgery (EACTS): The Task Force for the diagnosis and management of atrial fibrillation of the European Society of Cardiology (ESC) Developed with the special contribution of the European Heart Rhythm Association (EHRA) of the ESC. *Eur. Heart J.* **2021**, *42*, 373–498. [CrossRef]
9. Calkins, H.; Hindricks, G.; Cappato, R.; Kim, Y.H.; Saad, E.B.; Aguinaga, L.; Akar, J.G.; Badhwar, V.; Brugada, J.; Camm, J.; et al. 2017 HRS/EHRA/ECAS/APHRS/SOLAECE expert consensus statement on catheter and surgical ablation of atrial fibrillation. *Heart Rhythm* **2017**, *14*, e275–e444. [CrossRef]
10. Packer, D.L.; Mark, D.B.; Robb, R.A.; Monahan, K.H.; Bahnson, T.D.; Poole, J.E.; Noseworthy, P.A.; Rosenberg, Y.D.; Jeffries, N.; Mitchell, L.B.; et al. Effect of Catheter Ablation vs Antiarrhythmic Drug Therapy on Mortality, Stroke, Bleeding, and Cardiac Arrest Among Patients with Atrial Fibrillation: The CABANA Randomized Clinical Trial. *JAMA* **2019**, *321*, 1261–1274. [CrossRef]
11. Ruff, C.T.; Giugliano, R.P.; Braunwald, E.; Hoffman, E.B.; Deenadayalu, N.; Ezekowitz, M.D.; Camm, A.J.; Weitz, J.I.; Lewis, B.S.; Parkhomenko, A.; et al. Comparison of the efficacy and safety of new oral anticoagulants with warfarin in patients with atrial fibrillation: A meta-analysis of randomised trials. *Lancet* **2014**, *383*, 955–962. [CrossRef]
12. Bassiouny, M.; Saliba, W.; Rickard, J.; Shao, M.; Sey, A.; Diab, M.; Martin, D.O.; Hussein, A.; Khoury, M.; Abi-Saleh, B.; et al. Use of dabigatran for periprocedural anticoagulation in patients undergoing catheter ablation for atrial fibrillation. *Circ. Arrhyth. Electrophysiol.* **2013**, *6*, 460–466. [CrossRef]
13. Bin Abdulhak, A.A.; Khan, A.R.; Tleyjeh, I.M.; Spertus, J.A.; Sanders, S.U.; Steigerwalt, K.E.; Garbati, M.A.; Bahmaid, R.A.; Wimmer, A.P. Safety and efficacy of interrupted dabigatran for peri-procedural anticoagulation in catheter ablation of atrial fibrillation: A systematic review and meta-analysis. *Europace* **2013**, *15*, 1412–1420. [CrossRef] [PubMed]
14. Hohnloser, S.H.; Camm, A.J. Safety and efficacy of dabigatran etexilate during catheter ablation of atrial fibrillation: A meta-analysis of the literature. *Europace* **2013**, *15*, 1407–1411. [CrossRef] [PubMed]
15. Providência, R.; Marijon, E.; Albenque, J.P.; Combes, S.; Combes, N.; Jourda, F.; Hireche, H.; Morais, J.; Boveda, S. Rivaroxaban and dabigatran in patients undergoing catheter ablation of atrial fibrillation. *Europace* **2014**, *16*, 1137–1144. [CrossRef] [PubMed]
16. Armbruster, H.L.; Lindsley, J.P.; Moranville, M.P.; Habibi, M.; Khurram, I.M.; Spragg, D.D.; Berger, R.D.; Calkins, H.; Marine, J.E. Safety of novel oral anticoagulants compared with uninterrupted warfarin for catheter ablation of atrial fibrillation. *Ann. Pharm.* **2015**, *49*, 278–284. [CrossRef]
17. Rahman, H.; Khan, S.U.; DePersis, M.; Hammad, T.; Nasir, F.; Kaluski, E. Meta-analysis of safety and efficacy of oral anticoagulants in patients requiring catheter ablation for atrial fibrillation. *Cardiovasc. Revasc. Med.* **2019**, *20*, 147–152. [CrossRef]
18. Zhao, Y.; Lu, Y.; Qin, Y. A meta-analysis of randomized controlled trials of uninterrupted periprocedural anticoagulation strategy in patients undergoing atrial fibrillation catheter ablation. *Int. J. Cardiol.* **2018**, *270*, 167–171. [CrossRef] [PubMed]
19. Brockmeyer, M.; Lin, Y.; Parco, C.; Karathanos, A.; Krieger, T.; Schulze, V.; Heinen, Y.; Bejinariu, A.; Müller, P.; Makimoto, H.; et al. Uninterrupted anticoagulation during catheter ablation for atrial fibrillation: No difference in major bleeding and stroke between direct oral anticoagulants and vitamin K antagonists in an updated meta-analysis of randomised controlled trials. *Acta Cardiol.* **2021**, *76*, 288–295. [CrossRef] [PubMed]
20. Bejinariu, A.G.; Makimoto, H.; Wakili, R.; Mathew, S.; Kosiuk, J.; Linz, D.; Steinfurt, J.; Dechering, D.G.; Meyer, C.; Veltmann, C.; et al. One-Year Course of Periprocedural Anticoagulation in Atrial Fibrillation Ablation: Results of a German Nationwide Survey. *Cardiology* **2020**, *145*, 676–681. [CrossRef]
21. Ottóffy, M.; Mátrai, P.; Farkas, N.; Hegyi, P.; Czopf, L.; Márta, K.; Garami, A.; Balaskó, M.; Pótóné-Oláh, E.; Mikó, A.; et al. Uninterrupted or Minimally Interrupted Direct Oral Anticoagulant Therapy is a Safe Alternative to Vitamin K Antagonists in Patients Undergoing Catheter Ablation for Atrial Fibrillation: An Updated Meta-Analysis. *J. Clin. Med.* **2020**, *9*, 3073. [CrossRef] [PubMed]
22. van Vugt, S.; Westra, S.W.; Volleberg, R.; Hannink, G.; Nakamura, R.; de Asmundis, C.; Chierchia, G.B.; Navarese, E.P.; Brouwer, M.A. Meta-analysis of controlled studies on minimally interrupted vs. continuous use of non-vitamin K antagonist oral anticoagulants in catheter ablation for atrial fibrillation. *Europace* **2021**, *23*, 1961–1969. [CrossRef] [PubMed]
23. Rouse, B.; Chaimani, A.; Li, T. Network meta-analysis: An introduction for clinicians. *Intern. Emerg. Med.* **2017**, *12*, 103–111. [CrossRef] [PubMed]
24. Hutton, B.; Salanti, G.; Caldwell, D.M.; Chaimani, A.; Schmid, C.H.; Cameron, C.; Ioannidis, J.P.; Straus, S.; Thorlund, K.; Jansen, J.P.; et al. The PRISMA extension statement for reporting of systematic reviews incorporating network meta-analyses of health care interventions: Checklist and explanations. *Ann. Intern. Med.* **2015**, *162*, 777–784. [CrossRef] [PubMed]
25. Mehran, R.; Rao, S.V.; Bhatt, D.L.; Gibson, C.M.; Caixeta, A.; Eikelboom, J.; Kaul, S.; Wiviott, S.D.; Menon, V.; Nikolsky, E.; et al. Standardized bleeding definitions for cardiovascular clinical trials: A consensus report from the Bleeding Academic Research Consortium. *Circulation* **2011**, *123*, 2736–2747. [CrossRef] [PubMed]
26. Schulman, S.; Kearon, C.; Subcommittee on Control of Anticoagulation of the Scientific and Standardization Committee of the International Society on Thrombosis and Haemostasis. Definition of major bleeding in clinical investigations of antihemostatic medicinal products in non-surgical patients. *J. Thromb. Haemost.* **2005**, *3*, 692–694. [CrossRef] [PubMed]

27. Sterne, J.; Savović, J.; Page, M.J.; Elbers, R.G.; Blencowe, N.S.; Boutron, I.; Cates, C.J.; Cheng, H.Y.; Corbett, M.S.; Eldridge, S.M.; et al. RoB 2: A revised tool for assessing risk of bias in randomised trials. *BMJ* **2019**, *366*, l4898. [CrossRef] [PubMed]
28. Rücker, G.; Schwarzer, G. Resolve conflicting rankings of outcomes in network meta-analysis: Partial ordering of treatments. *Res. Synth. Methods* **2017**, *8*, 526–536. [CrossRef]
29. Rücker, G.; Schwarzer, G. Ranking treatments in frequentist network meta-analysis works without resampling methods. *BMC Med. Res. Methodol.* **2015**, *15*, 58. [CrossRef]
30. Krahn, U.; Binder, H.; König, J. A graphical tool for locating inconsistency in network meta-analyses. *BMC Med. Res. Methodol.* **2013**, *13*, 35. [CrossRef]
31. Higgins, J.P.; Thompson, S.G.; Deeks, J.J.; Altman, D.G. Measuring inconsistency in meta-analyses. *BMJ* **2003**, *327*, 557–560. [CrossRef] [PubMed]
32. Veroniki, A.A.; Vasiliadis, H.S.; Higgins, J.P.; Salanti, G. Evaluation of inconsistency in networks of interventions. *Int. J. Epidemiol.* **2013**, *42*, 332–345. [CrossRef] [PubMed]
33. White, I.R.; Barrett, J.K.; Jackson, D.; Higgins, J.P. Consistency and inconsistency in network meta-analysis: Model estimation using multivariate meta-regression. *Res. Synth. Methods* **2012**, *3*, 111–125. [CrossRef] [PubMed]
34. Egger, M.; Davey Smith, G.; Schneider, M.; Minder, C. Bias in meta-analysis detected by a simple, graphical test. *BMJ* **1997**, *315*, 629–634. [CrossRef] [PubMed]
35. Begg, C.B.; Mazumdar, M. Operating characteristics of a rank correlation test for publication bias. *Biometrics* **1994**, *50*, 1088–1101. [CrossRef]
36. Di Biase, L.; Burkhardt, J.D.; Santangeli, P.; Mohanty, P.; Sanchez, J.E.; Horton, R.; Gallinghouse, G.J.; Themistoclakis, S.; Rossillo, A.; Lakkireddy, D.; et al. Periprocedural stroke and bleeding complications in patients undergoing catheter ablation of atrial fibrillation with different anticoagulation management: Results from the Role of Coumadin in Preventing Thromboembolism in Atrial Fibrillation (AF) Patients Undergoing Catheter Ablation (COMPARE) randomized trial. *Circulation* **2014**, *129*, 2638–2644. [CrossRef]
37. Nin, T.; Sairaku, A.; Yoshida, Y.; Kamiya, H.; Tatematsu, Y.; Nanasato, M.; Inden, Y.; Hirayama, H.; Murohara, T. A randomized controlled trial of dabigatran versus warfarin for periablation anticoagulation in patients undergoing ablation of atrial fibrillation. *Pacing Clin. Electrophysiol.* **2013**, *36*, 172–179. [CrossRef]
38. Nogami, A.; Harada, T.; Sekiguchi, Y.; Otani, R.; Yoshida, Y.; Yoshida, K.; Nakano, Y.; Nuruki, N.; Nakahara, S.; Goya, M.; et al. Safety and Efficacy of Minimally Interrupted Dabigatran vs Uninterrupted Warfarin Therapy in Adults Undergoing Atrial Fibrillation Catheter Ablation: A Randomized Clinical Trial. *JAMA Netw. Open* **2019**, *2*, e191994. [CrossRef]
39. Cappato, R.; Marchlinski, F.E.; Hohnloser, S.H.; Naccarelli, G.V.; Xiang, J.; Wilber, D.J.; Ma, C.S.; Hess, S.; Wells, D.S.; Juang, G.; et al. Uninterrupted rivaroxaban vs. uninterrupted vitamin K antagonists for catheter ablation in non-valvular atrial fibrillation. *Eur. Heart J.* **2015**, *36*, 1805–1811. [CrossRef]
40. Kuwahara, T.; Abe, M.; Yamaki, M.; Fujieda, H.; Abe, Y.; Hashimoto, K.; Ishiba, M.; Sakai, H.; Hishikari, K.; Takigawa, M.; et al. Apixaban versus Warfarin for the Prevention of Periprocedural Cerebral Thromboembolism in Atrial Fibrillation Ablation: Multicenter Prospective Randomized Study. *J. Cardiovasc. Electrophysiol.* **2016**, *27*, 549–554. [CrossRef]
41. Calkins, H.; Willems, S.; Gerstenfeld, E.P.; Verma, A.; Schilling, R.; Hohnloser, S.H.; Okumura, K.; Serota, H.; Nordaby, M.; Guiver, K.; et al. Uninterrupted Dabigatran versus Warfarin for Ablation in Atrial Fibrillation. *N. Engl. J. Med.* **2017**, *376*, 1627–1636. [CrossRef] [PubMed]
42. Kimura, T.; Kashimura, S.; Nishiyama, T.; Katsumata, Y.; Inagawa, K.; Ikegami, Y.; Nishiyama, N.; Fukumoto, K.; Tanimoto, Y.; Aizawa, Y.; et al. Asymptomatic Cerebral Infarction During Catheter Ablation for Atrial Fibrillation: Comparing Uninterrupted Rivaroxaban and Warfarin (ASCERTAIN). *JACC Clin. Electrophysiol.* **2018**, *4*, 1598–1609. [CrossRef]
43. Kirchhof, P.; Haeusler, K.G.; Blank, B.; De Bono, J.; Callans, D.; Elvan, A.; Fetsch, T.; Van Gelder, I.C.; Gentlesk, P.; Grimaldi, M.; et al. Apixaban in patients at risk of stroke undergoing atrial fibrillation ablation. *Eur. Heart J.* **2018**, *39*, 2942–2955. [CrossRef] [PubMed]
44. Hohnloser, S.H.; Camm, J.; Cappato, R.; Diener, H.C.; Heidbüchel, H.; Mont, L.; Morillo, C.A.; Abozguia, K.; Grimaldi, M.; Rauer, H.; et al. Uninterrupted edoxaban vs. vitamin K antagonists for ablation of atrial fibrillation: The ELIMINATE-AF trial. *Eur. Heart J.* **2019**, *40*, 3013–3021. [CrossRef]
45. Yoshimura, A.; Iriki, Y.; Ichiki, H.; Oketani, N.; Okui, H.; Maenosono, R.; Namino, F.; Miyata, M.; Ohishi, M. Evaluation of safety and efficacy of periprocedural use of rivaroxaban and apixaban in catheter ablation for atrial fibrillation. *J. Cardiol.* **2017**, *69*, 228–235. [CrossRef] [PubMed]
46. Reynolds, M.R.; Allison, J.S.; Natale, A.; Weisberg, I.L.; Ellenbogen, K.A.; Richards, M.; Hsieh, W.H.; Sutherland, J.; Cannon, C.P. A Prospective Randomized Trial of Apixaban Dosing During Atrial Fibrillation Ablation: The AEIOU Trial. *JACC Clin. Electrophysiol.* **2018**, *4*, 580–588. [CrossRef]
47. Yu, H.T.; Shim, J.; Park, J.; Kim, T.H.; Uhm, J.S.; Kim, J.Y.; Joung, B.; Lee, M.H.; Kim, Y.H.; Pak, H.N. When is it appropriate to stop non-vitamin K antagonist oral anticoagulants before catheter ablation of atrial fibrillation? A multicentre prospective randomized study. *Eur. Heart J.* **2019**, *40*, 1531–1537. [CrossRef]

48. Nakamura, K.; Naito, S.; Sasaki, T.; Take, Y.; Minami, K.; Kitagawa, Y.; Motoda, H.; Inoue, M.; Otsuka, Y.; Niijima, K.; et al. Uninterrupted vs. interrupted periprocedural direct oral anticoagulants for catheter ablation of atrial fibrillation: A prospective randomized single-centre study on post-ablation thrombo-embolic and haemorrhagic events. *Europace* **2019**, *21*, 259–267. [CrossRef] [PubMed]
49. Nagao, T.; Suzuki, H.; Matsunaga, S.; Nishikawa, Y.; Harada, K.; Mamiya, K.; Shinoda, N.; Harada, K.; Kato, M.; Marui, N.; et al. Impact of periprocedural anticoagulation therapy on the incidence of silent stroke after atrial fibrillation ablation in patients receiving direct oral anticoagulants: Uninterrupted vs. interrupted by one dose strategy. *Europace* **2019**, *21*, 590–597. [CrossRef] [PubMed]
50. Ando, M.; Inden, Y.; Yoshida, Y.; Sairaku, A.; Yanagisawa, S.; Suzuki, H.; Watanabe, R.; Takenaka, M.; Maeda, M.; Murohara, T. Differences in prothrombotic response between the uninterrupted and interrupted apixaban therapies in patients undergoing cryoballoon ablation for paroxysmal atrial fibrillation: A randomized controlled study. *Heart Vessels* **2019**, *34*, 1533–1541. [CrossRef] [PubMed]
51. Yamaji, H.; Murakami, T.; Hina, K.; Higashiya, S.; Kawamura, H.; Murakami, M.; Kamikawa, S.; Hirohata, S.; Kusachi, S. Activated clotting time on the day of atrial fibrillation ablation for minimally interrupted and uninterrupted direct oral anticoagulation therapy: Sequential changes, differences among direct oral anticoagulants, and ablation safety outcomes. *J. Cardiovasc. Electrophysiol.* **2019**, *30*, 2823–2833. [CrossRef] [PubMed]
52. Yoshimoto, I.; Iriki, Y.; Oketani, N.; Okui, H.; Ichiki, H.; Maenosono, R.; Namino, F.; Miyata, M.; Ohishi, M. A randomized comparison of two direct oral anticoagulants for patients undergoing cardiac ablation with a contemporary warfarin control arm. *J. Interv. Card. Electrophysiol.* **2021**, *60*, 375–385. [CrossRef] [PubMed]
53. Connolly, S.J.; Ezekowitz, M.D.; Yusuf, S.; Eikelboom, J.; Oldgren, J.; Parekh, A.; Pogue, J.; Reilly, P.A.; Themeles, E.; Varrone, J.; et al. Dabigatran versus warfarin in patients with atrial fibrillation. *N. Engl. J. Med.* **2009**, *361*, 1139–1151. [CrossRef] [PubMed]
54. Patel, M.R.; Mahaffey, K.W.; Garg, J.; Pan, G.; Singer, D.E.; Hacke, W.; Breithardt, G.; Halperin, J.L.; Hankey, G.J.; Piccini, J.P.; et al. Rivaroxaban versus warfarin in nonvalvular atrial fibrillation. *N. Engl. J. Med.* **2011**, *365*, 883–891. [CrossRef] [PubMed]
55. Granger, C.B.; Alexander, J.H.; McMurray, J.J.; Lopes, R.D.; Hylek, E.M.; Hanna, M.; Al-Khalidi, H.R.; Ansell, J.; Atar, D.; Avezum, A.; et al. Apixaban versus warfarin in patients with atrial fibrillation. *N. Engl. J. Med.* **2011**, *365*, 981–992. [CrossRef]
56. Giugliano, R.P.; Ruff, C.T.; Braunwald, E.; Murphy, S.A.; Wiviott, S.D.; Halperin, J.L.; Waldo, A.L.; Ezekowitz, M.D.; Weitz, J.I.; Špinar, J.; et al. Edoxaban versus warfarin in patients with atrial fibrillation. *N. Engl. J. Med.* **2013**, *369*, 2093–2104. [CrossRef]
57. Müller, P.; Halbfass, P.; Szöllösi, A.; Dietrich, J.W.; Fochler, F.; Nentwich, K.; Roos, M.; Krug, J.; Schmitt, R.; Mügge, A.; et al. Impact of periprocedural anticoagulation strategy on the incidence of new-onset silent cerebral events after radiofrequency catheter ablation of atrial fibrillation. *J. Interv. Card. Electrophysiol.* **2016**, *46*, 203–211. [CrossRef]
58. Di Biase, L.; Lakkireddy, D.; Trivedi, C.; Deneke, T.; Martinek, M.; Mohanty, S.; Mohanty, P.; Prakash, S.; Bai, R.; Reddy, M.; et al. Feasibility and safety of uninterrupted periprocedural apixaban administration in patients undergoing radiofrequency catheter ablation for atrial fibrillation: Results from a multicenter study. *Heart Rhythm* **2015**, *12*, 1162–1168. [CrossRef]
59. Nakamura, K.; Naito, S.; Sasaki, T.; Minami, K.; Take, Y.; Goto, E.; Shimizu, S.; Yamaguchi, Y.; Suzuki, N.; Yano, T.; et al. Silent Cerebral Ischemic Lesions After Catheter Ablation of Atrial Fibrillation in Patients on 5 Types of Periprocedural Oral Anticoagulation—Predictors of Diffusion-Weighted Imaging-Positive Lesions and Follow-up Magnetic Resonance Imaging. *Circ. J.* **2016**, *80*, 870–877. [CrossRef]
60. Mao, Y.J.; Wang, H.; Huang, P.F. Peri-procedural novel oral anticoagulants dosing strategy during atrial fibrillation ablation: A meta-analysis. *Pacing Clin. Electrophysiol.* **2020**, *43*, 1104–1114. [CrossRef]
61. Vermeer, S.E.; Prins, N.D.; den Heijer, T.; Hofman, A.; Koudstaal, P.J.; Breteler, M.M. Silent brain infarcts and the risk of dementia and cognitive decline. *N. Engl. J. Med.* **2003**, *348*, 1215–1222. [CrossRef] [PubMed]
62. Gupta, A.; Giambrone, A.E.; Gialdini, G.; Finn, C.; Delgado, D.; Gutierrez, J.; Wright, C.; Beiser, A.S.; Seshadri, S.; Pandya, A.; et al. Silent Brain Infarction and Risk of Future Stroke: A Systematic Review and Meta-Analysis. *Stroke* **2016**, *47*, 719–725. [CrossRef]
63. Haines, D.E.; Stewart, M.T.; Barka, N.D.; Kirchhof, N.; Lentz, L.R.; Reinking, N.M.; Urban, J.F.; Halimi, F.; Deneke, T.; Kanal, E. Microembolism and catheter ablation II: Effects of cerebral microemboli injection in a canine model. *Circ. Arrhythmia Electrophysiol.* **2013**, *6*, 23–30. [CrossRef] [PubMed]
64. Takami, M.; Lehmann, H.I.; Parker, K.D.; Welker, K.M.; Johnson, S.B.; Packer, D.L. Effect of Left Atrial Ablation Process and Strategy on Microemboli Formation During Irrigated Radiofrequency Catheter Ablation in an In Vivo Model. *Circ. Arrhythmia Electrophysiol.* **2016**, *9*, e003226. [CrossRef] [PubMed]
65. Maury, P.; Belaid, S.; Ribes, A.; Voglimacci-Stephanopoli, Q.; Mondoly, P.; Blaye, M.; Mandel, F.; Monteil, B.; Carrié, D.; Galinier, M.; et al. Coagulation and heparin requirements during ablation in patients under oral anticoagulant drugs. *J. Arrhythmia* **2020**, *36*, 644–651. [CrossRef]
66. Martin, A.C.; Kyheng, M.; Foissaud, V.; Duhamel, A.; Marijon, E.; Susen, S.; Godier, A. Activated Clotting Time Monitoring during Atrial Fibrillation Catheter Ablation: Does the Anticoagulant Matter? *J. Clin. Med.* **2020**, *9*, 350. [CrossRef] [PubMed]

67. Martin, A.C.; Godier, A.; Narayanan, K.; Smadja, D.M.; Marijon, E. Management of Intraprocedural Anticoagulation in Patients on Non-Vitamin K Antagonist Oral Anticoagulants Undergoing Catheter Ablation for Atrial Fibrillation: Understanding the Gaps in Evidence. *Circulation* **2018**, *138*, 627–633. [CrossRef]
68. Pollack, C.V.; Reilly, P.A., Jr.; Eikelboom, J.; Glund, S.; Verhamme, P.; Bernstein, R.A.; Dubiel, R.; Huisman, M.V.; Hylek, E.M.; Kamphuisen, P.W.; et al. Idarucizumab for Dabigatran Reversal. *N. Engl. J. Med.* **2015**, *373*, 511–520. [CrossRef] [PubMed]
69. Connolly, S.J.; Milling, T.J., Jr.; Eikelboom, J.W.; Gibson, C.M.; Curnutte, J.T.; Gold, A.; Bronson, M.D.; Lu, G.; Conley, P.B.; Verhamme, P.; et al. Andexanet Alfa for Acute Major Bleeding Associated with Factor Xa Inhibitors. *N. Engl. J. Med.* **2016**, *375*, 1131–1141. [CrossRef]

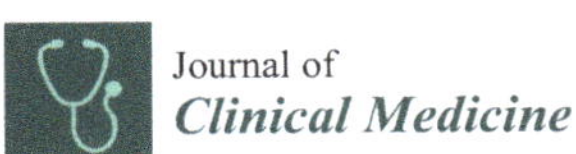
Journal of
Clinical Medicine

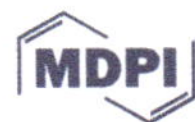

Article

Vascular Alterations Preceding Arterial Wall Thickening in Overweight and Obese Children

Sung-Ai Kim [1,*,†], Kyung Hee Park [2,†], Sarah Woo [3], Yoon Myung Kim [4], Hyun Jung Lim [5] and Woo-Jung Park [1]

1 Division of Cardiology, Department of Internal Medicine, Hallym Sacred Heart Hospital, Hallym University College of Medicine, Anyang 14068, Korea; cathpark@hallym.or.kr
2 Department of Family Medicine, Hallym Sacred Heart Hospital, Hallym University College of Medicine, Anyang 14068, Korea; beloved@hallym.or.kr
3 Department of Medical Science, Hallym University College of Medicine, Anyang 14068, Korea; hjejcross@naver.com
4 Department of Sports Industry Studies, Yonsei University International Campus, Incheon 21983, Korea; yoonkim@yonsei.ac.kr
5 Department of Medical Nutrition, Kyung Hee University, Yongin 17104, Korea; hjlim@khu.ac.kr
* Correspondence: 237419@hallym.or.kr; Tel.: +82-31-380-3977
† These authors contributed equally to this work as co-first author.

Abstract: Background: Childhood obesity is linked to adverse cardiovascular outcomes in adulthood. This study aimed to assess the impact of childhood obesity on the vasculature and to investigate whether vascular alteration precedes arterial wall thickening in childhood. Methods: A total of 295 overweight (body mass index [BMI] 85th to 95th percentile, $n = 30$) and obese (BMI $\geq$ 95th percentile, $n = 234$) children aged 7–17 years and 31 normal-weight controls with similar age and gender were prospectively recruited. We assessed anthropometric data and laboratory findings, and measured the carotid intima–media thickness (IMT), carotid artery (CA) diameter, M-mode-derived arterial stiffness indices, and velocity vector imaging parameters, including the CA area, fractional area change, circumferential strain, and circumferential strain rate (SR). Results: The mean $\pm$ standard deviation age of the participants was 10.8 $\pm$ 2.1 years; 172 (58%) children were male. Regarding structural properties, there was no difference in the IMT between the three groups. The CA diameter was significantly increased in obese children, whereas the CA area showed a significant increase beginning in the overweight stage. Regarding functional properties, contrary to β stiffness and Young's elastic modulus, which were not different between the three groups, the circumferential SR showed a significant decrease beginning in the overweight stage and was independently associated with BMI z-scores after adjusting for covariates. Conclusion: We have demonstrated that arterial stiffening and arterial enlargement precede arterial wall thickening, and that these vascular alterations begin at the overweight stage in middle childhood or early adolescence.

Keywords: obesity; childhood; vascular; stiffness

Citation: Kim, S.-A.; Park, K.H.; Woo, S.; Kim, Y.M.; Lim, H.J.; Park, W.-J. Vascular Alterations Preceding Arterial Wall Thickening in Overweight and Obese Children. *J. Clin. Med.* **2022**, *11*, 3520. https://doi.org/10.3390/jcm11123520

Academic Editor: Tomoaki Ishigami

Received: 24 May 2022
Accepted: 17 June 2022
Published: 19 June 2022

1. Introduction

Obesity leads to increased arterial stiffening and increased intima–media thickness (IMT), both of which have been linked to a pathological cascade of cardiovascular (CV) diseases [1]. Recently, childhood obesity has become a public health problem worldwide; its prevalence among children has been increasing due to a sedentary lifestyle and fast-food consumption [2]. As obese children are not only more likely to become obese adults but also have an increased risk of developing hypertension, dyslipidemia, type 2 diabetes mellitus, and future CV disease, childhood obesity will eventually be one of the most serious global health issues [3,4]. Large epidemiological studies have reported that childhood obesity is linked to adverse vascular alterations in adulthood [5–7]. Although the association between obesity and vascular alteration has been extensively investigated in adulthood, limited data exist on its impact on the vasculature in childhood. As surrogate markers of vascular alteration, both the IMT and arterial stiffness are known as independent predictors of future CV morbidity and mortality in adults, respectively [8]. However, in childhood, previous studies regarding the impact of obesity on IMT and arterial stiffness have yielded conflicting results, and not all studies have shown higher IMT and arterial stiffness in obese children [9–15]. Using the velocity vector imaging (VVI) technique to assess instantaneous vascular deformation, we previously quantified vascular alterations with aging [16] and demonstrated that the carotid artery (CA) could undergo functional alteration before the IMT increases in patients with hypertension [17]. In this study, we assessed vascular alterations using VVI in overweight and obese children and compared them to normal-weight children and sought to determine whether vascular alterations could be observed before arterial wall thickening in overweight and obese children.

2. Materials and Methods

2.1. Study Subjects

A total of 295 overweight (n = 30) and obese (n = 234) children aged 7–17 years (154 boys and 110 girls) and 31 sex- and age-matched normal-weight controls were prospectively recruited for the Intervention for Childhood and Adolescents Obesity via Activity and Nutrition (ICAAN) study through newspapers, broadcasts, posters, websites, and other social networking services. Overweight was defined as a BMI $\geq$ 85th percentile and <95th percentile for age- and sex-specific BMI according to the 2007 Korean National Growth Charts, while obesity was defined as a BMI $\geq$ 95th percentile for age and sex or a BMI $\geq$ 25 kg/m^2 [18,19]. This study was conducted according to the guidelines of the Declaration of Helsinki, and the study protocol was approved by the local ethics committee. Written informed consent was obtained from all participants and their parents or caregivers.

2.2. Anthropometric Data

Body weight was measured after a 10 h fast and voiding, with the participants barefoot and wearing indoor and lightweight clothing. Height was measured by a stadiometer (DS-103, DongSahn Jenix, Seoul, Korea) while the participants were barefoot. BMI was calculated (weight [kg]/height [m]^2) and converted into percentiles and z-scores based on the age- and sex-specific BMI of the 2007 Korean National Growth Charts [18].

2.3. Laboratory Test

Venous blood samples were obtained after 12 hours of fasting to determine the fasting plasma glucose (FPG), fasting plasma insulin, high-density lipoprotein cholesterol (HDL-C), low-density lipoprotein cholesterol (LDL-C), triglyceride (TG), aspartate aminotransferase (AST), alanine aminotransferase (ALT), and high-sensitivity C-reactive protein (hsCRP). FPG was measured using ultraviolet assay with hexokinase (Cobas 8000 C702, Roche, Mannheim, Germany). Insulin was measured using electrochemiluminescence immunoassay (Cobas 8000 e802, Roche, Mannheim, Germany). HDL-C and LDL-C were measured using a homogeneous enzymatic colorimetric test (Cobas 8000 C702, Roche, Mannheim, Germany). TG, AST, and ALT were measured using enzymatic assay (Cobas 8000 C702, Roche, Mannheim, Germany). hsCRP was measured using turbidimetric immunoassay (Cobas 8000 C702, Roche, Mannheim, Germany). The homeostasis model assessment for insulin resistance (HOMA-IR) was used to determine insulin sensitivity, and was calculated using the following formula: (FPG Level (mg/dL) $\times$ Fasting Plasma Insulin Level (uU/mL))/405. Adiponectin was measured using enzyme-linked immunosorbent assay (VersaMax ELISA Microplate Reader, Molecular Devices, San Jose, CA, USA).

2.4. Carotid Ultrasound and Vascular Parameters

Carotid ultrasound studies were performed by a single registered vascular technologist (S.H.P) who was blinded to the subject group assignment using a high-resolution B-mode ultrasound (Acuson Sequoia 512, Siemens Acuson, Mountain View, CA, USA) equipped with an 8 MHz linear-array transducer. Data were stored as digital cineloops for subsequent offline analysis, and a single experienced reader (S.A.K.) who was blinded to the subject's clinical status performed all measurements. The mean IMT was calculated as the average of three consecutive manual measurements at the far wall of the CA 1 cm proximal to the carotid bulb of both common carotid arteries (CCA) from leading edge (lumen–intima) to leading edge (media-adventitia) during end diastole. The average end-diastolic diameter (Dd, CA diameter) and peak systolic internal diameters (Ds) were assessed in three cycles as the distance between the intima–lumen interface at the near wall and the lumen–intima interface at the far wall of both CCAs (1 cm proximal to the beginning of the carotid bulb). The M-mode-derived CA stiffness indices were derived according to the following formula: β stiffness was determined as ln (Ps/Pd)/((Ds − Dd)/Dd) [20], where Ps and Pd are systolic and diastolic blood pressures. Young's elastic modulus (YEM) in $10^2 \times$ kPa/mm was calculated as [[Ps − Pd]/(Ds − Dd)] × (Dd/cIMT) [21]. Transverse images of both CCAs (1 cm proximal to the carotid bulb) were stored using acoustic capture for offline analysis with the VVI workstation (Syngo®, US Workplace, Siemens, Mountain View, CA, USA). VVI fundamentally uses a two-dimensional speckle-tracking method from which the blood–tissue border was traced manually over one frame of a cineloop and wherein the ultrasonic speckles automatically tracked vessel wall motion by dividing it into six segments.

VVI provides instantaneous quantitative measurements of vessel deformation throughout the cardiac cycle, including circumferential vessel area, fractional area change (FAC), circumferential strain and strain rate (SR). CA area was defined as minimal vessel area during the cardiac cycle and FAC was calculated by measuring the percent changes of the CA area [(maximal area) − (minimal area)/(minimal area)] × 100 (%). Circumferential strain (ε) represents the percent change (%) in length along the circumferential axis of CA and circumferential SR represents the temporal derivative of strain and describes the temporal change in strain (dε/dt, 1/s), producing a positive value in systole and a negative value in diastole. All CA measurements on both sides were averaged to obtain the mean values.

2.5. Statistical Analysis

Data are expressed as the mean ± standard deviation (SD) or as percentages. We compared the means of each continuous variable in the subject groups by one-way factorial analysis of variance with the post hoc test (Tukey). Analysis of covariance using the Bonferroni post hoc test was used to test the differences in the vascular parameters between the three groups while adjusting for covariates, such as age, sex, height, mean blood pressure, low-density lipoprotein (LDL)-cholesterol level, and homeostasis model assessment for insulin resistance (HOMA-IR). Multiple linear regression fit of the circumferential SR on the BMI z-score was generated by considering the effects of other covariates. All statistical analyses were performed using SPSS 24.0 (IBM Corp., Chicago, IL, USA) an open-source statistical package R version 3.6.3 (R Project for Statistical Computing, Vienna, Austria). Statistical significance was defined as $p < 0.05$.

3. Results

Overall, the mean ± SD age of all participants was 10.8 ± 2.1 years; 172 (58%) children were male. Table 1 presents the baseline characteristics of the study population and statistical differences between the groups.

Obese children had higher blood pressures, HOMA-IR, hsCRP, and LDL cholesterol levels and lower serum adiponectin levels than overweight and normal-weight children. Meanwhile, overweight children had higher levels of HOMA-IR compared to normal-weight children, although there were no differences in other variables between the groups.

In the structural evaluation of the CA (Table 2), there was no difference in IMT among the three groups ($p > 0.05$).

Table 1. Baseline characteristics.

	Normal Weight	Over Weight	Obese	p Value
Age, year	10.5 ± 2.4	10.5 ± 2.0	10.8 ± 2.1	0.685
Male, %	58	53	59	0.840
Height, cm	143 ± 13	145 ± 10	152 ± 12 **,‡	<0.001
Weight, kg	38.2 ± 11.8	49.9 ± 10.2 **	68.7 ± 18.1 **,‡	<0.001
BMI, kg/m^2	18.0 ± 2.4	23.3 ± 1.8 **	28.9 ± 4.1 **,‡	<0.001
BMI z-score	−0.13 ± 0.76	1.45 ± 0.17 **	2.38 ± 0.44 **,‡	<0.001
WC, cm	60.0 ± 7.3	74.7 ± 7.2 **	89.3 ± 10.6 **,‡	<0.001
HC, cm	78.3 ± 7.9	87.0 ± 6.7 **	98.3 ± 10.4 **,‡	<0.001
Systolic BP, mmHg	104 ± 11	107 ± 8.7	114 ± 9.6 **,‡	<0.001
Diastolic BP, mmHg	60 ± 6.0	63 ± 6.0	65 ± 8.0 **	0.003
Mean BP, mmHg	75 ± 6.8	78 ± 5.8	82 ± 7.5 **,†	<0.001
Heart rate, bpm	80 ± 11	79 ± 10	80 ± 12	0.909
Hemoglobin, mg/dL	13.9 ± 0.9	13.9 ± 0.8	13.7 ± 0.8	0.477
Creatinine, mg/dL	0.55 ± 0.13	0.53 ± 0.06	0.54 ± 0.10	0.729
Glucose, mg/dL	82 ± 10	86 ± 9.9	88 ± 7.6 **	0.001
AST, IU/L	27 ± 23	23 ± 8.5	27 ± 18	0.446
ALT, IU/L	16 ± 18	21 ± 21	37 ± 40 *	0.003
HOMA-IR	1.35 ± 0.75	2.89 ± 1.80 **	4.80 ± 2.79 **,‡	<0.001
hsCRP, mg/dL	0.47 ± 0.31	0.94 ± 0.83	2.17 ± 2.11 **,‡	<0.001
TG, mg/dL	78 ± 38	104 ± 51	114 ± 56 **	0.002
HDL-C, mg/dL	60 ± 13	56 ± 14	49 ± 11 **,‡	<0001
LDL-C, mg/dL	94 ± 20	105 ± 23	110 ± 25 **	0.003
Adiponectin, ug/mL	10.2 ± 4.0	9.4 ± 4.1	8.4 ± 3.2 **	0.012

* vs. normal < 0.05; ** vs. normal, <0.01; † vs. overweight < 0.05; ‡ vs. overweight < 0.01. BMI, body mass index; WC, waist circumference; HC, hip circumference; BP, blood pressure; AST, aspartate aminotransferase; ALT, alanine aminotransferase; HOMA-IR, homeostasis model assessment for insulin resistance; hsCRP, high-sensitivity C-reactive protein; TG, triglyceride; HDL-C, high-density lipoprotein cholesterol; LDL-C, low-density lipoprotein cholesterol.

Table 2. Structural and functional characteristics of the carotid artery.

	Normal Weight	Over Weight	Obese	p Value
M-mode-derived parameters				
Mean IMT, mm	0.44 ± 0.04	0.45 ± 0.05	0.45 ± 0.06	0.277
CA diameter, mm	5.05 ± 0.49	5.16 ± 0.51	5.58 ± 0.53 **,‡	<0.001
ß stiffness	4.15 ± 1.30	4.13 ± 1.77	4.53 ± 3.77	0.735
YEM, $10^2 \times$ kPa/mm	5.45 ± 1.65	5.51 ± 2.44	6.34 ± 5.05 ‡	0.443
VVI parameters				
CA area, mm^2	30.3 ± 5.0	34.0 ± 5.1 *	35.0 ± 5.6 **	<0.001
FAC, %	19.1 ± 4.2	17.9 ± 3.3	17.0 ± 3.6 **	0.007
Circumferential strain, %	6.50 ± 2.45	5.74 ± 1.64	5.67 ± 1.94	0.090
Circumferential SR, 1/s	0.68 ± 0.24	0.51 ± 0.21 **	0.44 ± 0.18 **	<0.001

* vs. normal < 0.05; ** vs. normal, <0.01; ‡ vs. overweight < 0.01. IMT, intima–media thickness; CA, carotid artery; YEM, Young's elastic modulus; VVI, velocity vector imaging; FAC, fractional area change; SR, strain rate.

The CA diameter in obese children was distinctly larger than that in normal-weight and overweight children, and there was no difference in the CA diameter between normal-weight and overweight children. Meanwhile, the CA area began to increase from the overweight stage. The CA of overweight children was significantly larger than that of normal-weight children but did not differ from obese children. Regarding the functional parameters of vascular elastic properties, M-mode-derived stiffness indices, such as β stiffness and YEM, were not significantly different among the three groups ($p > 0.05$). Meanwhile, the circumferential SR showed a significant decrease from the overweight stage (0.68 ± 0.24 1/s in normal-weight vs. 0.51 ± 0.21 1/s in overweight children, $p = 0.002$).

Figure 1 shows an example of VVI analysis in normal-weight (A), overweight (B) and obese children (C), respectively. As the BMI level increases, CA area gradually increases and both FAC and circumferential SR decrease in comparison with those of normal-weight children.

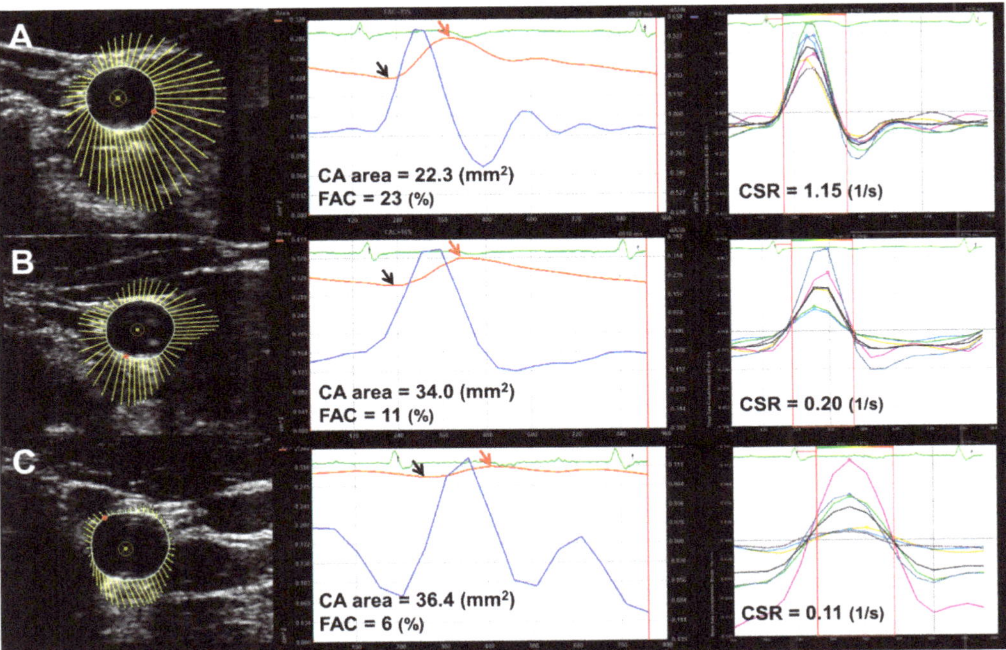

Figure 1. Velocity vector imaging analysis in normal-weight (**A**), overweight (**B**) and obese children (**C**). The red arrow points to maximal CA area and the black arrow points to minimal CA area during the cardiac cycle. CA area refers to minimal CA area (black arrow) and FAC was calculated by measuring the percent changes of the CA area [(maximal area) − (minimal area)/(minimal area)] × 100 (%). CSR refers to average value of peak CSRs of six segments during the systole. Compared to normal-weight children (**A**), overweight (**B**) and obese (**C**) children show an increase in CA area and a decrease in FAC and CSR. CA, carotid artery; FAC, fractional area change; CSR, circumferential strain rate.

In addition, when we compared the M-mode-derived parameters and VVI parameters between the groups after adjusting for age, sex, height, mean blood pressure, LDL cholesterol level, and HOMA-IR, respectively (Figure 2), the CA area and circumferential SR still showed significant changes beginning in the overweight stage in middle childhood or early adolescence.

Additionally, the circumferential SR showed a negative association with the BMI z-score, a linear estimate of obesity; this association remained significant after adjustment of covariates in the multiple linear regression analysis (adjusted $R^2 = 0.256$, $p < 0.001$, Figure 3).

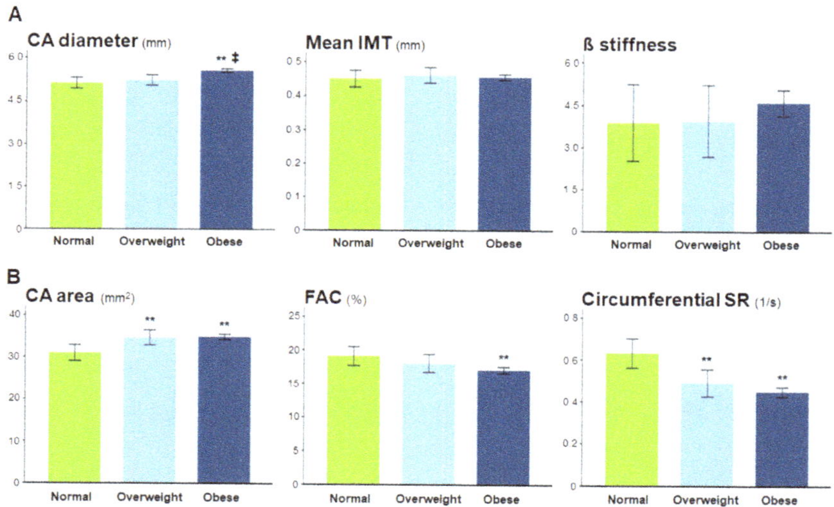

Figure 2. Comparison of M-mode-derived parameters and VVI parameters between the groups after adjusting for covariates including age, sex, height, mean blood pressure, LDL cholesterol and HOMA-IR. (**A**) M-mode-derived parameters; (**B**) VVI parameters. ** vs. normal, <0.01; ‡ vs. overweight < 0.01. CA, carotid artery; IMT, intima–media thickness; FAC, fractional area change; SR, strain rate; VVI, velocity vector imaging.

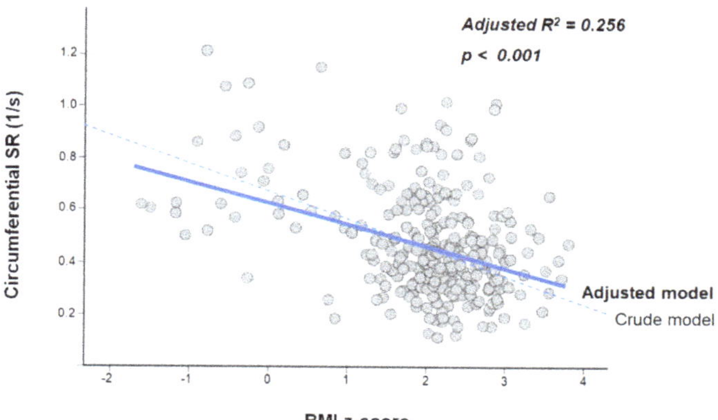

Figure 3. Multiple linear regression fit of the circumferential SR on the BMI z-score. SR, strain rate; BMI, body mass index.

4. Discussion

In this study, we demonstrated that even in childhood, arterial stiffening and enlargement, which occur in the overweight stage, precede arterial wall thickening. The circumferential SR, as a sensitive marker of arterial stiffness, significantly decreased in the early stages of obesity and showed a negative linear association with BMI z-score even after adjusting for covariates. Our results emphasize that interventions against childhood obesity should be initiated early to prevent the induction and irreversible progression of obesity-induced vascular complications.

The IMT is an established structural marker of subclinical arteriosclerosis [9,22]. Many studies in adults have demonstrated that obesity is independently associated with an increase in IMT [23–25]. Moreover, large longitudinal cohort studies have shown that childhood adiposity correlates with an increase in IMT later in adulthood [26,27]. However, some studies have reported the lack of association between BMI and IMT in childhood [9,11,28–33]. In middle childhood (mean age, 10 years; <12 years), BMI is not associated with IMT in obese and normal-weight children [11,28–30], whereas in adolescents (mean age, >12 years), BMI is positively associated with IMT [31–33]. This suggests that arterial wall damage begins later in childhood or in adolescence. Our results are also in line with those of previous reports of children aged 8–12 years that did not show a difference in the IMT between obese and normal-weight subjects [11,28–30]. Moreover, this study including overweight children, who were greater in number than obese children, showed that the IMTs in overweight and obese children were not different to those of normal-weight children, which suggests that the thickening of the arterial wall is limited by time in childhood obesity. In contrast, several studies with similar degree of obesity, age, and gender to this population have reported an increase in IMT in obese children compared with lean children [9,12,34]. These conflicting reports could be due to the differences in exposure duration to obesity, sample size, and racial and/or ethnic characteristics between studies [35,36]. Another possible explanation is that BMI or adiposity itself has no direct association with IMT, and that its effects are instead manifested through CV risk factors, such as age, hypertension, type 2 diabetes mellitus, and other metabolic complications [36,37]. It is also fundamentally linked to exposure duration to obesity.

In this study, we verified that arterial stiffening precedes wall thickening, and that arterial damage begins at the overweight stage in middle childhood or early adolescence. Although longitudinal processes linking obesity to vascular alteration are not fully understood, it is known that long-term exposure to hemodynamic stimuli and metabolic disturbance caused by obesity augments the arterial impedance and afterload of the heart, which eventually leads to an increase in CV morbidity and mortality [38]. In this study, overweight children showed higher insulin resistance than normal-weight children despite the comparable blood pressures and laboratory findings. Although the role of this metabolic disturbance in the process of arteriosclerosis remains unclear, abnormal glucose metabolism is associated with the accumulation of advanced end-glycation products that lead to arterial stiffening [39]. To assess arterial stiffness, we measured the instantaneous vessel deformational parameters (FAC, circumferential strain, and circumferential SR) using VVI as well as conventional M-mode-derived elastic moduli as β stiffness and YEM.

Although the M-mode-derived stiffness indices did not show any difference among the three groups, and the FAC and circumferential strain of overweight children were not significantly different from those of normal-weight children, only circumferential SR has proven its ability to independently confirm early vascular damage that began at the overweight stage and it showed a negative linear association with BMI z-score even after adjusting for covariates. M-mode derived stiffness indices as β-stiffness and YEM are calculated from CA diameter and blood pressures measured at peripheral artery. When interpreting the results, we should consider the facts that pulse pressure amplification may differ with obesity [40] and there is a time difference between the measurements of blood pressures and arterial diameter in pressure-related variables. These limitations may have affected the findings in this study.

Considering that the circumferential SR is the time rate of instantaneous circumferential deformation, it would have been a suitable indicator to reflect subtle vascular changes in these relatively healthy children, although the exact mechanisms cannot be clarified. Additionally, our results revealed the limitations of the M-mode-derived stiffness indices and the superiority of a two-dimensional approach by speckle tracking that enables instantaneous vessel wall motion in the entire circumference of vessel wall.

As a marker of structural change, we demonstrated that vessel area increases as obesity progresses, which is consistent with existing pediatric studies that reported that arterial diameters increase with obesity [41,42]. An increase in arterial diameter might be attributed to the fatiguing effects of tensile stress, which lead to fracture of load-bearing elastin fibers [43,44]. In this study, the CA area, measured by a two-dimensional approach, showed a significant increase from the overweight stage. These results reveal that arterial enlargement and stiffening occur before IMT progression and begin in the overweight stage in childhood. Considering the four large longitudinal cohort studies wherein people who were overweight or obese as children but were non-obese as adults had similar CV outcomes to those of people who were never obese [7], it is plausible that these vascular alterations in childhood are reversible and preventable through early intervention against obesity.

Our investigation has several limitations, including its cross-sectional observational study design, which does not allow causal or temporal inferences. A narrow age range in this population may limit generalizability to later adolescence, wherein the influence of pubertal development, with changes in body shape and adiposity, cannot be overlooked. It is unclear how much the duration of exposure to obesity might affect the degree of structural and functional vascular alterations in this population.

5. Conclusions

In conclusion, we demonstrated that vascular alterations such as arterial enlargement and arterial stiffening, represented by low circumferential SR, can occur before IMT progression even in the overweight stage in middle childhood or early adolescence. These results emphasize the importance of maintaining a normal body weight in childhood and the necessity of early intervention against childhood obesity to minimize the development of CV disease in adulthood.

Author Contributions: Conceptualization, S.-A.K.; data curation, S.-A.K., S.W. and K.H.P.; formal analysis, S.-A.K.; funding acquisition, K.H.P.; investigation, S.-A.K., Y.M.K., H.J.L. and K.H.P.; methodology, S.-A.K.; supervision, K.H.P. and W.-J.P.; validation, S.-A.K. and K.H.P. On behalf of the ICAAN study investigators: writing—original draft preparation, S.-A.K.; writing—review and editing, S.-A.K. and K.H.P. All authors have read and agreed to the published version of the manuscript.

Funding: This research was funded by the Korea Centers for Disease Control and Prevention, grant number 2016-ER6405.

Institutional Review Board Statement: The ICAAN study was conducted according to the guidelines of the Declaration of Helsinki and approved by the Hallym University Sacred Heart Hospital's Institutional Review Board (approval number: 2016-I135).

Informed Consent Statement: Informed consent was obtained from all subjects involved in the ICAAN study.

Data Availability Statement: The data presented in this study are available on request from the corresponding authors. The data are not publicly available due to privacy concerns.

Conflicts of Interest: The authors declare no conflict of interest.

References

1. Kass, D.A. Ventricular arterial stiffening: Integrating the pathophysiology. *Hypertension* **2005**, *46*, 185–193. [CrossRef] [PubMed]
2. Salas, X.R.; Buoncristiano, M.; Williams, J.; Kebbe, M.; Spinelli, A.; Nardone, P.; Rito, A.; Duleva, V.; Milanović, S.M.; Kunesova, M.; et al. Parental Perceptions of Children's Weight Status in 22 Countries: The WHO European Childhood Obesity Surveillance Initiative: COSI 2015/2017. *Obes Facts* **2021**, *14*, 658–674. [CrossRef] [PubMed]
3. Franks, P.W.; Hanson, R.L.; Knowler, W.C.; Sievers, M.L.; Bennett, P.H.; Looker, H.C. Childhood obesity, other cardiovascu-lar risk factors, and premature death. *N. Engl. J. Med.* **2010**, *362*, 485–493. [CrossRef] [PubMed]
4. Twig, G.; Yaniv, G.; Levine, H.; Leiba, A.; Goldberger, N.; Derazne, E.; Shor, D.B.-A.; Tzur, D.; Afek, A.; Shamiss, A.; et al. Body-Mass Index in 2.3 Million Adolescents and Cardiovascular Death in Adulthood. *N. Engl. J. Med.* **2016**, *374*, 2430–2440. [CrossRef] [PubMed]
5. Freedman, D.S.; Dietz, W.H.; Tang, R.; Mensah, G.; Bond, M.G.; Urbina, E.M.; Srinivasan, S.; Berenson, G.S. The relation of obesity throughout life to carotid intima-media thickness in adulthood: The Bogalusa Heart Study. *Int. J. Obes.* **2003**, *28*, 159–166. [CrossRef] [PubMed]
6. Koskinen, J.; Kähönen, M.; Viikari, J.S.; Taittonen, L.; Laitinen, T.; Rönnemaa, T.; Lehtimäki, T.; Hutri-Kähönen, N.; Pie-tikäinen, M.; Jokinen, E.; et al. Conventional cardiovascular risk factors and metabolic syndrome in predicting carotid intima media thickness progression in young adults: The Cardiovascular Risk in Young Finns Study. *Circulation* **2009**, *120*, 229–236. [CrossRef] [PubMed]

7. Juonala, M.; Magnussen, C.G.; Berenson, G.S.; Venn, A.; Burns, T.L.; Sabin, M.A.; Srinivasan, S.R.; Daniels, S.R.; Davis, P.H.; Chen, W.; et al. Childhood adiposity, adult adiposity, and cardiovascular risk factors. *N. Engl. J. Med.* **2011**, *365*, 1876–1885. [CrossRef]
8. Lorenz, M.W.; Markus, H.S.; Bots, M.L.; Rosvall, M.; Sitzer, M. Prediction of clinical cardiovascular events with carotid inti-ma-media thickness: A systematic review and meta-analysis. *Circulation* **2007**, *115*, 459–467. [CrossRef] [PubMed]
9. Iannuzzi, A.; Licenziati, M.R.; Acampora, C.; Salvatore, V.; Auriemma, L.; Romano, M.L.; Panico, S.; Rubba, P.; Trevisan, M. Increased Carotid Intima-Media Thickness and Stiffness in Obese Children. *Diabetes Care* **2004**, *27*, 2506–2508. [CrossRef] [PubMed]
10. Lamotte, C.; Iliescu, C.; Libersa, C.; Gottrand, F. Increased intima-media thickness of the carotid artery in childhood: A systematic review of observational studies. *Eur. J. Pediatr.* **2011**, *170*, 719–729. [CrossRef] [PubMed]
11. Tounian, P.; Aggoun, Y.; Dubern, B.; Varille, V.; Guy-Grand, B.; Sidi, D.; Girardet, J.-P.; Bonnet, D. Presence of increased stiffness of the common carotid artery and endothelial dysfunction in severely obese children: A prospective study. *Lancet* **2001**, *358*, 1400–1404. [CrossRef]
12. Yilmazer, M.M.; Tavli, V.; Carti, U.; Mese, T.; Guven, B.; Aydın, B.; Devrim, I.; Tavli, T.; Tavlı, T.; Aydin, B. Cardiovascular risk factors and noninvasive assessment of arterial structure and function in obese Turkish children. *Eur. J. Pediatr.* **2010**, *169*, 1241–1248. [CrossRef]
13. Whincup, P.H.; Gilg, J.A.; Donald, A.E.; Katterhorn, M.; Oliver, C.; Cook, D.G.; Deanfield, J.E. Arterial distensibility in adolescents: The influence of adiposity, the metabolic syndrome, and classic risk factors. *Circulation* **2005**, *112*, 1789–1797. [CrossRef]
14. Dangardt, F.; Osika, W.; Volkmann, R.; Gan, L.M.; Friberg, P. Obese children show increased intimal wall thickness and de creased pulse wave velocity. *Clin. Physiol. Funct. Imaging* **2008**, *28*, 287–293. [CrossRef]
15. Niboshi, A.; Hamaoka, K.; Sakata, K.; Inoue, F. Characteristics of brachial–ankle pulse wave velocity in Japanese children. *Eur. J. Pediatr.* **2006**, *165*, 625–629. [CrossRef]
16. Kim, S.-A.; Lee, K.H.; Won, H.-Y.; Park, S.; Chung, J.H.; Jang, Y.; Ha, J.-W. Quantitative Assessment of Aortic Elasticity With Aging Using Velocity-Vector Imaging and Its Histologic Correlation. *Arter. Thromb. Vasc. Biol.* **2013**, *33*, 1306–1312. [CrossRef] [PubMed]
17. Kim, S.-A.; Park, S.-H.; Jo, S.-H.; Park, K.-H.; Kim, H.-S.; Han, S.-J.; Park, W.-J.; Ha, J.-W. Alterations of carotid arterial mechanics preceding the wall thickening in patients with hypertension. *Atherosclerosis* **2016**, *248*, 84–90. [CrossRef] [PubMed]
18. Moon, J.S.; Lee, S.Y.; Nam, C.M.; Choi, J.M.; Choe, B.K.; Seo, J.W.; Oh, K.; Jang, M.J.; Hwang, S.S.; Yoo, M.H.; et al. 2007 Korean National Growth Charts: Review of developmental process and an outlook. *Korean J. Pediatr.* **2008**, *51*. [CrossRef]
19. Styne, D.M.; Arslanian, S.A.; Connor, E.L.; Farooqi, I.S.; Murad, M.H.; Silverstein, J.H.; Yanovski, J.A. Pediatric Obesity-Assessment, Treatment, and Prevention: An Endocrine Society Clinical Practice Guideline. *J. Clin. Endocrinol. Metab.* **2017**, *102*, 709–757. [CrossRef] [PubMed]
20. Hayashi, K.; Handa, H.; Nagasawa, S.; Okumura, A.; Moritake, K. Stiffness and elastic behavior of human intracranial and extracranial arteries. *J. Biomech.* **1980**, *13*, 175–184. [CrossRef]
21. O'Rourke, M. Arterial stiffness, systolic blood pressure, and logical treatment of arterial hypertension. *Hypertension* **1990**, *15*, 339–347. [CrossRef] [PubMed]
22. O'Leary, D.H.; Polak, J.F.; Kronmal, R.A.; Manolio, T.A.; Burke, G.L.; Wolfson, S.K., Jr. Carotid-artery intima and media thickness as a risk factor for myocardial infarction and stroke in older adults. *N. Engl. J. Med.* **1999**, *340*, 14–22. [CrossRef] [PubMed]
23. Park, J.; Kim, S.H.; Cho, G.Y.; Baik, I.; Kim, N.H.; Lim, H.E.; Kim, E.J.; Park, C.G.; Lim, S.Y.; Kim, Y.H.; et al. Obesity phenotype and cardiovascular changes. *J. Hypertens.* **2011**, *29*, 1765–1772. [CrossRef] [PubMed]
24. Blaha, M.J.; Rivera, J.J.; Budoff, M.J.; Blankstein, R.; Agatston, A.; O'Leary, D.H.; Cushman, M.; Lakoski, S.; Criqui, M.H.; Szklo, M.; et al. Association between obesity, high-sensitivity c-reactive protein $\geq$ 2mg/L, and subclinical atherosclerosis: Implications of JUPITER from the Multi-Ethnic Study of Atherosclerosis. Arteriosclerosis, thrombosis. *Vasc. Biol.* **2011**, *31*, 1430–1438. [CrossRef] [PubMed]
25. Reed, D.; Dwyer, K.M.; Dwyer, J.H. Abdominal obesity and carotid artery wall thickness. The Los Angeles Atherosclerosis Study. *Int. J. Obes.* **2003**, *27*, 1546–1551. [CrossRef] [PubMed]
26. Juonala, M.; Raitakari, M.; Viikari, J.S.; Raitakari, O.T. Obesity in youth is not an independent predictor of carotid IMT in adulthood: The Cardiovascular Risk in Young Finns Study. *Atherosclerosis* **2006**, *185*, 388–393. [CrossRef] [PubMed]
27. Freedman, D.S.; Patel, D.A.; Srinivasan, S.R.; Chen, W.; Tang, R.; Bond, M.G.; Berenson, G.S. The contribution of childhood obesity to adult carotid intima-media thick ness: The Bogalusa Heart Study. *Int. J. Obes.* **2008**, *32*, 749–756. [CrossRef]
28. Ayer, J.G.; Harmer, J.A.; Nakhla, S.; Xuan, W.; Ng, M.K.; Raitakari, O.T.; Marks, G.B.; Celermajer, D.S. HDL-Cholesterol, Blood Pressure, and Asymmetric Dimethylarginine Are Significantly Associated With Arterial Wall Thickness in Children. *Arter. Thromb. Vasc. Biol.* **2009**, *29*, 943–949. [CrossRef]
29. Geerts, C.C.; Evelein, A.M.; Bots, M.L.; van der Ent, C.K.; Grobbee, D.E.; Uiterwaal, C.S. Body fat distribution and early arterial changes in healthy 5-year-old children. *Ann. Med.* **2012**, *44*, 350–359. [CrossRef] [PubMed]
30. Whincup, P.H.; Nightingale, C.M.; Rapala, A.; Joysurry, D.; Prescott, M.; Donald, A.E.; Ellins, E.; Donin, A.; Masi, S.; Owen, C.G.; et al. 66 Ethnic differences in carotid intimal medial thickness and carotid-femoral pulse wave velocity are present in UK children. *Heart* **2011**, *97*, A41. [CrossRef]
31. Elkiran, O.; Yilmaz, E.; Koc, M.; Kamanli, A.; Ustundag, B.; Ilhan, N. The association between intima media thickness, central obesity and diastolic blood pressure in obese and owerweight children: A cross-sectional school-based study. *Int. J. Cardiol.* **2013**, *165*, 528–532. [CrossRef] [PubMed]

32. Ozguven, I.; Ersoy, B.; Ozguven, A.; Ozkol, M.; Onur, E. Factors affecting carotid intima media thickness predicts early atherosclerosis in overweight and obese adolescents. *Obesity Res. Clin. Pract.* **2010**, *4*, e1–e82. [CrossRef] [PubMed]
33. Caserta, C.A.; Pendino, G.M.; Alicante, S.; Amante, A.; Amato, F.; Fiorillo, M.; Messineo, A.; Polito, I.; Surace, M.; Surace, P.; et al. Body Mass Index, Cardiovascular Risk Factors, and Carotid Intima-Media Thickness in a Pediatric Population in Southern Italy. *J. Pediatr. Gastroenterol. Nutr.* **2010**, *51*, 216–220. [CrossRef] [PubMed]
34. Woo, K.S.; Chook, P.; Yu, C.; Sung, R.Y.T.; Qiao, M.; Leung, S.S.F.; Lam, C.W.K.; Metreweli, C.; Celermajer, D.S. Overweight in children is associated with arterial endothelial dysfunction and intima-media thickening. *Int. J. Obes.* **2004**, *28*, 852–857. [CrossRef] [PubMed]
35. Urbina, E. Noninvasive assessment of target organ injury in children with the metabolic syndrome. *J. CardioMetabolic Syndr.* **2006**, *1*, 277–281. [CrossRef]
36. Gao, Z.; Khoury, P.R.; McCoy, C.E.; Shah, A.S.; Kimball, T.R.; Dolan, L.M.; Urbina, E.M. Adiposity has no direct effect on carotid intima-media thickness in adolescents and young adults: Use of structural equation modeling to elucidate indirect & direct pathways. *Atherosclerosis* **2015**, *246*, 29–35. [CrossRef]
37. Osiniri, I.; Sitjar, C.; Soriano-Rodríguez, P.; Prats-Puig, A.; Casas-Satre, C.; Mayol, L.; de Zegher, F.; Ibánez, L.; Bassols, J.; López-Bermejo, A. Carotid Intima-Media Thickness at 7 Years of Age: Relationship to C-Reactive Protein Rather than Adiposity. *J. Pediatr.* **2012**, *160*, 276–280.e1. [CrossRef]
38. Giannattasio, C.; Failla, M.; Capra, A.; Scanziani, E.; Amigoni, M.; Boffi, L.; Whistock, C.; Gamba, P.; Paleari, F.; Mancia, G. Increased Arterial Stiffness in Normoglycemic Normotensive Offspring of Type 2 Diabetic Parents. *Hypertension* **2008**, *51*, 182–187. [CrossRef]
39. Aronson, D. Cross-linking of glycated collagen in the pathogenesis of arterial and myocardial stiffening of aging and diabetes. *J. Hypertens.* **2003**, *21*, 3–12. [CrossRef]
40. Ozcetin, M.; Celikyay, Z.R.; Celik, A.; Yilmaz, R.; Yerli, Y.; Erkorkmaz, U. The importance of carotid artery stiffness and in-creased intima-media thickness in obese children. *S. Afr. Med. J.* **2012**, *102*, 295–299. [CrossRef]
41. Şen, H.; Bakiler, A.R.; Aydoğdu, S.A.; Ünüvar, T.; Yenisey, Ç.; Özer, E.A. The mechanical properties and stiffness of aorta in obese children. *Turk. J. Pediatr.* **2013**, *55*, 309–314. [PubMed]
42. Charakida, M.; Jones, A.; Falaschetti, E.; Khan, T.; Finer, N.; Sattar, N.; Hingorani, A.; Lawlor, D.A.; Smith, G.D.; Deanfield, J.E. Childhood Obesity and Vascular Phenotypes: A Population Study. *J. Am. Coll. Cardiol.* **2012**, *60*, 2643–2650. [CrossRef] [PubMed]
43. Fonck, E.; Prod'Hom, G.; Roy, S.; Augsburger, L.; Rufenacht, D.A.; Stergiopulos, N. Effect of elastin degradation on carotid wall mechanics as assessed by a constituent-based biomechanical model. *Am. J. Physiol. Circ. Physiol.* **2007**, *292*, H2754–H2763. [CrossRef]
44. Eberth, J.; Gresham, V.C.; Reddy, A.K.; Popovic, N.; Wilson, E.; Humphrey, J.D. Importance of pulsatility in hypertensive carotid artery growth and remodeling. *J. Hypertens.* **2009**, *27*, 2010–2021. [CrossRef] [PubMed]

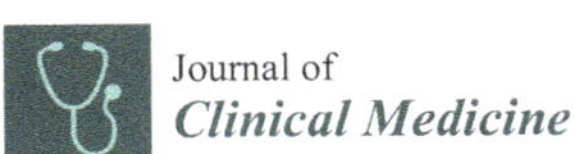
Journal of
Clinical Medicine

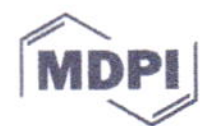

Article

The Prognostic Value of Cardiac Troponin I in Patients with or without Three-Vessel Disease Undergoing Complete Percutaneous Coronary Intervention

Zhi-Fan Li, Shuang Zhang, Hui-Wei Shi, Wen-Jia Zhang, Yong-Gang Sui, Jian-Jun Li, Ke-Fei Dou, Jie Qian and Na-Qiong Wu *

Cardiometabolic Center, National Center for Cardiovascular Diseases, Fuwai Hospital, Chinese Academy of Medical Science & Peking Union Medical College, Beijing 100037, China; lizajackson@foxmail.com (Z.-F.L.); tats246@163.com (S.Z.); 15770738175@163.com (H.-W.S.); wendyzhang0325@163.com (W.-J.Z.); fwsyg999@163.com (Y.-G.S.); lijianjun938@126.com (J.-J.L.); drdoukefei@126.com (K.-F.D.); qianjfw@163.com (J.Q.)
* Correspondence: fuwainaqiongwu@163.com; Tel.: +86-10-88396896

Abstract: Postprocedural cardiac troponin I (cTnI) elevation commonly occurs in patients undergoing percutaneous coronary intervention (PCI); however, its prognostic value remains controversial. This study aimed to investigate the prognostic value of peak postprocedural cTnI in cardiac patients with or without three-vessel disease (TVD) undergoing complete PCI. A total of 1237 consecutive patients (77% males, mean age 58 ± 10 years) with normal baseline cTnI levels were enrolled, 439 patients (77% males, 59 ± 10 years) with TVD, and 798 patients (77% males, 57 ± 10 years) with single- or double-vessel disease (non-TVD). The primary outcome was the occurrence of major adverse cardiovascular events (MACE), defined as a composite of non-fatal MI, non-fatal stroke, unplanned revascularization, re-hospitalization due to heart failure or severe arrhythmias, and all-cause death. During the median follow-up of 5.3 years, a total of 169 patients (13.7%) developed MACE, including 73 (16.6%) in the TVD group and 96 (12.0%) in the non-TVD group ($p = 0.024$). After adjustment, the multivariate Cox analysis showed that hypertension (HR 1.50; 95% CI: 1.01–2.20; $p = 0.042$), TVD (HR 1.44; 95% CI: 1.03–2.02; $p = 0.033$), and cTnI $\geq 70\times$ URL (HR 2.47; 95% CI: 1.28–4.78, $p = 0.007$) were independently associated with increased MACE during long-term follow-up. Further subgroup analyses showed that cTnI $\geq 70\times$ URL was an independent predictor of MACE in TVD patients (HR 3.32, 95% CI: 1.51–7.34, $p = 0.003$), but not in non-TVD patients (HR 1.01, 95%CI: 0.24–4.32, $p = 0.991$). In conclusion, elevation of post-PCI cTnI $\geq 70\times$ URL is independently associated with a high risk of MACE during long-term follow-up in patients with TVD, but not in those with non-TVD.

Keywords: percutaneous coronary intervention; cardiac troponin; three-vessel disease; prediction

Citation: Li, Z.-F.; Zhang, S.; Shi, H.-W.; Zhang, W.-J.; Sui, Y.-G.; Li, J.-J.; Dou, K.-F.; Qian, J.; Wu, N.-Q. The Prognostic Value of Cardiac Troponin I in Patients with or without Three-Vessel Disease Undergoing Complete Percutaneous Coronary Intervention. *J. Clin. Med.* **2022**, *11*, 3896. https://doi.org/10.3390/jcm11133896

Academic Editor: Tomoaki Ishigami

Received: 30 May 2022
Accepted: 30 June 2022
Published: 4 July 2022

1. Introduction

Cardiac troponin I (cTnI) is a sensitive marker of myocardial damage and necrosis, and is expressed only in myocardium [1]. Postprocedural cTnI elevation commonly occurs in patients with coronary heart disease (CAD) undergoing percutaneous coronary intervention (PCI) and may significantly relate to poor outcomes [2,3]. Current expert consensus states that elevated postoperative troponin is an important marker of procedure-related myocardial injury, even procedure-related myocardial infarction (MI), and different thresholds of troponin elevation define the degree of injury [4–7]. However, there is controversy over the predictive value of cTnI for the prognosis of patients undergoing PCI. Several studies have indicated that postprocedural cTn elevation is valuable for predicting of poor outcomes [8–13], whereas other studies have shown that it has no impact on prognosis even if the elevation is extremely high [14,15].

Three-vessel coronary artery disease (TVD) is a severe and complex type of CAD, defined as a lesion of >50% diameter stenosis (DS) in all three main epicardial coronary arteries, including the left anterior descending artery (LAD), the left circumflex artery (LCX), and the right coronary artery (RCA), with or without left main artery (LM) involvement. Patients with TVD have a higher risk of death and major adverse cardiac events (MACEs) [16–18]. In the SYNTAX (Synergy Between PCI With Taxus and Cardiac Surgery) trial, involving patients with TVD or LM, PCI-related myocardial damage was associated with all-cause mortality. However, this study only used creatine kinase–myocardial band (CK-MB) as a marker because cTnI was not collected [19]. More recently, studies on cTnI and post-PCI prognosis have been conducted in patients with acute myocardial infarction (AMI) [20], LM disease [21], chronic total occlusion (CTO) [22], and diabetes mellitus (DM) [23] who are undergoing PCI, but there is a lack of studies involving patients with TVD.

Here, our study focused on the predictive value of postprocedural cTnI for the long-term prognosis of patients undergoing complete PCI. Furthermore, our study explored variance in the prognostic performance of postprocedural cTnI between TVD and non-TVD patients and assessed the impact of different cTnI levels on outcomes in TVD patients.

2. Materials and Methods

2.1. Study Participants

We included consecutive CAD patients with normal preoperative cTnI levels who successfully underwent complete PCI at the Department of Cardiology, Fuwai Hospital, Chinese Academy of Medical Science between January 2011 and December 2013, and who consented for long-term follow-up. The inclusion criteria were as follows: (1) age <75 years; (2) acute coronary syndrome (ACS) or stable CAD with an indication for PCI; and (3) undergoing complete revascularization (CR). CR was defined by a combination of the operator's judgments of a patient's coronary angiography lesions and clinical manifestations (some patients had positive results in non-invasive examinations). TVD-CR was defined by the presence of >50% DS in the three coronary arteries (LAD, LCX, RCA), and the operator completed the revascularization treatment of lesions with interventional indications (i.e., segments >2.0 mm in diameter with ≥75% DS). The exclusion criteria were as follows: (1) the absence of postoperative cTnI measurements; (2) coronary stenosis with <50% DS in the main epicardial coronary arteries; (3) the presence of LM stenosis with >50% DS; (4) the presence of chronic total occlusion (CTO); (5) severe liver and kidney dysfunction; (6) combined cardiomyopathy or malignancies; (7) a left ventricular ejection fraction (LVEF) of <35%; (8) previous aorto-coronary bypass grafting surgery (CABG); and (9) the presence of valvular heart disease.

Baseline patient demographics, clinical and laboratory examinations, procedural characteristics, and medication at discharge were prospectively collected in a designed database by independent researchers. Risk factors, such as diabetes and hypertension, were determined based on medical record system queries or questionnaires. An echocardiogram was performed at the time of admission. This study was approved by the Fuwai Hospital Ethics Committee and was conducted in accordance with the Declaration of Helsinki. All participants provided written informed consent.

2.2. Procedural and Biomarker Assessment

PCI was performed by experienced interventionists according to standard clinical practices. The choice of PCI technique and stent type was at the discretion of the operators. Prior to PCI procedures, dual antiplatelet therapy (DAPT) was administered and continued for at least one year, according to AHA/ACC and ESC recommendations at the time of the index procedure [24–27]. Sufficient doses of dual antiplatelet medicines were administered before PCI procedures, and thereafter dual antiplatelet medicines were administered for at least 1 year.

Blood samples were routinely collected for cTnI testing before angiography (baseline cTnI level), within 8–24 h after PCI, and every morning thereafter during hospitalization. The patients' plasmid lipid profile, hemoglobin, and N-terminal pro-brain natriuretic peptide (NT-proBNP) levels were analyzed at the central chemistry laboratory. Standard cTnI levels were detected using a commercial chemiluminescence method through the Beckman Coulter (Brea, CA, USA) access immunoassay system and were normalized to the upper reference limit (URL). Patients with cTnI under 0.04 ng/mL (99th centile URL) were assessed as normal, as determined by the manufactures.

2.3. Follow-Up and Clinical Outcomes

Clinical follow-up information was collected from the patients' medical records on subsequent visits and from routine telephone or message-based surveys by research staff who were blinded to this study. All events were adjudicated by independent medical personnel who were not involved in the PCI procedure. The endpoint of interest was the occurrence of major adverse cardiovascular events (MACEs), defined as a composite of non-fatal MI, non-fatal stroke, unplanned revascularization, re-hospitalization due to heart failure or severe arrhythmias, and all-cause death.

2.4. Statistical Methods

Statistical analyses were performed using R version 4.1.1 (R Foundation for Statistical Computing, Vienna, Austria). The Shapiro–Wilk test was used to examine the normality of continuous variables. Data are reported as mean ± standard deviation (X ± SD) or median (interquartile range) for normal and non-normally distributed continuous variables, and as counts with percentages [n, (%)] for categorical variables. Differences between continuous variables were analyzed using the Student's unpaired t-test or Wilcoxon rank sum tests as appropriate, whereas differences between categorical variables were analyzed using the Chi-squared or Fischer's exact test depending on the size of the group.

The cumulative event-free survival data are presented graphically using the Kaplan–Meier method, and the differences among prespecified commonly used cTnI interval groups (<1×, 1–5×, 5–69×, and ≥70× URL) were compared using log-rank tests. Univariate and multivariate Cox regression analyses were used to investigate the impacts of the variables on long-term MACEs after PCI, with hazard ratios (HRs) and 95% confidence intervals (CIs). Age, sex, hypertension, DM, systolic blood pressure, LVEF, hemoglobin, and NT-proBNP were included in the adjusted models. Furthermore, the risk of MACEs in response to high cTnI levels and TVD and their interactions were tested. Similarly, Cox proportional hazard models were performed for TVD and non-TVD groups in order to assess the prognostic value of cTnI. All probability values were two-sided, and $p < 0.05$ was considered statistically significant.

3. Results

3.1. Study Population

A total of 1237 patients (77% males, mean age 58 ± 10 years) with normal preoperative cTnI levels were included in the study. Patients' baseline clinical characteristics, past history and comorbidities, laboratory results, and medication at discharge are shown in Table 1, and are stratified according to the presence or absence of TVD. Among these patients, 439 (35.5%) were diagnosed with TVD, 348 (28.1%) had single-vessel disease and 450 (36.3%) had double-vessel disease.

Compared to the non-TVD group, the TVD group were older (57 ± 10 vs. 59 ± 10 years, $p = 0.005$), had a higher proportion of patients with hypertension (61.6 vs. 68.2%, $p = 0.021$) and diabetes (25.5 vs. 33.8%, $p = 0.002$), and were more often discharged on beta-blockers (84.4 vs. 88.6%, $p = 0.044$). Furthermore, the TVD group had a significantly higher level of NT-proBNP and a significantly lower level of hemoglobin compared to the non-TVD group (555.8 [448.9706.7] vs. 579.75 [454.58,777.82] pg/mL, $p = 0.049$; 141.22 ± 14.37 vs. 143.09 ± 14.52 g/L, $p = 0.031$, respectively).

Table 1. Characteristics of the study population by the presence or absence of TVD.

Variables	All (n = 1237)	Non-TVD Group (n = 798)	TVD Group (n = 439)	p Value
Male, n (%)	952 (77.0)	614 (77.0)	338 (77.0)	0.984
Age ± SD, years	58 ± 10	57 ± 10	59 ± 10	0.005
BMI (Q1,Q3), kg/m^2	25.6 (23.7,27.7)	25.6 (23.6,27.7)	25.6 (23.9,27.8)	0.323
ACS, n (%)	868 (70.2)	557 (69.8)	311 (70.8)	0.750
Pre-PCI, n (%)	272 (22.0)	183 (23.0)	89 (20.3)	0.280
PAD, n (%)	7 (0.8)	2 (0.4)	5 (1.7)	0.117
Stroke, n (%)	51 (5.98)	30 (5.47)	21 (6. 9)	0.405
Hypertension, n (%)	787 (64.0)	489 (61.6)	298 (68.2)	0.021
Hyperlipidemia, n (%)	944 (76.7)	602 (75.9)	342 (78.1)	0.389
Diabetes mellitus, n (%)	350 (28.4)	202 (25.5)	148 (33.8)	0.002
Smoking history, n (%)	704 (57.2)	441 (55.5)	263 (60.2)	0.115
SBP (Q1,Q3), mmHg	120 (110,130)	120 (110,132)	120 (112,130)	0.496
LVEDD (Q1,Q3), mm	48 (45,50)	47 (45,50)	48 (45,50)	0.191
LVEF (Q1,Q3), %	65 (60,68)	65 (61,68)	64 (60,68)	0.058
TG (Q1,Q3), mmol/L	1.55 (1.13,2.14)	1.55 (1.10,2.14)	1.58 (1.16,2.20)	0.793
TC (Q1,Q3), mmol/L	4.03 (3.39,4.7)	4.02 (3.37,4.67)	4.04 (3.44,4.78)	0.283
HDL-C (Q1,Q3), mmol/L	1.02 (0.87,1.22)	1.02 (0.88,1.23)	1 (0.86,1.21)	0.302
LDL-C (Q1,Q3), mmol/L	2.31(1.80,2.92)	2.29 (1.77,2.88)	2.35 (1.87,2.99)	0.076
Lp(a) (Q1,Q3), mg/L	158.5 (68.18,353.23)	158.1 (63.23,337.25)	159.91 (73.68,363.56)	0.242
Hemoglobin ± SD, g/L	142.43 ± 14.49	143.09 ± 14.52	141.22 ± 14.37	0.031
NT-proBNP (Q1,Q3), pg/ml	561.5 (449.2,735.8)	555.8 (448.9,706.7)	579.75 (454.58,777.82)	0.049
Statins, n (%)	1214 (98.1)	782 (97.9)	432 (98.4)	0.515
Aspirin, n (%)	1233 (99.7)	792 (99.5)	438 (100)	0.336
Clopidogrel, n (%)	1224 (99.1)	787(98.9)	437 (99.5)	0.372
β-blockers, n (%)	1062 (85.9)	673 (84.4)	389 (88.6)	0.044
ACEI, n (%)	370 (30.0)	231 (29.0)	139 (31.7)	0.319
ARB, n (%)	342 (27.8)	208 (26.2)	134 (30.7)	0.089
cTnI < 1× URL, n (%)	499 (40.3)	342 (42.9)	157 (35.8)	
cTnI 1–5× URL, n (%)	392 (31.7)	247 (31.0)	145 (33.0)	0.055
cTnI 5–69× URL, n (%)	308 (24.9)	189 (23.7)	119 (27.1)	
cTnI ≥ 70× URL, n (%)	38 (3.1)	20 (2.5)	18 (4.1)	
MACE, n (%)	169 (13.7)	96 (12.0)	73 (16.6)	0.024
non-fatal MI, n (%)	24 (1.94)	14 (1.75)	10 (2.3)	0.523
non-fatal stroke, n (%)	34 (2.8)	21 (2.6)	13 (3.0)	0.734
unplanned revascularization, n (%)	86 (7.0)	49 (6.1)	37 (8.4)	0.130
re-hospitalization due to heart failure or severe arrhythmias, n (%)	5 (0.4)	4 (0.5)	1 (0.2)	0.797
all-cause death, n (%)	20 (1.6)	8 (1.0)	12 (2.7)	0.021

Notes: Data are expressed as mean + SD, median (Q1,Q3), or as number (%). TVD, three-vessel disease; BMI, body mass index; ACS, acute coronary syndrome; Pre-PCI, previous percutaneous coronary intervention; PAD, peripheral arterial disease; SBP, systolic blood pressure; LVEDD, left ventricular end diastolic diameter; LVEF, left ventricular ejection fraction; TG, triglyceride; TC, total cholesterol; HDL-C, high-density lipoprotein cholesterol; LDL-C, low-density lipoprotein cholesterol; Lp (a), lipoprotein (a); hs-CRP, hypersensitive C-reactive protein; NT-proBNP, N-terminal pro-B type natriuretic peptide; HbA1c, glycosylated hemoglobin A1 c; ACEI, Angiotensin converting enzyme inhibitors; ARB, Angiotension II receptor blockers; cTnI, cardiac troponin I; URL, upper reference limit; MACE, major adverse cardiovascular event.

cTnI elevation above the 1× URL occurred after 59.7% (738/1237) of the total number of procedures. In comparison with the non-TVD group, the TVD group had a higher proportion of 1× URL ≤ cTnI < 5× URL (31.0 vs. 33.0%), 5× URL ≤ cTnI < 70× URL (23.7 vs. 27.1%), and cTnI ≥ 70× URL (2.5 vs. 4.1%), and a lower proportion of cTnI < 1× URL (42.9 vs. 35.8%). However, the p-value did not reach significance (p = 0.055).

3.2. Outcome Analysis

A total of 169 (13.7%) patients developed MACEs after a median follow-up of 5.3 (4.5–5.5) years. The TVD group developed a significantly higher proportion of MACEs

(16.6 vs. 12.0%, $p = 0.024$) and all-cause death (2.7 vs. 1.0%, $p = 0.021$) compared to the non-TVD group.

The outcomes of different postoperative peak cTnI levels were explored. Patients with normal cTnI were considered the control group, whereas patients with elevated cTnI were divided into three groups (1× URL ≤ cTnI < 5× URL, 5× URL ≤ cTnI < 70× URL, and cTnI ≥ 70× URL). The relationships between peak postprocedural cTnI levels and MACEs are shown in Figure 1A. The Kaplan–Meier analysis showed that outcomes differed according to peak postprocedural cTnI levels, and that cTnI ≥ 70× URL was associated with 5-year MACEs (log-rank test $p = 0.012$). Univariate analyses between common clinical variables and MACEs were performed for the total patient cohort (Table 2). We found that the following variables had significant univariate associations: age (HR 1.02 [1.01,1.04], $p = 0.005$), hypertension (HR 1.56 [1.11,2.19], $p = 0.01$), diabetes mellitus (HR 1.55 [1.14,2.12], $p = 0.006$), TVD (HR 1.42 [1.04,1.92], $p = 0.026$), NT-proBNP (HR 1.00 [1.00,1.001], $p = 0.008$), and cTnI ≥ 70× URL (HR 2.09 [1.11–3.94], $p = 0.022$). After adjusting for all of the variables above, Cox multivariate analyses showed that hypertension (HR 1.50 [1.01–2.20], $p = 0.042$), TVD (HR 1.44 [1.03–2.02], $p = 0.033$), and cTnI ≥ 70× URL (HR 2.47 [1.28–4.78], $p = 0.007$) were associated with increased MACEs. We further divided the total population according to TVD and cTnI levels (70× URL) in Table 3. Among the four groups, patients with TVD and cTnI ≥ 70× URL had the highest risk of experiencing MACEs (50.0%). In the TVD group, those with cTnI ≥ 70× URL had an increased absolute and relative risk of MACEs compared to those with cTnI < 70× URL (HR 4.43, 95% CI: 2.13 to 9.24, $p < 0.001$). In contrast, the MACE risk difference in the non-TVD group was modest (HR 0.78, 95% CI: 0.19 to 3.20, $p = 0.731$). Interaction tests between TVD and the postprocedural peak cTnI level on the 5-year risk of MACE reached the significant cutoff value ($p = 0.05$). A sensitivity analysis for the interaction between TVD and cTnI ≥ 70× URL was performed according to clinical setting (ACS vs non-ACS). In the ACS subgroup (Supplementary Table S1), TVD patients with cTnI ≥ 70× URL were independently associated with a higher risk of MACE (HR: 5.30, 95% CI: 2.29–12.25, $p < 0.001$) (p for interaction = 0.04). However, in the non-ACS subgroup, the number of events was insufficient to analyze (Supplementary Table S2).

Table 2. Univariate and multivariate predictors of 5-year MACE in the total cohort assessed by Cox regression analysis.

Variables	Univariate Analysis		Multivariate Analysis	
	HR (95%CI)	*p* Value	HR (95%CI)	*p* Value
Age	1.02 (1.01,1.04)	0.005		0.199
Male	0.91 (0.64,1.29)	0.592		0.267
SBP	1.002 (0.992,1.013)	0.627		0.767
LVEF	1.003 (0.981,1.025)	0.802		0.515
Hypertension	1.56 (1.11,2.19)	0.01	1.50 (1.01–2.20)	0.042
Diabetes mellitus	1.55 (1.14,2.12)	0.006		0.533
TVD	1.42 (1.04,1.92)	0.026	1.44 (1.03–2.02)	0.033
Hemoglobin	0.99 (0.98,1)	0.195		0.736
NT-proBNP	1 (1,1.001)	0.008		0.141
cTnI < 1× URL	Ref		Ref	
1–5× URL	0.80 (0.55–1.15)	0.227		0.406
5–69× URL	0.76 (0.51–1.14)	0.183		0.044
≥70× URL	2.09 (1.11–3.94)	0.022	2.47 (1.28–4.78)	0.007

Notes: SBP, systolic blood pressure; LVEF, left ventricular ejection fraction; TVD, three-vessel disease; cTnI, cardiac troponin I; URL, upper reference limit.

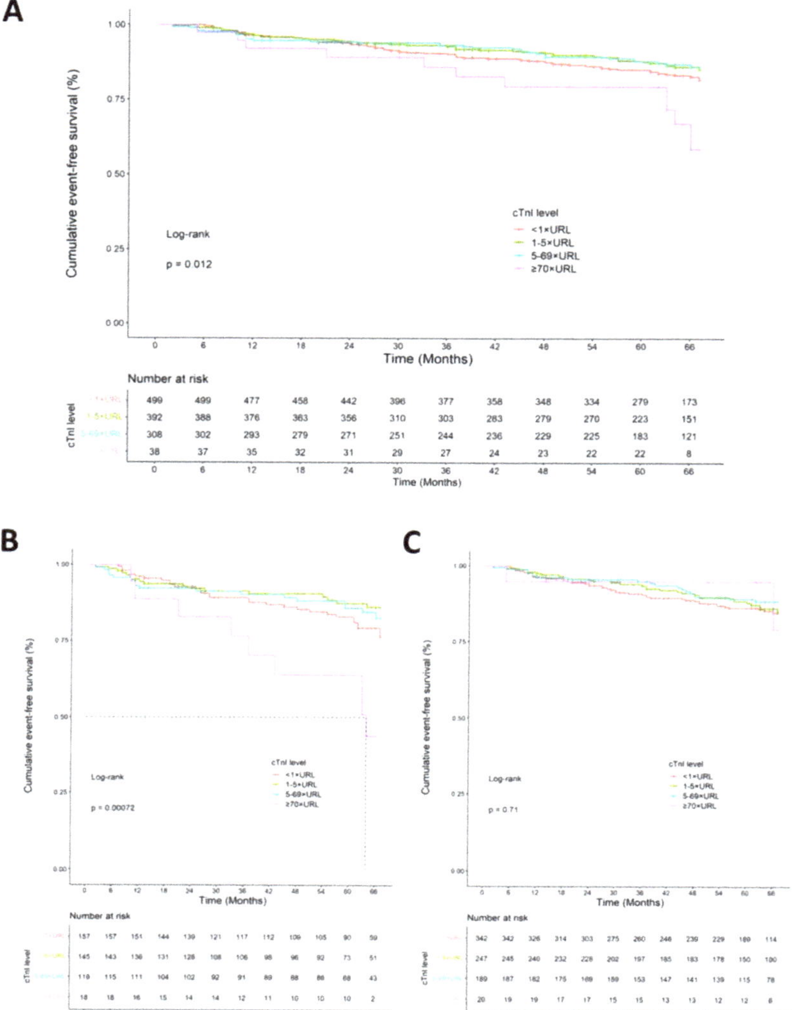

Figure 1. Cumulative Kaplan–Meier survival curve analysis of 5-year MACEs in total patients (**A**), TVD patients (**B**), and non-TVD patients (**C**) according to postprocedural cTnI levels. Notes: MACEs, major adverse cardiovascular events; cTnI, cardiac troponin I; URL, upper reference limit; TVD, three-vessel disease; non-TVD, non-three-vessel disease, including single-vessel disease and double-vessel disease.

Table 3. Effect modification of TVD on the predictive value of cTnI for 5-year MACE.

	cTnI < 70× URL (<2.8 ng/mL)		cTnI ≥ 70× URL (≥2.8 ng/mL)		Unadjusted		*p* Value * for Interaction	Adjusted †		*p* Value * for Interaction
	Total	Events (%)	Total	Events (%)	HR (95% CI)	*p* Value		HR (95% CI)	*p* Value	
Non-TVD	778	94 (12.1%)	20	2 (10.0%)	0.89 (0.23–3.60)	0.868	Ref	0.78 (0.19–3.20)	0.731	Ref
TVD	421	64 (15.2%)	18	9 (50.0%)	3.61 (1.80–7.27)	<0.001	0.08	4.43 (2.13–9.24)	<0.001	0.05

Notes: TVD, three-vessel disease; cTnI, cardiac troponin I; URL, upper reference limit; HR, hazard ratio; CI, confidence interval; * *p* value for the interaction test represents the interaction of cTnI level (≥70× URL vs. <70× URL) and participant group (Non-TVD vs. TVD) on MACE. † Adjusted for age, sex, systolic blood pressure, left ventricular end-diastolic volume, hypertension, diabetes mellitus, hemoglobin, and NT-proBNP. The cTnI <70× URL group is the reference group.

We further analyzed prognosis for different cTnI thresholds among TVD and non-TVD patients. In the TVD cohort, the Kaplan–Meier survival curve showed significantly lower event-free survival in patients with cTnI ≥ 70× URL compared to patients with normal postoperative peak cTnI (<1× URL) (log-rank $p < 0.001$) (Figure 1B). The log-rank test showed no significant difference for patients with 5× URL ≤ cTnI < 70× URL ($p = 0.4$) and 1× URL ≤ cTnI < 5× URL ($p = 0.1$). The multivariate Cox regression analysis, adjustedfor the covariates discussed above, showed that only cTnI ≥ 70× URL was associated with a significantly higher rate of MACE during long-term follow-up when compared with the reference cTnI value (HR 3.32; 95%CI: 1.51–7.34; $p = 0.003$) (Table 4). However, such an association was not present for non-TVD patients with any range of post-PCI peak cTnI (Figure 1C). The Cox regression analysis for a single adverse event showed that unplanned revascularization had a significantly higher HR in the TVD group with cTnI ≥ 70× URL (HR 4.94, 95%CI: 1.83–13.30, $p = 0.002$) compared to the reference group (Supplementary Table S3).

Table 4. Univariate and Multivariate Cox analysis of the predictive value of cTnI for 5-year MACE among TVD and non-TVD patients.

	Unadjusted HR (95% CI)	*p* Value	Adjusted HR * (95% CI)	*p* Value
TVD < 1× URL	Reference		Reference	
1–5× URL	0.64 (0.35–1.16)	0.139	0.61 (0.32–1.15)	0.126
5–69× URL	0.75 (0.41–1.36)	0.349	0.63 (0.33–1.20)	0.163
≥70× URL	2.91 (1.38–6.14)	0.005	3.32 (1.51–7.34)	0.003
Non-TVD < 1× URL	Reference		Reference	
1–5× URL	0.89 (0.56–1.41)	0.622	1.11 (0.67–1.84)	0.682
5–69× URL	0.73 (0.43–1.25)	0.250	0.58 (0.30–1.12)	0.106
≥70× URL	0.80 (0.19–3.29)	0.754	1.01 (0.24–4.32)	0.991

Notes: TVD, three-vessel disease; cTnI, cardiac troponin I; URL, upper reference limit; HR, hazard ratio; CI, confidence interval; * adjusted for age, sex, systolic blood pressure, left ventricular end-diastolic volume, hypertension, diabetes mellitus, hemoglobin, and NT-proBNP.

4. Discussion

To the best of our knowledge, there have been no previous studies exploring the prognostic value of elevated cTnI in a population of TVD patients undergoing complete PCI. This is the first study unveiling the potential prognostic differences of post-PCI cTnI elevation in patients with and without TVD. In this study examining the predictive value of post-PCI cTnI for long-term prognosis in patients with or without TVD, the major findings were: (1) significant elevations in post-PCI peak cTnI levels (cTnI ≥ 70× URL) were independently associated with an increased risk of long-term MACEs in patients with TVD, but not in those with non-TVD; and (2) elevations in post-PCI peak cTnI < 70× URL were not prognostically significant.

Cardiac troponin is widely used in the diagnosis of myocardial injury and is significantly associated with increased MACEs and mortality [5,28,29]. The routine assessment of cardiac biomarkers 8 to 12 h after PCI is advised, according to the American College of Cardiology/American Heart Association (ACC/AHA) guidelines for PCI (class II-b recommendation) [26]. Troponin I elevation frequently occurs in patients undergoing PCI [14,30]. In our study, the overall percentage of cTnI elevation was 59.7%, and the incidence was higher in TVD patients (64.2%). As a sensitive and specific biomarker reflecting myocardial injury, assessment of cTnI has been commonly recommended to define procedure-related myocardial injury and periprocedural MI (PMI). The 3rd Universal Definition of Myocardial Infarction (UDMI) identifies cTn as the biomarker used to define PCI-related MI (type 4a MI), and CK-MB is used only if cTn is unavailable [4]. The 4th UDMI defines PMI only by troponin levels [5]. Myocardial injury is defined by the standalone detection of postprocedural cTn elevation above the 99th percentile URL [4,5]. The European Association of Percutaneous Cardiovascular Interventions (EAPCI) proposed that a >5-fold increase in post-PCI cTn values is a prognostically relevant "major" periprocedural myocardial injury [6]. The definition of type 4a MI is not only based on the same cutoff threshold (cTn > 5× URL), but also requires at least one clinical correlate, including ischemic electrocardiogram changes, flow-limiting angiographic complications, and/or supporting evidence obtained from imaging [5,6]. In contrast, groups of interventional cardiologists from the Society of Cardiovascular Angiography and Interventions (SCAI) strongly preferred CK-MB > 10 times the upper limit of normal (ULN, similar to URL) as a PMI threshold, otherwise cTn > 70× ULN. Based on SCAI, the Academic Research Consortium-2 (ARC-2) recommended that post-PCI MI be defined as cTn > 35× ULN with ancillary criteria or cTn > 70× ULN for isolated biomarker elevation [7]. Therefore, in this study, we set threshold intervals of isolated cTnI elevation (<1× URL, 1–5× URL, 5–70× URL, ≥70× URL) based on expert recommendations for myocardial injury, major perioperative myocardial injury, and PMI.

Previous research exploring the relationship between post-PCI troponin elevation and clinical prognosis has produced inconsistent results [14,31,32]. In our study, we found that 13.7% of patients developed MACEs after a median follow-up of 5.3 years. Furthermore, we found a positive association between large cTnI elevation and MACEs. This result is in accordance with a meta-analysis conducted by Nienhuis et al., who found that post-PCI troponin elevation was significantly associated with increased mortality (4.4% vs. 3.3%, $p = 0.001$; OR 1.35) and incidence of death or nonfatal MI (8.1% vs. 5.2%, $p < 0.001$; OR 1.59) [31]. A recent meta-analysis that pooled all prospective trials (11 studies, 13,932 patients) indicated that elevated cTnI after elective PCI was associated with an increase in all-cause mortality compared with non-elevated cTnI (OR 1.42, 95% CI 1.19 to 1.69, $p < 0.001$), and for every 3 × 99th percentile URL increment of cTnI, the pooled risk of death increased by 33% (95% CI 1.15 to 1.53, $p < 0.001$) [32]. In this study, we used the experts' suggested cutoff values for the prognostic significance of post-PCI cTnI elevation. As shown in the Kaplan–Meier survival curves, the event-free survival rate was apparently lower when the post-PCI cTnI ratio was no less than 70× URL. Similarly, univariate and multivariate Cox analyses indicated that patients with cTnI ≥ 70× URL were at a significantly higher risk of experiencing MACEs. For patients with normal cTnI (<99th percentile URL), post-PCI 1× URL ≤ cTnI < 5× URL, and 5× URL ≤ cTnI < 70× URL, we found no difference in event-free survival among them. In this regard, our study is consistent with a recent pooled analysis of 4362 elective PCI patients with normal baseline conventional cTn levels. This pooled analysis found a significant association between subsequent 1-year all-cause mortality and post-PCI cTn ≥ 70× URL (adjusted OR, 5.97 95% CI 1.65 to 21.59, $p = 0.023$). Among a total of 9081 patients (including patients with hs-cTn data), 1-year all-cause mortality was strongly associated with the lesser threshold of post-PCI cTn elevation (either hs-cTn or conventional cTn ≥ 5× URL) [33]. Another pooled analysis of 13,452 stable CAD patients undergoing elective PCI compared 1-year mortality in patients with different cTn cutoff values (normal, 1 ≤ cTn < 3, 3 ≤ cTn < 5, 5 ≤ cTn < 10, 10 ≤ cTn < 20, 20 ≤ cTn < 35, 35 ≤ cTn < 70, and ≥70 times ULN). Although cTn ≥ 70× ULN was associated with increased risk of mortality as indicated by the Kaplan–Meier curves, the Cox multivariate analysis showed that the mortality rate did not increase, irrespective of any level of cTn elevation [14]. Discordance may be due to the use of different models for multivariate analysis, a wider primary end-point and a longer follow-up time in our study, and variance in the population. Of note, most patients included in this pooled analysis had single-vessel disease (78%), whereas only 28.2% of the patients in our study had single-vessel disease.

TVD confers higher rates of mortality and an increased risk of MACEs compared with non-TVD, and is regarded as a severe condition [34,35]. A meta-analysis showed that complete revascularization for TVD significantly reduced the risk of all-cause mortality compared to incomplete revascularization [36]. In this study, all patients underwent complete PCI for clinical benefit, and 439 patients (35.5%) were diagnosed with TVD. A study by Tsai et al. reported that TVD was an independent predictor for the time-dependent occurrence of MACEs in patients with elective PCI after a mean follow-up period of 32 months. The researchers believed that multifactorial occurrence—including TVD—facilitated the association of stent implantation with MACEs [37]. Similarly, the results from our multivariate Cox analysis also showed that TVD was associated with a higher risk of MACEs. Previous studies have reported that the number of target vessels in PCI play a crucial role in the elevation of cardiac enzymes, and multi-vessel PCI could increase the risk of sustained periprocedural myocardial injury or PMI [9,38]. In our population, TVD patients had a higher proportion of post-PCI cTnI elevation. Moreover, cTnI $\geq 70\times$ URL was also an independent predictor of MACEs. Therefore, we further tested and confirmed the interaction between TVD and a high post-PCI cTnI cutoff ($70 \times$ URL). We suggest that the effect of TVD should be carefully considered in future prognostic studies of cardiac biomarkers.

Postprocedural cardiac enzyme elevation was frequently detected after complex PCI (i.e., CTO, LM, or multivessel PCI), whereas the prognostic impact of cTn remained controversial [13,39]. In this study, we included TVD and non-TVD patients, and found that postoperative cTnI elevation is an independent prognostic value for long-term prognosis only in TVD patients as these patients had a significantly higher occurrence of MACEs when their cTnI levels surpass $70\times$ URL. On the other hand, for non-TVD patients or for those with mild cTnI elevation, our study suggests that there are no significant adverse effects on long-term prognosis. Since delayed-enhancement MRI verified the degree of post-PCI cTnI elevation that correlated directly with the extent of new irreversible myocardial injury [40], patients with higher cTnI elevation were presumed to have more severe perioperative myocardial necrosis. Thus, we speculated that a large range of PCI-induced myocardial injury indicated by cTnI $\geq 70\times$ URL, rather than minor necrosis, would produce a poor prognosis, according to our results. Therefore, the routine measurement of cTnI may be helpful for risk stratification and for the postprocedural management of patients undergoing PCI. Increased awareness of the prognostic value of cTn may contribute to the early detection of high-risk patients and the prevention of postoperative adverse events. Further large-scale prospective trials are needed to confirm the contribution of post-PCI elevated cTnI to prognosis in different patients with more clinically relevant variables.

5. Limitations

The present study has several potential limitations. Firstly, we used a single-center, observational study design which included a relatively low rate of MACEs. This may limit the power of our analysis and the generalizability of our results. Secondly, although we attempted to adjust for multiple covariates, data was unavailable for some confounders (e.g., operative data, postprocedural echo data, and risk scores), which may also affect the results. Thirdly, the perioperative levels of other biomarkers, such as CK-MB, cardiac troponin T, and high-sensitivity troponin, were not collected for most patients in our center, but this complied with the standard practice for elective PCI. Thus, the prognostic values provided by cardiac biomarkers remains important for future research, and large prospective trials with more biomarker assessment and hard endpoints (e.g., cardiac death) are required.

6. Conclusions

In this observational study, we found the frequent occurrence of cTnI elevation in CAD patients who underwent complete PCI. Elevation in post-PCI cTnI $\geq 70\times$ 99th percentile URL is independently associated with a high risk of MACEs during long-term follow-up for patients with TVD, but not for those with non-TVD. Elevation in post-PCI cTnI $< 70 \times$ 99th percentile URL has no prognostic value regarding the risk of MACEs during follow-up for both TVD and non-TVD patients.

Supplementary Materials: The following are available online at https://www.mdpi.com/article/10.3390/jcm11133896/s1, Table S1: Effect modification of TVD on the predictive value of cTnI for 5-year MACE in ACS patients, Table S2: The effect of TVD on the predictive value of cTnI for 5-year MACE in non-ACS patients, Table S3: Multivariate Cox analysis of the prognostic value of cTnI for 5-year MACE and single outcomes of the TVD and Non-TVD patients.

Author Contributions: N.-Q.W.: conception/design. W.-J.Z., Y.-G.S., J.-J.L., K.-F.D. and J.Q.: provision of study materials. S.Z., H.-W.S. and Z.-F.L.: collection and/or assembly of data. Z.-F.L.: data analysis, interpretation, and manuscript writing. All authors have read and agreed to the published version of the manuscript.

Funding: This study was supported by the CAMS Innovation Fund for Medical Sciences (CIFMS) (2021-I2M-1-008).

Institutional Review Board Statement: The study was conducted in accordance with the Declaration of Helsinki, and approved by the Ethics Committee of Fuwai Hospital (protocol code 2013-442, and date of approval: 29 May 2013.

Informed Consent Statement: Informed consent was obtained from all subjects involved in the study.

Data Availability Statement: Not applicable.

Acknowledgments: In this section, you can acknowledge any support given which is not covered by the author contribution or funding sections. This may include administrative and technical support, or donations in kind (e.g., materials used for experiments).

Conflicts of Interest: The authors declare no conflict of interest.

References

1. Keller, T.; Zeller, T.; Peetz, D.; Tzikas, S.; Roth, A.; Czyz, E.; Bickel, C.; Baldus, S.; Warnholtz, A.; Frohlich, M.; et al. Sensitive troponin I assay in early diagnosis of acute myocardial infarction. *N. Engl. J. Med.* **2009**, *361*, 868–877. [CrossRef] [PubMed]
2. Seto, A.H. Does "Myocardial Injury" Matter Post-PCI? *JACC. Cardiovasc. Interv.* **2019**, *12*, 1963–1965. [CrossRef] [PubMed]
3. Gollop, N.D.; Dhullipala, A.; Nagrath, N.; Myint, P.K. Is periprocedural CK-MB a better indicator of prognosis after emergency and elective percutaneous coronary intervention compared with post-procedural cardiac troponins? *Interact. Cardiovasc. Thorac. Surg.* **2013**, *17*, 867–871. [CrossRef] [PubMed]
4. Thygesen, K.; Alpert, J.S.; Jaffe, A.S.; Simoons, M.L.; Chaitman, B.R.; White, H.D.; Executive Group on behalf of the Joint European Society of Cardiology/American College of Cardiology/American Heart Association/World Heart Federation. Third Universal Definition of Myocardial Infarction. *Circulation* **2012**, *126*, 2020–2035. [CrossRef]
5. Thygesen, K.; Alpert, J.S.; Jaffe, A.S.; Chaitman, B.R.; Bax, J.J.; Morrow, D.A.; White, H.D.; Executive Group on behalf of the Joint European Society of Cardiology/American College of Cardiology/American Heart Association/World Heart Federation Task Force for the Universal Definition of Myocardial Infarction. Fourth Universal Definition of Myocardial Infarction (2018). *J. Am. Coll. Cardiol.* **2018**, *72*, 2231–2264. [CrossRef] [PubMed]
6. Bulluck, H.; Paradies, V.; Barbato, E.; Baumbach, A.; Botker, H.E.; Capodanno, D.; De Caterina, R.; Cavallini, C.; Davidson, S.M.; Feldman, D.N.; et al. Prognostically relevant periprocedural myocardial injury and infarction associated with percutaneous coronary interventions: A Consensus Document of the ESC Working Group on Cellular Biology of the Heart and European Association of Percutaneous Cardiovascular Interventions (EAPCI). *Eur. Heart J.* **2021**, *42*, 2630–2642. [CrossRef]
7. Garcia-Garcia, H.M.; McFadden, E.P.; Farb, A.; Mehran, R.; Stone, G.W.; Spertus, J.; Onuma, Y.; Morel, M.A.; van Es, G.A.; Zuckerman, B.; et al. Standardized End Point Definitions for Coronary Intervention Trials: The Academic Research Consortium-2 Consensus Document. *Eur. Heart J.* **2018**, *39*, 2192–2207. [CrossRef]
8. Huang, Z.S.; Zheng, Z.D.; Zhang, J.W.; Tang, L.L.; Zhou, L.L.; Li, S.H.; Xie, X.J.; Dong, R.M.; Zhu, J.M.; Liu, J.L. Association of major adverse cardiovascular events and cardiac troponin-I levels following percutaneous coronary intervention: A three-year follow-up study at a single center. *Eur. Rev. Med. Pharmacol. Sci.* **2020**, *24*, 3981–3992. [CrossRef]

9. Zhou, Y.; Chen, Z.; Ma, J.; Chen, A.; Lu, D.; Wu, Y.; Ren, D.; Zhang, C.; Dai, C.; Zhang, Y.; et al. Incidence, predictors and clinical significance of periprocedural myocardial injury in patients undergoing elective percutaneous coronary intervention. *J. Cardiol.* **2020**, *76*, 309–316. [CrossRef]
10. Ghersin, I.; Zahran, M.; Azzam, Z.S.; Suleiman, M.; Bahouth, F. Prognostic value of cardiac troponin levels in patients presenting with supraventricular tachycardias. *J. Electrocardiol.* **2020**, *62*, 200–203. [CrossRef]
11. Ferreira, R.M.; de Souza, E.S.N.A.; Salis, L.H.A.; da Silva, R.R.M.; Maia, P.D.; Horta, L.F.B.; Salles, E.F.; Nunes, H.M.P.; de Oliveira, J.B.M.; Domingues, Y.P.S.; et al. Troponin I elevation and all-cause mortality after elective percutaneous coronary interventions. *Cardiovasc. Revascularization Med. Incl. Mol. Interv.* **2017**, *18*, 255–260. [CrossRef] [PubMed]
12. Zeljković, I.; Manola, Š.; Radeljić, V.; Delić Brkljačić, D.; Babacanli, A.; Pavlović, N. Routinely Available Biomarkers as Long-term Predictors of Developing Systolic Dysfunction in Completely Revascularized Patients with Acute ST Elevation Myocardial Infarction. *Acta Clin. Croat.* **2019**, *58*, 95–102. [CrossRef] [PubMed]
13. Gregson, J.; Stone, G.W.; Ben-Yehuda, O.; Redfors, B.; Kandzari, D.E.; Morice, M.C.; Leon, M.B.; Kosmidou, I.; Lembo, N.J.; Brown, W.M.; et al. Implications of Alternative Definitions of Peri-Procedural Myocardial Infarction After Coronary Revascularization. *J. Am. Coll. Cardiol.* **2020**, *76*, 1609–1621. [CrossRef] [PubMed]
14. Garcia-Garcia, H.M.; McFadden, E.P.; von Birgelen, C.; Rademaker-Havinga, T.; Spitzer, E.; Kleiman, N.S.; Cohen, D.J.; Kennedy, K.F.; Camenzind, E.; Mauri, L.; et al. Impact of Periprocedural Myocardial Biomarker Elevation on Mortality Following Elective Percutaneous Coronary Intervention. *JACC. Cardiovasc. Interv.* **2019**, *12*, 1954–1962. [CrossRef]
15. Sun, S.; Ou, Y.; Shi, H.; Luo, J.; Luo, X.; Shen, Y.; Chen, Y.; Liu, X.; Zhu, Z.; Shen, W. Myocardial damage associated with elective percutaneous coronary intervention in Chinese patients: A retrospective study. *J. Int. Med. Res.* **2020**, *48*, 300060520907783. [CrossRef]
16. Zeymer, U.; Vogt, A.; Zahn, R.; Weber, M.A.; Tebbe, U.; Gottwik, M.; Bonzel, T.; Senges, J.; Neuhaus, K.L.; Arbeitsgemeinschaft Leitende Kardiologische Krankenhausärzte (ALKK). Predictors of in-hospital mortality in 1333 patients with acute myocardial infarction complicated by cardiogenic shock treated with primary percutaneous coronary intervention (PCI); Results of the primary PCI registry of the Arbeitsgemeinschaft Leitende Kardiologische Krankenhausarzte (ALKK). *Eur. Heart J.* **2004**, *25*, 322–328. [CrossRef]
17. Watanabe, Y.; Sakakura, K.; Taniguchi, Y.; Adachi, Y.; Noguchi, M.; Akashi, N.; Wada, H.; Momomura, S.I.; Fujita, H. Determinants of In-Hospital Death in Acute Myocardial Infarction with Triple Vessel Disease. *Int. Heart J.* **2016**, *57*, 697–704. [CrossRef]
18. de Waha, S.; Eitel, I.; Desch, S.; Fuernau, G.; Poss, J.; Schuler, G.; Thiele, H. Impact of multivessel coronary artery disease on reperfusion success in patients with ST-elevation myocardial infarction: A substudy of the AIDA STEMI trial. *Eur. Heart J. Acute Cardiovasc. Care* **2017**, *6*, 592–600. [CrossRef]
19. Hara, H.; Serruys, P.W.; Takahashi, K.; Kawashima, H.; Ono, M.; Gao, C.; Wang, R.; Mohr, F.W.; Holmes, D.R.; Davierwala, P.M.; et al. Impact of Peri-Procedural Myocardial Infarction on Outcomes After Revascularization. *J. Am. Coll. Cardiol.* **2020**, *76*, 1622–1639. [CrossRef]
20. Zhao, X.; Wang, Y.; Liu, C.; Zhou, P.; Sheng, Z.; Li, J.; Zhou, J.; Chen, R.; Chen, Y.; Zhao, H.; et al. Association between Variation of Troponin and Prognosis of Acute Myocardial Infarction before and after Primary Percutaneous Coronary Intervention. *J. Interv. Cardiol.* **2020**, *2020*, 4793178. [CrossRef]
21. Wang, H.Y.; Xu, B.; Dou, K.; Guan, C.; Song, L.; Huang, Y.; Zhang, R.; Xie, L.; Zhang, M.; Yan, H.; et al. Implications of Periprocedural Myocardial Biomarker Elevations and Commonly Used MI Definitions After Left Main PCI. *JACC. Cardiovasc. Interv.* **2021**, *14*, 1623–1634. [CrossRef] [PubMed]
22. Song, L.; Wang, Y.; Guan, C.; Zou, T.; Sun, Z.; Xie, L.; Zhang, R.; Dou, K.; Yang, W.; Wu, Y.; et al. Impact of Periprocedural Myocardial Injury and Infarction Definitions on Long-Term Mortality After Chronic Total Occlusion Percutaneous Coro nary Intervention. *Circ. Cardiovasc. Interv.* **2021**, *14*, e010923. [CrossRef] [PubMed]
23. Leutner, M.; Tscharre, M.; Farhan, S.; Taghizadeh Waghefi, H.; Harreiter, J.; Vogel, B.; Tentzeris, I.; Szekeres, T.; Fritzer-Szekeres, M.; Huber, K.; et al. A Sex-Specific Analysis of the Predictive Value of Troponin I and T in Patients With and Without Diabetes Mellitus After Successful Coronary Intervention. *Front. Endocrinol.* **2019**, *10*, 105. [CrossRef] [PubMed]
24. Fihn, S.D.; Gardin, J.M.; Abrams, J.; Berra, K.; Blankenship, J.C.; Dallas, A.P.; Douglas, P.S.; Foody, J.M.; Gerber, T.C.; Hinderliter, A.L.; et al. 2012 ACCF/AHA/ACP/AATS/PCNA/SCAI/STS Guideline for the diagnosis and management of patients with stable ischemic heart disease: A report of the American College of Cardiology Foundation/American Heart Association Task Force on Practice Guidelines, and the American College of Physicians, American Association for Thoracic Surgery, Preventive Cardiovascular Nurses Association, Society for Cardiovascular Angiography and Interventions, and Society of Thoracic Surgeons. *J. Am. Coll. Cardiol.* **2012**, *60*, e44–e164. [CrossRef]
25. Task Force, M.; Montalescot, G.; Sechtem, U.; Achenbach, S.; Andreotti, F.; Arden, C.; Budaj, A.; Bugiardini, R.; Crea, F.; Cuisset, T.; et al. 2013 ESC guidelines on the management of stable coronary artery disease: The Task Force on the management of stable coronary artery disease of the European Society of Cardiology. *Eur. Heart J.* **2013**, *34*, 2949–3003. [CrossRef]
26. Levine, G.N.; Bates, E.R.; Blankenship, J.C.; Bailey, S.R.; Bittl, J.A.; Cercek, B.; Chambers, C.E.; Ellis, S.G.; Guyton, R.A.; Hollenberg, S.M.; et al. 2011 ACCF/AHA/SCAI Guideline for Percutaneous Coronary Intervention: A report of the American College of Cardiology Foundation/American Heart Association Task Force on Practice Guidelines and the Society for Cardiovascular Angiography and Interventions. *Circulation* **2011**, *124*, e574–e651. [CrossRef]

27. Hamm, C.W.; Bassand, J.P.; Agewall, S.; Bax, J.; Boersma, E.; Bueno, H.; Caso, P.; Dudek, D.; Gielen, S.; Huber, K.; et al. ESC Guidelines for the management of acute coronary syndromes in patients presenting without persistent ST-segment elevation: The Task Force for the management of acute coronary syndromes (ACS) in patients presenting without persistent ST-segment elevation of the European Society of Cardiology (ESC). *Eur. Heart J.* **2011**, *32*, 2999–3054. [CrossRef]
28. Everett, B.M.; Brooks, M.M.; Vlachos, H.E.; Chaitman, B.R.; Frye, R.L.; Bhatt, D.L.; Group, B.D.S. Troponin and Cardiac Events in Stable Ischemic Heart Disease and Diabetes. *N. Engl. J. Med.* **2015**, *373*, 610–620. [CrossRef]
29. Sze, J.; Mooney, J.; Barzi, F.; Hillis, G.S.; Chow, C.K. Cardiac Troponin and its Relationship to Cardiovascular Outcomes in Community Populations-A Systematic Review and Meta-analysis. *Heart Lung Circ.* **2016**, *25*, 217–228. [CrossRef]
30. Idris, H.; Lo, S.; Shugman, I.M.; Saad, Y.; Hopkins, A.P.; Mussap, C.; Leung, D.; Thomas, L.; Juergens, C.P.; French, J.K. Varying definitions for periprocedural myocardial infarction alter event rates and prognostic implications. *J. Am. Heart Assoc.* **2014**, *3*, e001086. [CrossRef]
31. Nienhuis, M.B.; Ottervanger, J.P.; Bilo, H.J.; Dikkeschei, B.D.; Zijlstra, F. Prognostic value of troponin after elective percutaneous coronary intervention: A meta-analysis. *Catheter. Cardiovasc. Interv. Off. J. Soc. Card. Angiogr. Interv.* **2008**, *71*, 318–324. [CrossRef] [PubMed]
32. Li, Y.; Pei, H.; Bulluck, H.; Zhou, C.; Hausenloy, D.J. Periprocedural elevated myocardial biomarkers and clinical outcomes following elective percutaneous coronary intervention: A comprehensive dose-response meta-analysis of 44,972 patients from 24 prospective studies. *EuroIntervention* **2020**, *15*, 1444–1450. [CrossRef] [PubMed]
33. Silvain, J.; Zeitouni, M.; Paradies, V.; Zheng, H.L.; Ndrepepa, G.; Cavallini, C.; Feldman, D.N.; Sharma, S.K.; Mehilli, J.; Gili, S.; et al. Procedural myocardial injury, infarction and mortality in patients undergoing elective PCI: A pooled analysis of patient-level data. *Eur. Heart J.* **2021**, *42*, 323–334. [CrossRef] [PubMed]
34. Min, J.K.; Dunning, A.; Lin, F.Y.; Achenbach, S.; Al-Mallah, M.; Budoff, M.J.; Cademartiri, F.; Callister, T.Q.; Chang, H.J.; Cheng, V.; et al. Age- and sex-related differences in all-cause mortality risk based on coronary computed tomography angiography findings results from the International Multicenter CONFIRM (Coronary CT Angiography Evaluation for Clinical Outcomes: An International Multicenter Registry) of 23,854 patients without known coronary artery disease. *J. Am. Coll. Cardiol.* **2011**, *58*, 849–860. [CrossRef]
35. Schulman-Marcus, J.; Hartaigh, B.O.; Gransar, H.; Lin, F.; Valenti, V.; Cho, I.; Berman, D.; Callister, T.; DeLago, A.; Hadamitzky, M.; et al. Sex-Specific Associations Between Coronary Artery Plaque Extent and Risk of Major Adverse Cardiovascular Events: The CONFIRM Long-Term Registry. *JACC Cardiovasc. Imaging* **2016**, *9*, 364–372. [CrossRef]
36. Ando, T.; Takagi, H.; Grines, C.L. Complete versus incomplete revascularization with drug-eluting stents for multi-vessel disease in stable, unstable angina or non-ST-segment elevation myocardial infarction: A meta-analysis. *J. Interv. Cardiol.* **2017**, *30*, 309–317. [CrossRef]
37. Tsai, I.T.; Wang, C.P.; Lu, Y.C.; Hung, W.C.; Wu, C.C.; Lu, L.F.; Chung, F.M.; Hsu, C.C.; Lee, Y.J.; Yu, T.H. The burden of major adverse cardiac events in patients with coronary artery disease. *BMC Cardiovasc. Disord.* **2017**, *17*, 1. [CrossRef]
38. Chen, Z.W.; Yang, H.B.; Chen, Y.H.; Ma, J.Y.; Qian, J.Y.; Ge, J.B. Impact of multi-vessel therapy to the risk of periprocedural myocardial injury after elective coronary intervention: Exploratory study. *BMC Cardiovasc. Disord.* **2017**, *17*, 69. [CrossRef]
39. Lo, N.; Michael, T.T.; Moin, D.; Patel, V.G.; Alomar, M.; Papayannis, A.; Cipher, D.; Abdullah, S.M.; Banerjee, S.; Brilakis, E.S. Periprocedural myocardial injury in chronic total occlusion percutaneous interventions: A systematic cardiac biomarker evaluation study. *JACC. Cardiovasc. Interv.* **2014**, *7*, 47–54. [CrossRef]
40. Selvanayagam, J.B.; Porto, I.; Channon, K.; Petersen, S.E.; Francis, J.M.; Neubauer, S.; Banning, A.P. Troponin elevation after percutaneous coronary intervention directly represents the extent of irreversible myocardial injury: Insights from cardiovascular magnetic resonance imaging. *Circulation* **2005**, *111*, 1027–1032. [CrossRef]

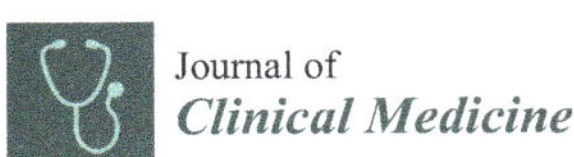

Journal of
Clinical Medicine

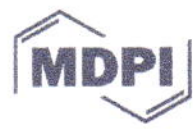

Article

Upper-Arm SBP Decline Associated with Repeated Cuff-Oscillometric Inflation Significantly Correlated with the Arterial Stiffness Index

Noriyuki Kawaura [1], Rie Nakashima-Sasaki [1], Hiroshi Doi [2], Kotaro Uchida [1], Takuya Sugawara [1], Sae Saigo [3], Kaito Abe [1], Kentaro Arakawa [1], Koichi Tamura [1], Kiyoshi Hibi [4] and Tomoaki Ishigami [1,*]

1 Department of Medical Science and Cardiorenal Medicine, Yokohama City University Graduate School of Medicine, Yokohama 236-0004, Japan
2 Kawasaki Saiwai Clinic, Kawasaki 212-0016, Japan
3 Department of Cardiology, Kanagawa Cardiovascular and Respiratory Center, Yokohama 236-0051, Japan
4 Department of Cardiology, Yokohama City Medical Center, Yokohama 232-0024, Japan
* Correspondence: tommmish@hotmail.com or tommmis@yokohama-cu.ac.jp; Tel.: +81-45-787-2635; Fax: +81-45-701-3738

Abstract: We evaluated the clinical significance of the new non-invasive vascular indices to explore their potential utility using repeated cuff-oscillometric inflation. In 250 consecutive outpatients, we performed a cross-sectional, retrospective, single-center, observational study to investigate sequential differences in arterial stiffness using blood pressure, arterial velocity pulse index (AVI), and arterial pressure volume index (API) with repeated measurements. Males accounted for 62.7% of the patients, and the mean age was 68.1 ± 12.1 years. The mean systolic blood pressure (SBP) and diastolic blood pressure (DBP) of the first reading in repeated measurements were 133.07 ± 21.20 mmHg and 73.94 ± 13.56 mmHg, respectively. The mean AVI and API were 23.83 ± 8.30 and 31.12 ± 7.86, respectively. In each measurement of these parameters, although DBP and AVI did not show significant changes throughout repeated measurements, SBP and API decreased significantly according to the measurement orders. Furthermore, changes in SBP and API were significantly correlated in several of the models. In this study, it was concluded that upper-arm SBP decline associated with repeated cuff-oscillometric inflation was significantly correlated with the arterial stiffness index. The findings of this study will allow clinicians to easily recognize the progression of atherosclerosis through regular, routine practice. In conclusion, this study suggests that changes in repeated SBP measurements may be predictive of arterial stiffness and atherosclerosis.

Keywords: arterial stiffness; atherosclerosis; non-invasive; cuff-oscillometric; repeated measurements; blood pressure change

Citation: Kawaura, N.; Nakashima-Sasaki, R.; Doi, H.; Uchida, K.; Sugawara, T.; Saigo, S.; Abe, K.; Arakawa, K.; Tamura, K.; Hibi, K.; et al. Upper-Arm SBP Decline Associated with Repeated Cuff-Oscillometric Inflation Significantly Correlated with the Arterial Stiffness Index. *J. Clin. Med.* **2022**, *11*, 6455. https://doi.org/10.3390/jcm11216455

Academic Editors: Jose Luis Sanchez-Quesada and Alessandro Delitala

Received: 8 September 2022
Accepted: 24 October 2022
Published: 31 October 2022

1. Introduction

Atherosclerosis is the common result of the advanced progression of diseases based on diet and exercise in daily life, such as hypertension (HT), diabetes, dyslipidemia (DL), or lifestyle-related diseases. Consequently, atherosclerosis can lead to fatal cardiovascular events, and it is necessary to salvage and counteract life-threatening diseases such as acute myocardial infarction and acute cerebral infarction. Even if fatality can be avoided, it is a strong limiting factor for healthy life expectancy as it can cause serious sequelae with disability and result in the need for permanent nursing care [1–3].

To date, the mainstream countermeasures against atherosclerotic events have been the establishment of a life-saving emergency system that concentrates medical resources on the disease and its symptoms that develop in an acute catastrophe and the control of population risk through public and personal hygiene by controlling blood pressure (BP), blood sugar, and lipids, which are risk factors for the disease. The former requires not only enormous social costs, including human and medical resources and costs, for unpredictable lethal events but also poses other challenges, such as regional disparities among nationwide healthcare services that can and cannot supply them and inappropriate work overload for healthcare personnel [4,5]. The latter is expected to have a uniform effect with no regional differences; however, its results for medical care may take a long time to achieve, and there is also the problem of lack of certainty. Therefore, since atherosclerosis is a disease caused by an abnormal biological process, its control and suppression require both molecular and cellular level understanding of its pathogenesis and technological innovations [6]. Current oncology has made substantial progress with a successful inventory of various molecular target biologics [7]. Additionally, earlier diagnosis and detection of unaware subclinical atherosclerosis with less invasive clinical devices are necessary to adequately monitor disease progression, which is necessary for novel drug discovery in these areas [3].

Recent technological innovations have made it possible for us to use the AVE-1500 (Shisei Datum, Tokyo, Japan), which can easily measure indices reflecting arterial stiffness and central arterial pressure with little physical burden using the cuff-oscillometric method. The AVE-1500 can measure the arterial pressure volume index (API), an index reflecting arterial stiffness, and the arterial velocity pulse index (AVI), an index reflecting central arterial pressure. Several studies have clarified the relationship between these indices and arterial stiffness [8,9].

HT is one of the most important lifestyle-related diseases that causes atherosclerosis. Guidelines for the management of HT have been established by various academic societies worldwide. It is frequently observed that repeated measurement of BP changes its value; therefore, the guidelines recommend using an average of two or three measurements on a single occasion [10–12]. Repeated cuff-oscillometric inflation is necessary to measure the BP two or three times on a single occasion, and it is frequently noted that BP changes were observed throughout the measurements. Our analyses aimed to reveal the regularity of BP changes with repeated cuff-oscillometric inflation at BP measurements.

It is unknown how repeated cuff-oscillometric inflations with BP measurement are related to arterial stiffness and central arterial pressure and how changes to the API and AVI will be brought about by repeated cuff-oscillometric inflations. Therefore, in the present study, we evaluated the clinical significance of the new non-invasive vascular indices, AVI and API, in outpatients with various clinical backgrounds to explore the potential utility of these two indices by using repeated cuff-oscillometric inflation in actual clinical settings.

2. Materials and Methods

2.1. Study Design and Population

We performed a cross-sectional, retrospective, observational study at the Yokohama City University Hospital in Japan. The study protocol was registered and approved by the ethics committee of Yokohama City University Hospital in 2015 (B150701005) with notifications for guaranteed withdrawal of participants on the website providing means of "opt-out," and due to the non-invasive observational study design, we did not request additional informed consent from the participants.

We used a multifunctional BP monitoring device, AVE-1500 (Shisei Datum, Tokyo, Japan), to evaluate the AVI and API in 250 consecutive outpatients in the Department of Medical Science and Cardiorenal Medicine between May 2013 and March 2015. Patients who had atrial fibrillation were excluded from the study. Medical records were reviewed to collect data for each patient's profile, general status, medical history, laboratory data, and concomitant medications. HT was defined as systolic BP (SBP) of $\geq$140 mmHg, diastolic BP (DBP) of $\geq$90 mmHg, or ongoing medical treatment for HT. DL was defined as a low-density lipoprotein (LDL) cholesterol level of $\geq$140 mg/dl, triglyceride level of $\geq$150 mg/dl, high-density lipoprotein (HDL) cholesterol level of $\leq$40 mg/dl, or ongoing medical treatment for DL. Chronic heart failure was defined as a B-type natriuretic peptide level of $\geq$40 pg/mL caused by cardiovascular disease. Valvular heart disease was defined as valve regurgitation/stenosis of at least a moderate degree. Plasma glucose and triglyceride levels were measured using casual blood sampling without overnight fasting.

2.2. AVI and API

Both AVI and API are novel arterial indices measurable by a multifunctional BP monitoring device, AVE-1500 (Shisei Datum, Tokyo, Japan), with cuff-oscillometric-based technologies. The AVI is an index of the characteristics of the pulse waveform at high cuff pressures above the maximum BP. Recent findings have revealed that central arterial stiffness and characteristics are strongly reflected in the pulse wave in this pressure region [8,9]. This pulse wave has an increased late systolic waveform and a steeper falling curve thereafter, owing to an increase in the reflected wave due to aging, stiffening, and increased peripheral resistance. However, the ejection phase is not affected by the reflected wave, and as a result, the pulse wave amplitude differentiated from the ejection phase increases only the velocity change during brachial artery diastole (cardiac systole) out of the absolute value of the bottom of the valley of differentiated waveforms between pulse wave and time (Vr) and velocity change during brachial artery relaxation (cardiac diastole), and the value of the pulse waveform characteristics (Vr/first peak of the differentiated waveform between pulse wave and time (Vf)) become an index that varies with the magnitude of the reflected wave [13].

The API is an index of arterial pressure–volume characteristics derived from the arterial volume change resulting from cuff pressure relative to the internal and external pressure difference (BP–cuff pressure) applied to the arterial wall. Previous studies have shown that softer vessels show more rapid changes in arterial volume with changes in cuff pressure and that the degree of the slope of this curve varies primarily with the stiffness of the vessel's media and adventitia. API has developed and indexed a method to stably evaluate the differences in this characteristic [9].

The AVE-1500 (Shisei Datum, Tokyo, Japan) is a newly developed device that can non-invasively evaluate arterial stiffness and endothelial dysfunction of the central arteries (AVI) and peripheral arteries (API) using a cuff-oscillometric method in a single BP measurement. AVI and API were measured using an AVE-1500 with the participants in the supine position. Finally, the AVE-1500 can evaluate the conventional SBP, DBP, API, AVI, and pulse rate in a single measurement.

Measurements were taken at least thrice for each participant in a quiet temperature-controlled room (24.0–26.8 °C). The average measurements for API and AVI at the time of participant enrollment were used for subsequent analyses.

2.3. Statistical Analysis

Data are shown as the mean ± standard deviation for continuous variables and as frequencies and percentages for categorical variables. Analysis for time-series measurements was compared using repeated measures analysis of variance and Friedman rank sum test, with additional analysis using the Holm method. Statistical significance was set at $p < 0.05$. The relationships between AVI and API and all other variables were analyzed using a linear regression model and Pearson's correlation coefficient. Statistical analysis was performed using R version 4.1.2 (The R Foundation for Statistical Computing, Vienna, Austria).

3. Results

3.1. Baseline Characteristics

Of the 250 enrolled participants, 236 who met the inclusion criteria and did not have missing key data were analyzed. The baseline patient characteristics are shown in Table 1. Of the patients, 62.7% were males, with an overall mean age of 68.1 ± 12.1 years. This study included 158 patients with HT (67.0%), 48 with diabetes (20.3%), and 109 with DL (46.2%). The mean creatinine (Cr) and estimated glomerular filtration rate were 0.98 ± 1.01 mg/dl and 69.26 ± 23.72 mL/min/1.73 m^2, respectively. In Table 2, the antihypertensive drugs were renin–angiotensin system inhibitors (121 patients, 51.3%), calcium-channel antagonists (119 patients, 50.4%), β-blockers (71 patients, 30.1%), and diuretics (54 patients, 22.9%). The mean SBP and DBP of the first measurement were 133.1 ± 21.2 mmHg and 73.9 ± 13.6 mmHg, respectively (Table 3). The mean AVI and API of the first measurement were 23.8 ± 8.3 and 31.1 ± 7.9, respectively. The total number of BP, AVI, and API measurements was 2452; therefore, an average of 9.89 measurements per person were performed.

Table 1. Baseline characteristics.

	Male (*n* = 148)	Female (*n* = 88)	Total (*n* = 236)
Age (years)	68.0 ± 12.1	68.2 ± 12.1	68.1 ± 12.1
Hypertension (%)	99 (66.9)	59 (67.1)	158 (67.0)
Diabetes (%)	38 (25.7)	10 (11.4)	48 (20.3)
Dyslipidemia (%)	70 (47.3)	39 (44.3)	109 (46.2)
IHD (%)	28 (18.9)	6 (6.8)	34 (14.4)
ASO (%)	11 (7.4)	4 (4.6)	15 (6.4)
VHD (%)	11 (7.4)	10 (11.4)	21 (8.9)
OMI (%)	12 (8.1)	4 (4.6)	16 (6.8)
CHF (%)	20 (13.5)	10 (11.4)	30 (12.7)
Cardiomyopathy (%)	5 (3.4)	4 (4.6)	9 (3.8)
PH (%)	1 (0.7)	3 (3.4)	4 (1.7)
AF (%)	29 (19.6)	7 (8.0)	36 (15.3)
PM/ICD (%)	2 (1.4)	0 (0)	2 (0.85)
COPD (%)	5 (3.4)	0 (0)	5 (2.1)
Smoking			
Current (%)	24 (16.2)	7 (8.0)	31 (13.2)
Past (%)	61 (41.2)	6 (6.8)	67 (28.4)
Never (%)	63 (42.6)	75 (85.2)	138 (58.4)
Laboratory data			
Creatinine (mg/dL)	1.12 ± 1.20	0.73 ±0.46	0.98 ± 1.01
eGFR (mL/min/1.73 m^2)	67.45 ± 21.96	72.43 ± 26.34	69.26 ± 23.72
Uric acid (mg/dL)	5.90 ± 1.46	5.01 ± 1.35	5.58 ± 1.49
Plasma glucose (mg/dL)	130.29 ± 34.35	116.92 ± 32.07	125.84 ± 34.07
HbA1c (%)	6.10 ± 0.84	6.15 ± 1.00	6.11 ± 0.89
CRP (mg/dL)	0.32 ± 0.75	0.49 ± 1.25	0.38 ± 0.96
TG (mg/dL)	143.63 ± 80.09	152.28 ± 95.43	146.49 ± 85.35
HDL-C (mg/dL)	59.10 ± 16.30	66.58 ± 22.38	61.54 ± 18.79
LDL-C (mg/dL)	105.27 ± 34.80	115.47 ± 35.78	108.85 ± 35.38
T-Cho (mg/dL)	181.37 ± 37.64	204.55 ± 44.24	189.29 ± 41.36
BNP (pg/mL)	121.06 ± 230.01	62.6 ± 106.4	99.93 ± 196.27

Data are presented as the mean ± standard deviation or *n* (%). IHD, ischemic heart disease; ASO, arteriosclerosis obliterans; VHD, valvular heart disease; OMI, old myocardial infarction; CHF, chronic heart disease; PH, pulmonary hypertension; AF, atrial fibrillation; PM/ICD, pacemaker/implantable cardioverter-defibrillator; COPD, chronic obstructive pulmonary disease; eGFR, estimated glomerular filtration rate; HbA1c, glycosylated hemoglobin; CRP, C-reactive protein; TG, triglyceride; HDL-C, high-density lipoprotein cholesterol; LDL-C, low-density lipoprotein cholesterol; T-Cho, total cholesterol; BNP, brain natriuretic peptide.

Table 2. Medications at baseline.

	Male **(n = 148)**	**Female** **(n = 88)**	**Total** **(n = 236)**
RAS inhibitors (%)	79 (53.4)	42 (47.7)	121 (51.3)
Ca antagonists (%)	72 (48.7)	47 (53.4)	119 (50.4)
β-blockers (%)	48 (32.4)	23 (26.1)	71 (30.1)
Diuretics (%)	32 (21.6)	22 (25.0)	54 (22.9)
α-blockers (%)	1 (0.7)	1 (1.1)	2 (0.9)
Nitrites (%)	16 (10.8)	8 (9.1)	24 (10.2)
Biguanides (%)	7 (4.7)	3 (3.4)	10 (4.2)
Statins (%)	60 (40.5)	39 (44.3)	99 (42.0)
Bezafibrates (%)	7 (4.7)	2 (2.3)	9 (3.8)
EPA (%)	6 (4.1)	1 (1.1)	7 (3.0)
Ezetimibe (%)	6 (4.1)	3 (3.4)	9 (3.8)
Sulfonylureas (%)	11 (7.4)	1 (1.1)	12 (5.1)
α-glucosidase inhibitors (%)	13 (8.8)	0 (0)	13 (4.3)
Thiazolidine (%)	6 (4.1)	1 (1.1)	7 (3.0)
DPP-4 inhibitors (%)	17 (11.5)	6 (6.8)	23 (9.8)
GLP-1 analogs (%)	2 (1.4)	0 (0)	2 (0.9)
Insulin (%)	8 (5.4)	2 (2.3)	10 (4.2)
Aspirin (%)	46 (31.1)	18 (20.5)	64 (27.1)
Thienopyridine (%)	15 (10.1)	3 (3.4)	18 (7.6)
Cilostazol (%)	6 (4.1)	4 (4.6)	10 (4.2)
Sarpogrelate (%)	1 (0.7)	0 (0)	1 (0.4)
Dipyridamole (%)	0 (0)	0 (0)	0 (0)
Prostaglandin (%)	3 (2.0)	1 (1.1)	4 (1.7)

Data are presented as the mean ± standard deviation or n (%). RAS, renin-angiotensin system; Ca, calcium; EPA, eicosapentaenoic acid; DPP-4, dipeptidyl-peptidase-4; GLP-1, glucagon-like peptide-1.

Table 3. Measurements of Blood pressure, AVI and API at baseline.

	Male **(n = 148)**	**Female** **(n = 88)**	**Total** **(n = 236)**
SBP (mmHg)	131.9 ± 19.8	135.2 ± 23.4	133.1 ± 21.2
DBP (mmHg)	75.3 ± 34.4	71.7 ± 14.4	73.9 ± 13.6
AVI	22.9 ± 8.4	25.4 ± 7.9	23.8 ± 8.3
API	29.3 ± 6.9	34.2 ± 8.5	31.1 ± 7.9
Pulse rate (/min)	73.5 ± 12.4	75.2 ± 14.4	74.1 ± 13.2
Measurements of AVI and API			
Total number	1545	907	2452
Total visits	300	496	796
Per visit per person	3.02	3.12	3.04

Data are presented as the mean ± standard deviation or n (%). SBP, systolic blood pressure; DBP, diastolic blood pressure; AVI, arterial velocity pulse index; API, arterial pressure volume index.

3.2. Changes in BP, API, and AVI with Repeated Measurements

The results of the repeated measurements of BP (SBP/DBP), AVI, and API are shown in Table 4 and Figure 1. The average of the first SBP measurement in repeated measurements (SBP01) was 136.6 mmHg, the second (SBP02) was 133.6 mmHg, and the third (SBP03) was 131.9 mmHg. The average of each measurement of DBP, AVI, and API is also shown in Table 4. In each measurement, although DBP and AVI did not show significant changes throughout the measurements, SBP and API decreased significantly according to the measurement orders, as shown in Figure 1.

Table 4. The average of each measurement in repeated measurements.

	First Measurement	Second Measurement	Third Measurement
SBP	136.6± 20.4	133.6 ± 19.8	131.9 ± 18.2
DBP	74.5 ± 13.8	74.0 ± 12.7	73.7 ± 13.0
AVI	23.8 ± 8.2	24.1 ± 7.8	24.2 ± 7.7
API	32.5 ± 8.8	31.1 ± 6.5	30.5 ± 6.4

SBP, systolic blood pressure; DBP, diastolic blood pressure; AVI, arterial velocity pulse index; API, arterial pressure volume index.

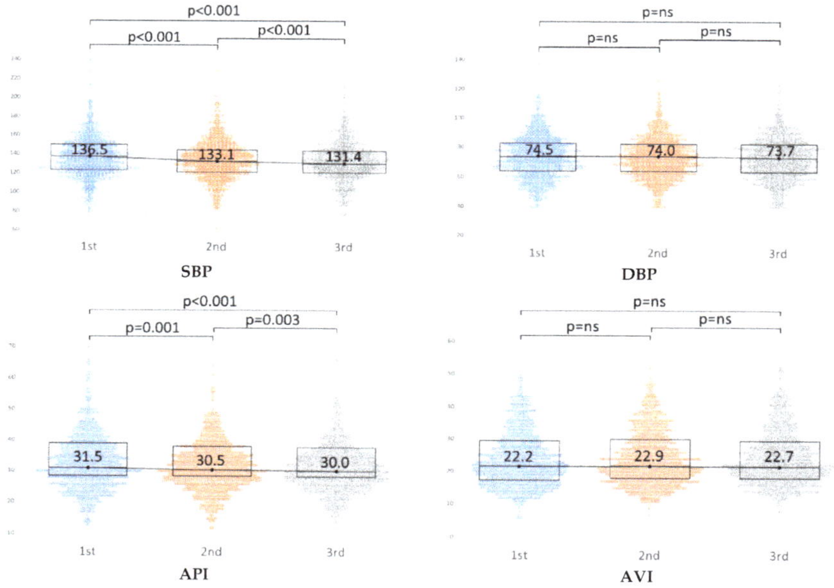

Figure 1. Changes in the repeated measurements of blood pressure (BP) (SBP/DBP), AVI, and API. The value of BP is represented in mmHg. Significant changes are indicated by $p < 0.05$. SBP, systolic blood pressure; DBP, diastolic blood pressure; AVI, arterial velocity pulse index; API, arterial pressure volume index.

3.3. Regression Analysis of the Relationship between Novel Vascular Indices and Clinical Characteristics

Univariate and multivariate analyses of SBP change, defined as "ΔSBP = (SBP01 − SBP03)/SBP01, were conducted to determine the association between each clinical parameter and measure (Tables 5 and 6). In the univariate analysis of the SBP change, sex and Cr were significant in this model, and in the multivariate analysis, sex was significant (Table 5). The same model was adapted for the API. Regarding the API change, in the univariate analysis, age, diabetes mellitus (DM), sex, and Cr were significant in this model, whereas in the multivariate analysis, only age, DM and Cr were significant (Table 6). ΔSBP and ΔAPI were significantly correlated (Figure 2). Moreover, another three models (models 1 and 2: ΔSBP = (SBP01 − SBP03)/SBP01, models 3 and 4: ΔSBP = (SBP01 − SBP03)/mean SBP, models 1 and 3 included hemodialysis patients; models 2 and 4 did not include hemodialysis patients) were created and analyzed to ensure that the analysis was accurate for the phenomenon that occurred. In the univariate analysis of the changes in SBP, sex, Cr, smoker and LDL were significant in some models, and in the multivariate analysis, LDL was significant in one model and sex was significant in all models. Regarding the changes in API, in the univariate analysis, age, diabetes mellitus (DM), sex, Cr, and ischemic heart disease (IHD) were significant in some models, whereas in the multivariate analysis, only age and DM were significant in all models. In all models, ΔSBP and ΔAPI were significantly correlated.

Table 5. Multivariate regression results with SBP change.

Independent Variables	Standardized Regression Estimate	95%CI		*p*
Sex	0.0261	0.0081	0.0440	0.005 *
Creatinine	−0.0058	−0.0134	0.0019	0.14

Multivariate regression results with SBP change were analyzed. SBP change was defined as (SBP01 − SBP03)/SBP01. The adopted independent variables were significant in the univariate regression analysis. Hypertension was excluded from the analysis because of its presumed strong relationship with SBP. Adjusted R-squared 0.044, F-statistic 6.238, *p*-value 0.002. SBP, systolic blood pressure; SBP01 (03), first (third) SBP measurement in the repeated measurements. * $p < 0.05$.

Table 6. Multivariate regression results with API change.

Independent Variables	Standardized Regression Estimate	95%CI		*p*
Age	−0.0020	−0.0038	−0.0003	0.020 *
Diabetes	−0.0578	−0.1105	−0.0050	0.032 *
Sex	0.0248	−0.0200	0.0695	0.276
Creatinine	−0.0189	−0.0378	−0.00001	0.050

Multivariate regression results with API change were analyzed. API change was defined as (API01 − API03)/API01. The adopted independent variables were significant in the univariate regression analysis. Adjusted R-squared 0.060, F-statistic 4.63, *p*-value 0.001. API, arterial pressure volume index; API01 (03), first (third) API measurement in the repeated measurements. * $p < 0.05$.

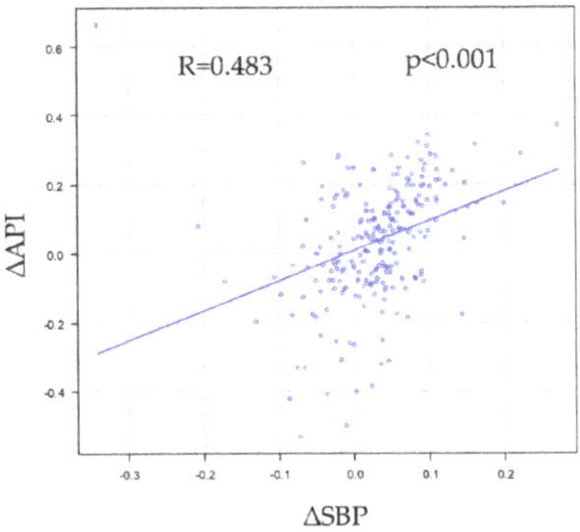

Figure 2. Correlations between SBP change (ΔSBP) and API change (ΔAPI). ΔSBP was defined as (SBP01 − SBP03)/SBP01, and the same model was adapted for the API (ΔAPI = (API01 − API03)/API01). ΔSBP and ΔAPI significantly correlated (R = 0.483, $p < 0.001$). API, arterial pressure volume index; SBP, systolic blood pressure; SBP01 (API01), first SBP (API) measurement in repeated measurements; SBP03 (API03), third SBP (API03) measurement in the repeated measurements.

4. Discussion

The AVE-1500 is a newly developed medical device that can simultaneously measure BP and evaluate peripheral arterial stiffness and central arterial pressure [14,15]. In the present study, we used the AVE-1500 to measure API, an index of peripheral arterial stiffness, and AVI, an index of central arterial pressure, not in a single measurement but in repeated BP measurements, and showed the relationship between these changes. We also investigated the relationship between these changes and each of the parameters associated with atherosclerosis. In the repeated measurements of BP and API/AVI, the changes in SBP and API showed a similar regression that decreased by measurement thrice. In the univariate analysis of the changes in SBP, sex, smoking, Cr, and LDL were significant in some models, and in the multivariate analysis, LDL was significant in one model and sex was significant in all models. Regarding the changes in API, in the univariate analysis, age, DM, sex, Cr, and IHD were significant in some models, while in the multivariate analysis, only age and DM were significant in all models.

Several studies have reported changes with repeated BP measurements on a single occasion. Some reports have suggested that the second measurement is lower than the first, and the third measurement is lower than the second [16,17]. Other reports have indicated that the measurement interval has some influence on changes in repeated BP measurements [18]. Our study also showed a significant stepwise decrease in the first, second, and third measurements, similar to previous reports. On the other hand, some reports have suggested that BP variability can be attributed to psychological effects and regression to the mean, in addition to baroreflex effects [19,20]. The current guidelines for HT in most societies recommend measuring BP at least twice on a single occasion [10–12].

In previous studies that investigated the relationship between BP and API/AVI on single measurements, almost all the studies we examined showed significant correlations between SBP and API [21–24]. In most of these studies, the strength of the correlation was moderate, while some studies showed a strong correlation. Although regression analysis has also shown significant results in several studies, all of them were based on single measurements. The correlation between SBP and API in a single measurement was also significant in the present study. Moreover, to further explore the relationship between these two variables, we focused on the changes in SBP and API, which showed a linear decreasing type with statistical significance in repeated measurements, and analyzed the relationship between them. To analyze the changes in SBP and API, two models were used: one in which the change was divided by the first measurement and the other in which the change was divided by the average of the three measurements to ensure that the analysis was accurate for the phenomenon that occurred. The results showed that in both models, there was a significant correlation between the changes in SBP and API.

The results of the analyses of the relationship between the changes in API and SBP with repeat measurements and some variables in the four models showed that SBP and API were related to variables known to be associated with arterial stiffness and atherosclerosis. Although previous studies have examined SBP and API using single measurements (not repeated measurements), significant correlations were noted for age, the prevalence of diabetes, smoking, and sex, and the results were consistent with those of the present study [9,21–23].

Although there have been several previous reports on the comparison of BP and API/AVI with risk factors for atherosclerosis in single measurements, to the best of our knowledge, this is the first report of a study investigating the relationship between BP and API/AVI with changes in repeated measurements. Prior to the development of the AVE-1500, BP and vascular stiffness indices such as API/AVI were evaluated separately with different devices to measure them; therefore, the relationship between them was undetermined. However, with the new development of the AVE-1500 BP and pulse wave meter, both can now be compared simultaneously, making it possible to better determine the relationship between BP and central artery index and arterial stiffness. Although the relationship between SBP and API in a single measurement has already been reported in previous studies because of the availability of simultaneous measurements, we confirmed that the relationship was stronger by adding evaluation with repeated measurements in the present study. The reason for the strong relationship between SBP and API may be that API is an index of arterial stiffness, as mentioned above, as well as an index of arterial volume change from the viewpoint of the measurement principle; therefore, it is appropriate from the measurement principle that the changes in API show a strong relation to the changes in SBP. In other words, this study suggests that changes in repeated SBP measurements may be predictive of arterial stiffness and atherosclerosis. However, we cannot conclude whether "SBP decline with repeated cuff-oscillometric pressure" can be used as a substitute for arterial stiffness in this study alone, and we can only propose a hypothesis. It is necessary to examine it from a different perspective, for example, by comparing it with other stiffness modalities.

The present study has some limitations. The study was cross-sectional and retrospective, and the sample size was relatively small. In addition, the participants of this study were outpatients of a cardiorenal division. Therefore, future research is required, and we believe that this study only proves the concept of a voluminous subject. However, we have concluded that we might be able to take arterial stiffness and stiffness one step further in the present study by using the new device AVE-1500. The authors should discuss the results and how they can be interpreted from the perspective of previous studies and the working hypotheses. These findings and their implications should be discussed in the broadest possible context. Future research directions may also be highlighted.

5. Conclusions

In conclusion, this study suggests that changes in repeated SBP measurements may be predictive of arterial stiffness and atherosclerosis.

Author Contributions: Conceptualization, N.K. and T.I.; methodology, N.K. and T.I.; software, N.K. and T.I.; validation, R.N.-S., H.D., K.U., T.S., S.S., K.A. (Kaito Abe), K.A. (Kentaro Arakawa), K.T., K.H., N.K. and T.I.; formal analysis, K.A. (Kaito Abe); investigation, R.N.-S., H.D., N.K. and T.I.; resources, R.N.-S., H.D., N.K. and T.I.; data curation, R.N.-S., H.D., S.S., N.K. and T.I.; writing—original draft preparation, N.K. and T.I.; writing—review and editing, N.K. and T.I.; visualization, N.K. and T.I.; supervision, T.I.; project administration, N.K. and T.I.; All authors have read and agreed to the published version of the manuscript.

Funding: This research received no external funding.

Institutional Review Board Statement: The study was conducted according to the guidelines of the Declaration of Helsinki, and approved by the Yokohama City University Hospital Institutional Review Board (IRB) ethics committee (protocol code B150701005 and 7 August 2015).

Informed Consent Statement: Informed consent was obtained from all the subjects involved in the study.

Data Availability Statement: The data presented in this study are available upon request from the corresponding author. The data are not publicly available due to privacy regulations.

Conflicts of Interest: The authors declare no conflict of interest.

References

1. Lee, H.Y.; Oh, B.H. Aging and arterial stiffness. *Circ. J.* **2010**, *74*, 2257–2262. [CrossRef] [PubMed]
2. Singhal, A. Endothelial dysfunction: Role in obesity-related disorders and the early origins of CVD. *Proc. Nutr. Soc.* **2005**, *64*, 15–22. [CrossRef] [PubMed]
3. Nabel, E.G.; Braunwald, E. A tale of coronary artery disease and myocardial infarction. *N. Engl. J. Med.* **2012**, *366*, 54–63. [CrossRef] [PubMed]
4. Rajaram, V.; Pandhya, P.; Patel, S.; Peter, M.M.; Goldin, M. Role of surrogate markers in assessing patients with diabetes mellitus and the metabolic syndrome and in evaluating lipid-lowering therapy. *Am. J. Cardiol.* **2004**, *93*, 32–48. [CrossRef] [PubMed]
5. Birmpili, P.; Johal, A.; Li, Q.; Waton, S.; Chetter, I.; Boyle, J.R.; Cromwell, D. Factors associated with delays in revascularization in patients with chronic limb-threatening ischaemia: Population-based cohort study. *Br. J. Surg.* **2021**, *108*, 951–959. [CrossRef]
6. Falk, E. Pathogenesis of Atherosclerosis Viewpoint. *J. Am. Coll. Cardiol.* **2006**, *47* (Suppl. 8), C7–C12. [CrossRef]

7. Yamamoto, Y.; Kanayama, N.; Nakayama, Y. Current status, issues and future prospects of personalized medicine for each disease. *J. Pers. Med.* **2022**, *12*, 444. [CrossRef]
8. Liang, F.; Takagi, S.; Himeno, R.; Liu, H. A computational model of the cardiovascular system coupled with an upper-arm oscillometric cuff and its application to studying the suprasystolic cuff oscillation wave, concerning its value in assessing arterial stiffness. *Comput. Methods Biomech. Biomed. Eng.* **2013**, *16*, 141–145. [CrossRef]
9. Komine, H.; Asai, Y.; Yokoi, T.; Yoshizawa, M. Non-invasive assessment of arterial stiffness using oscillometric blood pressure measurement. *Biomed. Eng. Online* **2012**, *11*, 6. [CrossRef]
10. Mancia, G.; Fagard, R.; Narkiewicz, K.; Redón, J.; Zanchetti, A.; Böhm, M.; Christiaens, T.; Cifkova, R.; De Backer, G.; Dominiczak, A. 2013 ESH/ESC guidelines for the management of arterial hypertension: The task force for the management of arterial hypertension of the European society of hypertension (ESH) and of the European society of cardiology (ESC). *Eur. Heart J.* **2013**, *34*, 2159–2219. [CrossRef]
11. Whelton, P.K.; Carey, R.M.; Aronow, W.S.; Casey, D.E., Jr.; Collins, K.J.; Dennison Himmelfarb, C.; DePalma, S.M.; Gidding, S.; Jamerson, K.A.; Jones, D.W. ACC/AHA/AAPA/ABC/ACPM/AGS/APhA/ASH/ASPC/NMA/PCNA guideline for the prevention, detection, evaluation, and management of high blood pressure in adults: A report of the American college of cardiology/American heart association task force on clinical practice guidelines. *Hypertension* **2017**, *71*, e13. [PubMed]
12. Umemura, S.; Arima, H.; Arima, S.; Asayama, K.; Dohi, Y.; Hirooka, Y.; Horio, T.; Hoshide, S.; Ikeda, S.; Ishimitsu, T.; et al. The Japanese Society of Hypertension Guidelines for the Management of Hypertension (JSH 2019). *Hypertens. Res.* **2019**, *42*, 1235–1481. [CrossRef] [PubMed]
13. Sueta, D.; Yamamoto, E.; Tanaka, T.; Hirata, Y.; Sakamoto, K.; Tsujita, K. The accuracy of central blood pressure waveform by novel mathematical transformation of non-invasive measurement. *Int. J. Cardiol.* **2015**, *189*, 244–246. [CrossRef] [PubMed]
14. Sasaki-Nakashima, R.; Kino, T.; Chen, L.; Doi, H.; Ishigami, T. Successful prediction of cardiovascular risk by new non-invasive vascular indexes using suprasystolic cuff oscillometric waveform analysis. *J. Cardiol.* **2017**, *69*, 30–37. [CrossRef] [PubMed]
15. Doi, H.; Ishigami, T.; Nakashima-Sasaki, R.; Kino, T.; Chen, L. New non-invasive indexes of arterial stiffness are significantly correlated with severity and complexity of coronary atherosclerosis. *Clin. Exp. Hypertens.* **2018**, *41*, 187–193. [CrossRef]
16. Kawabe, H.; Saito, I.; Saruta, T. Influence of repeated measurement on one occasion, on successive days, and on workdays on home blood pressure values. *Clin. Exp. Hypertens.* **2005**, *27*, 215–222. [CrossRef]
17. Eguchi, K.; Kuruvilla, S.; Ogedegbe, G.; Gerin, W.; Schwartz, J.E.; Pickering, T.G. What is the optimal interval between successive home blood pressure readings using an automated oscillometric device? *J. Hypertens.* **2009**, *27*, 1172. [CrossRef]
18. Imamura, M.; Asayama, K.; Sawanoi, Y.; Shiga, T.; Saito, K.; Ohkubo, T. Effects of measurement intervals on the values of repeated auscultatory blood pressure measurements. *Clin. Exp. Hypertens.* **2020**, *42*, 105–109. [CrossRef]
19. van Loo, J.M.; Peer, P.G.; Thien, T.A. Twenty-five minutes between blood pressure readings: The influence on prevalence rates of isolated systolic hypertension. *J. Hypertens.* **1986**, *4*, 631–635. [CrossRef]
20. Reeves, R.A. The rational clinical examination: Does this patient have hypertension? How to measure blood pressure. *JAMA* **1995**, *273*, 1211–1218. [CrossRef]
21. Okamoto, M.; Nakamura, F.; Musha, T.; Kobayashi, Y. Association between novel arterial stiffness indices and risk factors of cardiovascular disease. *BMC Cardiovasc. Disord.* **2016**, *16*, 211. [CrossRef] [PubMed]
22. Zhang, Y.; Yin, P.; Xu, Z.; Xie, Y. Non-Invasive Assessment of Early Atherosclerosis Based on New Arterial Stiffness Indices Measured with an Upper-Arm Oscillometric Device. *Tohoku J. Exp. Med.* **2017**, *241*, 263–270. [CrossRef] [PubMed]
23. Komatsu, S.; Tomiyama, H.; Kimura, K.; Matsumoto, C.; Shiina, K.; Yamashina, A. Comparison of the clinical significance of single cuff-based arterial stiffness parameters with that of the commonly used parameters. *J. Cardiol.* **2017**, *69*, 678–683. [CrossRef] [PubMed]
24. Kobayashi, R.; Iwanuma, S.; Ohashi, N.; Hashiguchi, T. New indices of arterial stiffness measured with an upper-arm oscillometric device in active versus inactive women. *Physiol. Rep.* **2018**, *6*, e13574. [CrossRef]

MDPI
St. Alban-Anlage 66
4052 Basel
Switzerland
Tel. +41 61 683 77 34
Fax +41 61 302 89 18
www.mdpi.com

Journal of Clinical Medicine Editorial Office
E-mail: jcm@mdpi.com
www.mdpi.com/journal/jcm

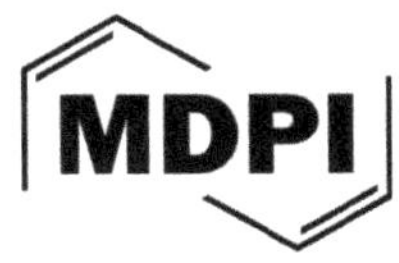

www.ingramcontent.com/pod-product-compliance
Lightning Source LLC
LaVergne TN
LVHW070906170726
843515LV00005B/718

* 9 7 8 3 0 3 6 5 7 7 3 0 2 *